Homelessness Prevention and Intervention in Social Work

Heather Larkin • Amanda Aykanian
Calvin L. Streeter
Editors

Homelessness Prevention and Intervention in Social Work

Policies, Programs, and Practices

Springer

Editors
Heather Larkin
School of Social Welfare
University at Albany (SUNY)
Albany, NY, USA

Amanda Aykanian
School of Social Welfare
University at Albany (SUNY)
Albany, NY, USA

Calvin L. Streeter
School of Social Work
University of Texas at Austin
Austin, TX, USA

Additional material to this book can be downloaded from http://extras.springer.com

ISBN 978-3-030-03726-0   ISBN 978-3-030-03727-7 (eBook)
https://doi.org/10.1007/978-3-030-03727-7

Library of Congress Control Number: 2019933104

This Springer imprint is published by the registered company Springer Nature Switzerland AG
The registered company address is: Gewerbestrasse 11, 6330 Cham, Switzerland

Preface

In examining curricula across schools of social work for the National Homelessness Social Work Initiative (NHSWI), we found that homelessness was covered sporadically and inconsistently—at times left out altogether. We saw this as an opportunity to develop a text that could be used as the foundation for a dedicated course on homelessness and that would inspire educators to integrate homelessness content throughout course offerings. Homelessness-related content is an important and valuable contribution to social work curriculum for multiple reasons.

First, we believe homelessness fits squarely within the professional charge of social work. The NASW Code of Ethics prioritizes helping people in need, addressing social problems, and pursuing social change to better the lives of vulnerable and oppressed individuals and groups. Homelessness is a complex social problem that is disproportionately experienced by some of the most vulnerable and oppressed groups in our society. And, the experience of homelessness itself commonly results in further marginalization.

Second, social workers possess the skills needed to end homelessness, which makes them an important asset in the broad system of services and supports for people experiencing homelessness. Homelessness can result from a range of individual, familial, community, policy, and system factors. In turn, ending homelessness requires multifaceted efforts to strengthen services, improve systems, and alleviate the societal conditions that put people at risk. Therefore, viewing clients and client systems through social work's person-in-environment perspective helps to more fully understand and respond to the varied causes and consequences of homelessness. Thus, adequately preparing social workers to lead efforts to end homelessness will strengthen the homeless services workforce.

Finally, homelessness intersects with many other social problems and impacts a range of client groups. It is associated with individual-level concerns (e.g., substance use, mental health problems, and chronic health issues), interpersonal conflict (e.g., domestic violence, family rejection), societal failings (e.g., poverty, lack of affordable housing), and involvement in complex systems (e.g., criminal justice, foster care, child welfare). Further, while people experiencing homelessness often engage with homeless-specific services, they also frequently access mainstream services. Therefore, social workers commonly work with clients who have a history of homelessness or who are currently at high risk for experiencing homelessness.

Keeping these points in mind, we recognized the need to strengthen the social work curriculum in a way that better prepares social workers to help clients experiencing homelessness and pursue efforts to end homelessness. This book was written in collaboration with faculty and students from several partner schools of the National Center for Excellence in Homeless Services. And, it is one of multiple curricular resources developed through the NHSWI to support social work educators interested in integrating homelessness content into their course offerings and degree programs.

We aimed to cover a broad range of topics in this book to give students insight into the far-reaching implications of homelessness for the people, groups, and systems with which they will engage as social workers. However, we were admittedly unable to cover the full depth and breadth of homelessness and have consciously kept the book's focus almost entirely on the United States. Thus, we see this book as an introduction to homelessness and as a resource that will hopefully spark further reading and research into areas not fully covered in these pages.

How to Use This Book

Our goal is for this book to be of use in multiple ways. As a complete volume, it can serve as the foundational text for a full course on homelessness or as a companion text for courses that more broadly concern poverty in the United States. We are particularly hopeful that it will inspire social work educators to develop homelessness courses in programs that have historically lacked one. The broad range of topics covered and the supplementary materials that accompany each chapter (i.e., discussion questions, activities, and suggested readings) are intended to support this process.

This book is also useful for educators interested in integrating homelessness content into other courses, such as those that address evidence-based practice or working with youth. A single chapter could be used to facilitate drawing connections between the course topic and homelessness. Educators may even choose to adapt the example discussion questions and activities to deepen this connection, and the suggested readings provide interested students with opportunities to further explore the topic.

Outside of the classroom, we hope this book serves as an educational resource for social work educators, social workers, and other helping professionals. It is useful for those looking to expand their knowledge about homelessness, whether they seek a general overview of the topic or a more in-depth look at responses to homelessness or practice approaches for working with people experiencing homelessness.

Organization

This book is organized into three parts, each containing multiple chapters. The organization is intended to create a progression from understanding the causes and consequences of homelessness to understanding individual and community responses to homelessness, to understanding approaches to meeting the service needs of people experiencing homelessness.

Part I: Characteristics and Service Needs of People Experiencing Homelessness is intended to ground readers in the topic as preparation for moving through the subsequent parts. Chapter 1 provides an overview of what homelessness looks like today and the historical and political contexts that shaped its emergence and evolution over time. It also introduces different approaches for defining homelessness and estimating the number of people experiencing homelessness in a community and nationally. Chapter 2 offers a comprehensive look at the intersection of trauma and homelessness, including a discussion of opportunities to prevent or alleviate the consequences of early childhood adversity. Chapter 3 takes a close look at the relationship between homelessness and health concerns, specifically highlighting the significant health disparities found among the homeless population. It shows how health problems can create a susceptibility to homelessness as well as how they can be caused or exacerbated by homelessness. Chapter 4 concludes this section with a broad discussion of the complex and varied needs of people experiencing homelessness, shedding light on some of the challenges for designing comprehensive service systems.

Part II: Individual, Community, and System Responses to Homelessness covers a range of topics related to perceptions of homelessness and actions taken in response to homelessness. It includes responses that are potentially problematic as well as efforts to prevent or end homelessness. Chapter 5 overviews policy and political responses in the realm of affordable housing, including how housing policy has evolved over time. Chapter 6 draws on discourse analysis to illustrate how the public, communities, systems, and homeless people themselves construct and reinforce different narratives of homelessness. Chapter 7 looks at the various community-based responses to homelessness over time, with a specific focus on strategic planning and federally mandated approaches to implementing services and monitoring progress. Chapter 8 shows how community factors influence responses to homelessness by comparing two cities—New York and Los Angeles. It also includes a discussion of the emergence of Housing First. Chapter 9 focuses on how negative perceptions of homelessness can result in problematic policies that criminalize homelessness and behaviors associated with it. Finally, Chap. 10 introduces the emerging trend of Pay for Success funding models that communities are using to garner private investments to support housing and other services.

The chapters in *Part III: Homelessness Service Delivery* cover several topics related to designing and implementing services and supports for people experiencing homelessness. Relevant challenges to service delivery are also discussed. Chapter 11 presents an in-depth description of Critical Time Intervention, an evidence-based practice designed to prevent homelessness. Chapter 12 discusses the potential of multisectoral collaborations for ending homelessness, highlighting two examples of business sector collaborations. Chapter 13 introduces how a trauma-informed approach can be used within homeless services and the potential challenges that can emerge. Chapter 14 highlights the important role of street outreach within a comprehensive homeless service system. Chapter 15 is the first of three chapters that center on young people experiencing homelessness. It discusses approaches to homeless counts, research, and assessments when working with youth. Chapter 16 uses positive youth development and empowerment practice frameworks to illustrate the value and importance of incorporating youth voices into service planning and implementation processes. And, Chap. 17 discusses homelessness in higher education and the special considerations it warrants for defining homelessness and creating appropriate supports. Finally, Chap. 18 orients readers to the experiences and perspectives of providers on the front lines of homeless services, revealing the challenges and successes faced in their day-to-day work.

No matter how students, teachers, and practitioners choose to use this resource, we feel confident they will find good reading, discussion questions, and activities to help them better understand the complex nature of homelessness in the United States. We have learned a great deal from reading and editing the work of the expert contributors, and we hope others will find this book equally enjoyable and stimulating.

Albany, NY, USA Heather Larkin
Albany, NY, USA Amanda Aykanian
Austin, TX, USA Calvin L. Streeter

Contents

Part I
Characteristics and Service Needs of People Experiencing Homelessness

Chapter 1
Homelessness in America: An Overview

Kathi R. Trawver, Stephen Oby, Lauren Kominkiewicz, Frances Bernard Kominkiewicz, and Kelsey Whittington

The term *homeless* is frequently used to describe a person's stigma-filled identity. However, homelessness is more accurately understood as a state or experience, rather than a personal trait, which is impacted by multiple social, cultural, and economic factors. To meet Social Work's Grand Challenge of Ending Homelessness, it is critical to understand these factors (Henwood et al. 2015; Larkin et al. 2016). This chapter provides a broad overview of homelessness in America by first defining homelessness and its history and policies. The chapter goes on to report homelessness prevalence and describes groups that experience particularly high rates of homelessness. The chapter concludes with a discussion about the consequences of homelessness and the significant impacts homelessness has on individuals and families.

Electronic supplementary material: The online version of this chapter (https://doi.org/10.1007/978-3-030-03727-7_1) contains supplementary material, which is available to authorized users.

K. R. Trawver (✉)
University of Alaska Anchorage, Anchorage, AK, USA
e-mail: krtrawver@alaska.edu

S. Oby
University at Albany, Albany, NY, USA
e-mail: soby@albany.edu

L. Kominkiewicz
Children's Legal Services of San Diego, San Diego, CA, USA

F. B. Kominkiewicz
Saint Mary's College, Notre Dame, IN, USA
e-mail: kominkie@saintmarys.edu

K. Whittington
VA Palo Alto Health Care System, Palo Alto, CA, USA

H. Larkin et al. (eds.), *Homelessness Prevention and Intervention in Social Work*, https://doi.org/10.1007/978-3-030-03727-7_1

History of Homelessness in the United States

While the deinstitutionalization movement of the 1960s that prompted thousands of individuals diagnosed with serious mental illness to be released from state psychiatric hospitals to the community is often identified as the beginning of homelessness as we know it today, the causes and history of homelessness in the United States are more complex and long-standing. Throughout history, there have been systemic and personal factors identified as contributing to homelessness in the United States. Systemic issues include poverty, economic recession and depression, wars, inadequate income, lack of jobs and high unemployment rates, lack of affordable housing, immigration of people without resources, natural disasters, and lack of access to health, behavioral health, and other social services. Personal factors include individual or family health crises and illnesses, trauma, domestic violence, mental illness, and addiction (National Coalition for the Homeless 2017a; National Law Center on Homelessness and Poverty 2015).

Early Homelessness in America

Homelessness has always been a part of American history, beginning with early Colonial times. In fact, as early as 1640, Boston peace officers were charged with arresting people disparagingly referred to as "vagrants" or "vagabonds." By the late 1700s, individuals known as "sturdy beggars" were common sights throughout early American cities, such as Baltimore and Philadelphia (Kusmer 2002, p. 29). Homelessness continued to grow substantially through America's early urbanization and industrial development era of the early 1800s, and, by the 1820s and 1830s, the Industrial Revolution had lured people from their farms to the cities in search of much needed employment.

By the 1840s and 1850s, city homeless populations had grown so substantially that many northeastern cities began providing overnight housing for homeless individuals in sections of police stations termed "tramp rooms," and several independent charities began to organize their efforts to impact the problems associated with homelessness (Kusmer 2002). According to Kusmer (2002), while slavery had somewhat moderated homelessness across the south, post-Civil War America (1865) saw many soldiers flock to the cities in search of work. This was also the period that saw the development of a counterculture of men who rode the railroads, referred to pejoratively as "hobos" and "tramps." In response, many cities developed "tramp rooms" and other cheap congregate lodging close to the railroads, like the infamous Bowery in New York City, resulting in city-dwelling residents moving out of city centers to newly developing suburbs to avoid individuals who were homeless (Kusmer 2002).

Following the Great Depression, the high unemployment of the 1930s and countless numbers of business and rural farm failures, millions of people across America lost their housing due to evictions and bank foreclosures related to the economic system crisis (DePastino 2004). As the number of homeless Americans grew, many industrial cities further developed high-density housing, or missions, in city areas often referred to as skid rows. For example, by 1932, city shelters in Chicago housed more people in 1 day (20,000) than they had in any given year during the 1920s (Hoch 2004). This is also the era during which devastated families relied on soup lines and began to migrate from the east coast westward in search of work (Kusmer 2002).

Deinstitutionalization

While the deinstitutionalization movement was not the beginning of American homelessness, it marks an era of expansive growth and early recognition of homelessness as a social problem. With the development of psychotropic medications and the Civil Rights Movement, President John F. Kennedy signed the landmark Community Mental Health Act in 1962, which provided funds to develop community-based programs to serve individuals with serious mental illness as they were released from languishing in psychiatric hospitals and other institutions. While community mental health programs were established, between the coinciding Vietnam War and developing economic crises, the programs were never fully funded to meet the extensive treatment and support service needs of institutionally discharged individuals. Some researchers suggest that deinstitutionalization resulted in "transinstitutionalization," simply moving seriously mentally ill individuals from hospital care to jails, streets, and shelters (Primeau et al. 2013).

Establishment of the US Department of Housing and Urban Development

On the tail of the Civil Rights Movement, the US Department of Housing and Urban Development (HUD) was established "to create strong, sustainable, inclusive communities and quality affordable homes for all" (HUD 2017b, para 1). HUD oversees a wide range of programs related to community development, community planning, and housing, and it is the primary funder of federal homelessness programs and services. Because it is a federal agency, HUD's activities have evolved over time with shifting and expanding legislation.

Fair Housing Act

Shortly after HUD was established, the Fair Housing Act, which prohibited housing discrimination, was passed by Congress as part of the Civil Rights Act of 1968 (Wong 2009). Under the Fair Housing Act, it is unlawful "to refuse to sell or rent after the making of a bona fide offer, or to refuse to negotiate for the sale or rental of, or otherwise make unavailable or deny, a dwelling to any person because of race, color, religion, sex, familial status, or national origin" (42 USC § 3604(a) 2006a). It is also unlawful "to discriminate in the sale or rental, or to otherwise make unavailable or deny, a dwelling to any buyer or renter because of a handicap of— (A) that buyer or renter; (B) a person residing in or intending to reside in that dwelling after it is so sold, rented, or made available; or (C) any person associated with that buyer or renter" (42 USC § 3604(f)(1) 2006b).

Although the Fair Housing Act protection scope includes any "dwelling," its protection is not clearly delineated for homeless shelters, tent cities, substance abuse treatment locations, or other nontraditional sleeping environments (Wong 2009). Discriminatory policies in admissions to shelters may result in some homeless individuals being denied housing in shelters when they request it (Cheyne 2009). Unfortunately, statistics are not maintained regarding the number of individuals who are denied access based on the admission criteria of shelters, how many individuals can locate another shelter facility, and if they locate another shelter, the quality of that shelter that was located (Cheyne 2009).

The McKinney-Vento Homeless Assistance Act

The first legislation that specifically addressed homelessness, and is still today considered to be the primary and most significant federal policy focusing on homelessness (Canfield et al. 2017), was passed by Congress in 1987. Originally named The Stewart B. McKinney Homeless Assistance Act of 1987, it was later renamed The McKinney-Vento Homeless Assistance Act (MVA). The MVA removed many of the bureaucratic structures that discriminated against homeless individuals, such as permanent address requirements for benefit eligibility applications (Losinksi et al. 2013). Moreover, it provided funding for shelters, transitional housing, nutrition programs, and mobile healthcare as well as granting additional flexibility for schools to use funding to help homeless children (Losinksi et al. 2013). Under provisions of the MVA, schools are required to enroll students who self-identify as homeless within 48 hours without requiring proof of residency or immunization records (42 USC § 11431.723(d & f)).

The MVA secures the rights of children by mandating states who receive funds to "ensure that each child of a homeless individual and each homeless youth has equal access to the same free, appropriate public education, including a public preschool education, as provided to other children and youths," noting that "[h]omelessness is not a sufficient reason to separate students from the mainstream school environment" (42 USC § 11431(1) & (3)). These guidelines impact children who are considered homeless under the MVA and encompass children sharing housing with other persons in an emergency or transitional shelter (42 USC § 11434a(2) (A-B)). Programs authorized under the MVA were designed to ensure equal educational access to homeless children. Under the McKinney-Vento Education of Home Children and Youth (EHCY) passed in 1987, children were identified as homeless to remove the barriers that impacted their ability to succeed in school (Cunningham et al. 2010).

Establishment of HUD's Community Continuums of Care (CoCs)

The MVA was amended by the HEARTH Act of 2009, which combined most of the homeless assistance programs established under the MVA into a single grant program called the Continuum of Care (CoC) program. A CoC is a community-driven model to plan and fund homeless services through coordination, collaboration, and strategic use of fiscal resources. CoCs are responsible to develop a long-term community homelessness strategic plan and year-round planning. A lead agency submits funding requests to HUD on behalf of the entire CoC for community permanent housing, transitional housing, supportive services, homeless prevention, and the homeless management information system (HUD 2017d).

To fulfill CoC requests for funding to address homelessness, $2.25 billion is requested in the 2018 fiscal year President's budget for Homeless Assistance Grants (HAG) through Community Planning and Development Homeless Assistance Grants (HUD 2017c). This request includes $1.988 billion for the CoC Program, which serves over 750,000 people experiencing homelessness annually (HUD 2017c), and $255 million to assist over 350,000 individuals in emergency shelter annually through the Emergency Solutions Grants (ESG) (HUD 2017c). These allocations allow HUD to continue to provide homelessness prevention, emergency shelter, rapid rehousing, transitional housing, and permanent supportive housing (HUD 2017c).

HUD has been the primary resource for data on homelessness by requiring COCs to conduct Point-in-Time (PIT) counts that tally the sheltered and unsheltered individuals on one night each January (Wilkins et al. 2016). Accurate counts help track homelessness rates and support creating new programs where they are most needed. This is exemplified by recent efforts to foster permanent supportive housing (PSH) programs that subsidize housing with matching ongoing, supportive services (Byrne et al. 2014). PSH programs have been linked to steep declines in chronic homelessness over time (Byrne et al. 2014). Therefore, understanding the value of data can be a feedback tool for future funding to fight homelessness.

Federally Funded Housing and Services

HUD is the primary funder of federal homeless services and administers multiple housing programs for low-income and homeless populations. While HUD's homelessness assistance is primarily funded through the COC program, communities may also supplement with funds from other mechanisms (e.g., block grants).

Federal housing programs are perhaps the most well known and most relied upon solutions in addressing homelessness in the United States, reaching about 5 million low-income households (Center on Budget and Policy Priorities 2017). In a recent report, the Urban Institute (Kingsley 2017) outlined two of the most common federal housing programs: public housing and rental subsidies. Public housing, sometimes referred to as "housing projects" and which are owned and managed by local public housing entities, were built in response to inadequate living conditions for many Americans beginning in the 1930s. As physical infrastructure became less of a concern than affordability, an emphasis on subsidized rental opportunities arose in the 1960s, with privately owned subsidized housing and housing vouchers—the most common of which is known as Section 8 (now called Housing Choice Vouchers)—enabling low-income households to access long-term housing more affordably. While these two programs are joined by a range of disparate programs and tax credits representing a broad spectrum of federal housing assistance, federal housing programs are vulnerable to critiques including ineffectiveness, failure to fulfill their initial purpose, and a lack of coordination across programs (Landis and McClure 2010).

Permanent Housing

Permanent housing is defined as community-based housing without a designated length of stay in which formerly homeless individuals and families live as independently as possible. In permanent housing, a program participant must be the tenant on a lease (or sublease) for an initial term of at least 1 year that is renewable and is terminable only for cause. Further, leases (or subleases) must be renewable for a minimum term of 1 month (HUD n.d., para 3).

Through community COCs, HUD funds two types of permanent housing: permanent supportive housing and rapid rehousing.

Permanent Supportive Housing

Permanent supportive housing is an intervention for individuals experiencing homelessness or at risk for homelessness that combines permanent independent housing with individualized support services. These supports may include case management, treatment for substance abuse or psychiatric health conditions, and obtaining and maintaining employment. In this model, service providers participate in the maintenance of housing on an ongoing basis, collaborating with landlords and property managers to ensure continued housing and assisting in the resolution of crises or other housing-related concerns. The combination of personal support and targeted support services distinguishes permanent supportive housing programs from other housing-based interventions (Rog et al. 2014).

A meta-analysis suggests that permanent supportive housing reduces homelessness, increases housing stability, reduces emergency room use and hospitalizations, and increases consumer satisfaction (Rog et al. 2014). However permanent supportive housing at this time may refer to a broad range of housing programs with varying standards and philosophies, making meaningful analysis of permanent supportive housing difficult. Clearer guidelines and program interventions, as seen in the Housing First model, are warranted to clarify the value of this housing intervention.

Rapid Rehousing

Rapid rehousing is a community-level strategy aimed at addressing homelessness informed by the Housing First approach. The central tenet of rapid rehousing is the speedy connection of homeless individuals to permanent housing through the use of time-limited financial support and individualized support services. This approach aims to provide practical and immediate solutions to those challenges related to the experience of homelessness to reduce how long the period of homelessness lasts while also avoiding a near-term return to homelessness. Rapid rehousing is premised on the idea that most experiences of homelessness are related to a crisis, financial or otherwise, that leads to loss of housing; that most homeless individuals and families are not unlike others living in poverty in that they can maintain housing without long-term support; that prolonged exposure to homelessness is characterized by a series of very dangerous risk factors; and that, given the dearth of resources available to address the problem of homelessness, effective and short-term strategies should be utilized wherever possible (HUD 2015a).

Transitional Housing

HUD also funds transitional housing programs that provide support services and move families and individuals into interim housing for up to 24 months. The goal of transitional housing programs is to provide supports that enable residents to move into permanent housing (HUD n.d.).

Supportive Services

General services to conduct outreach and engage individuals and families who are homeless and unsheltered funded by HUD are referred to as supportive services. These services may be mobile, street based, or office based. The goal of supportive services is to engage people experiencing homelessness in available services, supports, and housing (HUD n.d.).

Homelessness Prevention

HUD funds are also available through community COCs to provide homeless prevention services to individuals and families at risk of experiencing homelessness, such as short-term rental assistance, relocation services, and/or a move to permanent housing. The goal of homeless prevention services is to avoid homelessness before it occurs (HUD n.d.).

Criminalization of Homelessness

Homelessness has historically been associated with deviance and immorality. Negative perceptions of homeless people and behaviors associated with homelessness and vagrancy (e.g., panhandling and public intoxication) have fueled efforts to manage homelessness through police intervention since the early 1900s, stemming from vagrancy laws common in the decades prior. Recently, there has been a significant increase in the number of communities that have passed laws making it illegal to carry out daily activities that individuals who are homeless must perform to survive, such as sleeping or sitting down in public, urinating in public, camping in public, loitering, panhandling, living in vehicles, and sharing food (National Law Center on Homelessness and Poverty [NLCHP] 2016). From 2006 to 2016, there was a 69% increase in bans on camping citywide, a 31% increase in bans on sleeping in public, and a 143% increase in bans on living in a vehicle (NLCHP 2016). Violations of these laws have resulted in individuals receiving tickets, being fined, and even being arrested. In addition to being problematic policy that perpetuates a stigmatized view of homeless people, criminalization tactics increase homeless people's involvement with the criminal justice system, which can limit access to housing, voting, education, benefits, and employment and contribute to homelessness (see Chap. 9 for more on the criminalization of homelessness).

Natural Disasters

Natural disasters have historically played a significant factor in displacing people from their homes, resulting in homelessness across all segments of society. Examples include the 1871 Chicago fire, the 1900 Galveston hurricane, the 1906 San Francisco earthquake, and the massive flooding of the Mississippi River in the 1920s from Ohio through New Orleans that displaced over 1.3 million people (Kusmer 2002). More recent disasters include the following: (1) Hurricane Katrina, which displaced over 400,000 people from New Orleans and the Mississippi Gulf Coast in 2005 (Whoriskey 2006); (2) Hurricane Harvey, which displaced over 10,000 people from their homes in 2017 (Fausset and Robertson 2017); and severe fires in Sonoma County, CA, in 2017, which were estimated to have resulted in more than 10,000 people losing their housing.

Defining and Estimating Homelessness

While poverty and a lack of safe and affordable housing underlie all types of homelessness, there is a diversity in experiences of homelessness. To define and describe types of homelessness, effectively target services to people experiencing homelessness, and set eligibility requirements for specific homeless services and assistance programs, multiple typologies of homelessness have been developed.

In lives that are marked by instability, verifying homelessness is another rule that must be followed to access assistance but can create barriers to services if a person is unable to provide sufficient evidence or documentation. Eligibility for federal programs is determined based on meeting definition criteria, and service providers are required to maintain records that establish whether the agency has complied with homeless definitions (HUD 2015b). In practice, the procedure asks clients to prove that they have been homeless for the appropriate periods and/or number of times (HUD 2015b).

Despite the downsides to creating a rigid definition for homelessness, gathering data within the confines of a definition of homelessness allows legislators to obtain a snapshot of how homelessness is affected by public funding and already available resources (Wilkins et al. 2016). How homelessness is defined also has direct implications for the kinds of services offered and who is eligible to receive them. However, consistently defining homelessness can be challenging. There are several different federal definitions of homelessness utilized by HUD, the US Department of Health and Social Services, the US Department of Veterans Affairs, and the Social Security Administration, and each state sets its own definition as well (National Health Care for the Homeless Council 2017). The following provides an overview of some of the key federal definitions of homelessness.

HEARTH Act Definitions

The Homeless Emergency Assistance and Rapid Transition to Housing (HEARTH) Act (§896), and its 2012 update, includes four broad categories of homelessness:

1. People who are living in a place not meant for human habitation, in emergency shelter, and in transitional housing or are exiting an institution where they temporarily resided
2. People who are losing their primary nighttime residence, which may include a motel or hotel or a doubled-up situation, within 14 days and lack resources or support networks to remain in housing
3. Families with children or unaccompanied youth who are unstably housed and likely to continue in that state
4. People who are fleeing or attempting to flee domestic violence, have no other residences, and lack the resources or support networks to obtain other permanent housing

US Department of Housing and Urban Development Definitions

Another way homelessness categories are defined is based on the number of homeless episodes a person has experienced and their total length of time spent homeless. Using this approach, homelessness typically considers one's risk of becoming homeless and chronically homeless. This categorization is the approach used by HUD to describe homelessness in the United States, such as in its Annual Homelessness Assessment Report to Congress, and to define eligibility standards for the services and housing it funds.

At Risk of Homelessness

Individuals and families who do not meet homeless definitions under the HEARTH Act but whose economic and housing circumstances indicate significant housing instability (e.g., has an annual income below 30% of median area income, is living with someone else due to economic hardship, has received an eviction notice) are considered *at risk of homelessness.* Additionally, unaccompanied children and youth and families with children and youth are considered at risk of homelessness if they qualify as homeless under at least one federal definition (HUD 2012). In practice, "at risk" is sometimes referred to by researchers and advocates as *housing insecure*, and the designation applies to individuals and families, unaccompanied children and youth, and families with children/youth (HUD 2012).

Chronic Homelessness

Currently, HUD defines a chronically homelessness individual as someone who (1) experiences a disability; (2) lives in a place not meant for human habitation, a safe haven, an emergency shelter, or in an institutional care facility; and (3) has lived there for at least 12 months or on four or more separate occasions during the prior 3 years for a total of at least 12 months. Families are considered chronically homeless when the adult head of the household meets the definition of a chronically homeless individual.

Homeless

Currently, HUD groups the homeless definitions for their programs into the following four categories (United States Interagency on Homelessness 2018).

1. *Literally Homeless*: Individual or family who lacks a fixed, regular, and adequate nighttime residence, meaning:
   - (i) Has a primary nighttime residence that is a public or private place not meant for human habitation
   - (ii) Is living in a publicly or privately operated shelter designated to provide temporary living arrangements (including congregate shelters, transitional housing, and hotels and motels paid for by charitable organizations or by federal, state, and local government programs)
   - (iii) Is exiting an institution where (s)he has resided for 90 days or less and who resided in an emergency shelter or place not meant for human habitation immediately before entering that institution
2. *Imminent Risk of Homelessness*: Individual or family who will imminently lose their primary nighttime residence, provided that:
   - (i) Residence will be lost within 14 days of the date of application for homeless assistance.
   - (ii) No subsequent residence has been identified.
   - (iii) The individual or family lacks the resources or support networks needed to obtain other permanent housing.
3. *Homeless Under Other Federal Statutes*: Unaccompanied youth under 25 years of age or families with children and youth, who do not otherwise qualify as homeless under this definition, but who:
   - (i) Are defined as homeless under the other listed federal statutes
   - (ii) Have not had a lease, ownership interest, or occupancy agreement in permanent housing during the 60 days prior to the homeless assistance application
   - (iii) Have experienced persistent instability as measured by two moves or more during the preceding 60 days
   - (iv) Can be expected to continue in such status for an extended period of time due to special needs or barriers

4. *Fleeing/Attempting to Flee Domestic Violence*: Any individual or family who:
   (i) Is fleeing or attempting to flee their housing or the place they are staying because of domestic violence, dating violence, sexual assault, stalking, or other dangerous or life-threatening conditions related to violence that has taken place in the house or has made them afraid to return to the house, including trading sex for housing, trafficking, physical abuse, violence (or perceived threat of violence) because of the youth's sexual orientation
   (ii) Has no other residence
   (iii) Lacks the resources or support networks to obtain other permanent housing

Children, Youth, and Transitional Age Youth

To further complicate matters, there are also several definitions utilized to describe youth and transitional age youth who experience homelessness that vary based on age and housing situations. While many young people experience homelessness within a family unit, youths who are not in the physical custody of a parent or guardian are termed by the MVA (42 USC § 11434a(6)) as *unaccompanied youth.* The Runaway and Homeless Youth Act, the US Department of Education, and HUD (see Category Three above) all offer slightly different definitions. The Runaway and Homeless Youth Act (42 USC §5732a) provides for community-based runaway and homeless youth projects, including temporary shelter. Depending on its programs, eligible youth seeking shelter must be age 21 and under, while those eligible for home-based services are limited to ages 16 to 21 and under some conditions age 22. The US Department of Education (2004) defines homeless children and youths as individuals who lack a fixed, regular, and adequate nighttime residence (within the meaning of section 11302(a)(1) of this title) and includes the following:

(i) Children and youths who are sharing the housing of other persons due to loss of housing, economic hardship, or a similar reason; are living in motels, hotels, trailer parks, or camping grounds due to the lack of alternative adequate accommodations; are living in emergency or transitional shelters; are abandoned in hospitals; or are awaiting foster care placement
(ii) Children and youths who have a primary nighttime residence that is a public or private place not designed for or ordinarily used as a regular sleeping accommodation for human beings (within the meaning of section 11302(a)(2)(C) of this title)
(iii) Children and youths who are living in cars, parks, public spaces, abandoned buildings, substandard housing, bus or train stations, or similar settings
(iv) Migratory children (as such term is defined in section 6399 of title 20) who qualify as homeless for the purposes of this subtitle because the children are living in circumstances described in clauses (i) through (iii) (42 USC § 11434a(2))

General Homelessness Definition

One comprehensive general definition of homelessness is found in Title 42 (The Public Health and Welfare) of the US Code (§11302):

1. An individual who lacks a fixed, regular, and adequate nighttime residence
2. An individual who has a primary nighttime residence that is a public or private place not designed for or ordinarily used as a regular sleeping accommodation for human beings, including a car, park, abandoned building, bus or train station, airport, or camping ground
3. An individual or family living in a supervised publicly or privately operated shelter designated to provide temporary living arrangements (including hotels and motels paid for by Federal, State, or local government programs for low-income individuals or by charitable organizations, congregate shelters, and transitional housing)
4. An individual who resided in a shelter or place not meant for human habitation and who is exiting an institution where he or she temporarily resided
5. An individual or family who:

   (a) Will imminently lose their housing, including housing they own, rent, or live in without paying rent, are sharing with others, and rooms in hotels or motels not paid for by Federal, State, or local government programs for low-income individuals or by charitable organizations as evidenced by (i) a court order resulting from an eviction action that notifies the individual or family that they must leave within 14 days; (ii) the individual or family having a primary nighttime residence that is a room in a hotel or motel and where they lack the resources necessary to reside there for more than 14 days; or (iii) credible evidence indicating that the owner or renter of the housing will not allow the individual or family to stay for more than 14 days, and any oral statement from an individual or family seeking homeless assistance that is found to be credible shall be considered credible evidence for purposes of this clause; (iv) has no subsequent residence identified; and (v) lacks the resources or support networks needed to obtain other permanent housing

6. Unaccompanied youth and homeless families with children and youth defined as homeless under other Federal statutes who

   (a) Have experienced a long-term period without living independently in permanent housing
   (b) Have experienced persistent instability as measured by frequent moves over such period
   (c) Can be expected to continue in such status for an extended period of time because of chronic disabilities, chronic physical health or mental health conditions, substance addiction, histories of domestic violence or childhood abuse, the presence of a child or youth with a disability, or multiple barriers to employment

The fact that homelessness has no official definition but rather is defined in closely related, yet substantively different, ways has significant implications for how we can fully understand the size and scope of homelessness. More importantly, because these definitions classify the types of services and supports available to a person or family experiencing homelessness, it is imperative that service providers understand their impact on client services.

Estimating Homelessness in the United States

The first known census of individuals experiencing homelessness was conducted in 1933 (Kusmer 2002). Since then, obtaining a reliable and accurate census count to document the number and location of individuals and families who experience homelessness remains a nearly impossible task. The following are just some of the challenges faced when trying to accurately estimate homelessness: locating individuals and families who are homeless but are not engaged in services, finding individuals who do not self-identify as experiencing homelessness (e.g., couch surfing, temporarily staying with family, temporarily down on their luck), the transitory nature of homelessness, and the use of narrow or inconsistent definitions of homelessness.

Currently, the best available estimate of the prevalence of homelessness within the United States is derived from annual community homeless unduplicated Point-in-Time (PIT) counts that are required of every community receiving federal homelessness services funds from HUD. PIT counts were first initiated in 2005 and are conducted once each year during one designated 24-hour period in January to estimate a community's number of homeless individuals, families, and unaccompanied homeless youth. Although the PIT count is required to occur once in January, communities can opt to conduct additional counts throughout the year.

HUD requires each funded community to conduct annual PIT *sheltered counts* that utilize client records drawn from the emergency shelter and transitional housing program's electronic Homeless Information Management System (HMIS) to identify the number and characteristics of homeless residents on the identified January date. On odd-numbered years, HUD also requires PIT *unsheltered counts*. Unsheltered counts rely on a variety of outreach workers and community volunteers to canvas each community to locate and identify individuals who are not staying in shelters or transitional housing programs and are living in places that are not meant for permanent human habitation (e.g., cars, camps, sidewalks). Many communities conduct more frequent sheltered and unsheltered counts throughout the year to more regularly track community housing and homelessness trends and identify emerging community needs (National Alliance to End Homelessness 2016). The PIT counts also identify whether included individuals and families experience chronic homelessness are homeless because of fleeing a domestic violence situation, experience disabilities, are a parenting youth, have a chronic substance abuse issue or severe mental illness, have HIV/AIDS, or are a veteran.

Current Estimates of Homelessness

The Annual Homeless Assessment Report (AHAR) is a report that HUD provides to Congress each year that offers a national estimate of homelessness. The AHAR also includes demographic, special populations, service delivery, and community housing inventory counts. This data is drawn from shelter data systems (i.e., Homeless Information Management System) and annual Point-in-Time and Housing Inventory Counts (HUD 2018).

Table 1.1 displays data from the 2017 PIT counts (HUD 2017a). On a single night in January 2017, a total of 553,742 individuals were counted as homeless. Overall, there was a slightly higher representation of males compared to females, transgender, or others in sheltered settings (55%), but that difference was markedly higher in the unsheltered count (71%). Most of the individuals counted (64%) were sheltered, staying in some type of emergency shelter or transitional housing. Unaccompanied homeless youth (i.e., under age 18) and transitional age youth (i.e., age 18–24) accounted for 49,799 (8.9%) of the counted individuals. A total of 95,419 (16.9%) individuals met the HUD defined criteria of chronic homelessness.

As shown in Fig. 1.1, while the number of counted individuals who experienced homelessness steadily declined between 2012 and 2016, it increased by almost 7% between 2016 and 2017. Since 2014, unsheltered individuals and those who met the definition of chronic homelessness have both increased, and the number of sheltered individuals has decreased. While the overall number of counted individuals and families experiencing homelessness has decreased by 4.5% over the last 5 years, several population groups saw increases from 2016 to 2017 in both number and percentage of the overall homeless population, including unaccompanied youth (+39.5%), victims of domestic violence (+27.5%), chronically homeless (+10.9%), persons living with HIV/AIDS (+10.1%), persons with severe mental illness (+3.8%), and veterans (+1.5%). Decreases were seen in the number of people reporting a chronic substance abuse issue (−5.5%) and children of parenting youth (−8.7%) (HUD 2016a, 2017a).

Homeless Data Limitations and Strengths

While annual PIT counts currently provide the most accurate and consistent data regarding homelessness in the United States, the resulting data are not without significant limitations that must be considered when relying on these findings. First, PIT count definitions and count methodology have varied from year to year and across communities, potentially creating issues with reliability and validity over time (National Alliance to End Homelessness 2016). Second, unsheltered counts have even more variability in collection methods and data collected and are reliant on the numbers of people, typically unpaid volunteers, canvassing a community and locating homeless individuals to count. Finally, counts are conducted

Table 1.1 HUD 2017 Point-in-Time Count Data, including all States, territories, Puerto Rico, and District of Columbia (HUD 2016a, 2017a)

	Emergency shelter	Transitional housing	Unsheltered	Total
Total homeless persons counted	**262,430*	*98,437*	**192,875*	**563,742*
Summary by household (HHs) type				
HHs without children	*134,017	50,860	*160,785	*345,662
HHs with at least one adult and one child	*37,951	14,878	5142	57,971
HHs with only children	1573	535	*2409	*4517
Total homeless HHs	**173,541*	*66,273*	**168,336*	**408,150*
Age				
Persons in HHs without children	**139,141*	*51,674*	**173,156*	**363,971*
Persons age 18–24	11,103	6788	820,139	*38,030
Persons over age 24	*128,038	44,886	*53,017	*325,941
Persons in HHs with at least one adult and one child	**121,587*	*46,136*	*16,938*	*184,661*
Children under age 18	*72,648	28,312	8759	109,719
Persons age 18–24	*9900	3951	*1557	15,408
Persons over age 24	*39,039	13,873	6662	59,534
HHs with only children	**1702*	*627*	**2781*	**5110*
Gender				
Female	117,126	43,480	55,103	215,709
Male	144,472	54,463	136,103	335,038
Transgender	709	391	992	2092
Other	123	103	667	903
Race				
Black or African American	128,721	38,768	57,448	224,937
White	106,543	47,946	106.490	260,979
Asian	2571	1132	3057	6796
American Indian or Alaska Native	6228	2496	8072	16,796
Native Hawaiian or other Pacific Islander	2807	1678	4040	8525
Multiple races	15,560	6417	13,768	35,745
Subpopulations				
Chronically homeless	*31,711	*898	*62,810	*95,419
Severely mentally ill	40,538	18,189	*53,175	*111,902
Chronic substance abuse	27,909	18,953	42,471	89,333
Veterans	10,504	14,186	*15,366	*40,056
HIV/AIDS	4494	2507	*3170	*10,171
Victims of domestic violence	*34,801	*14,276	*38,252	*87,329
Unaccompanied youth	*11,417*	*7125*	**22,257*	**49,799*
Unaccompanied youth under 18	1614	508	*2667	*4789
Unaccompanied youth 18–24	9803	6617	*19,590	*36,010
Parenting youth (24 and under)	5892	2967	*577	*9436
Children of parenting youth	7336	4097	719	12,152

Note. *Indicates an increase in numbers from 2016 PIT count

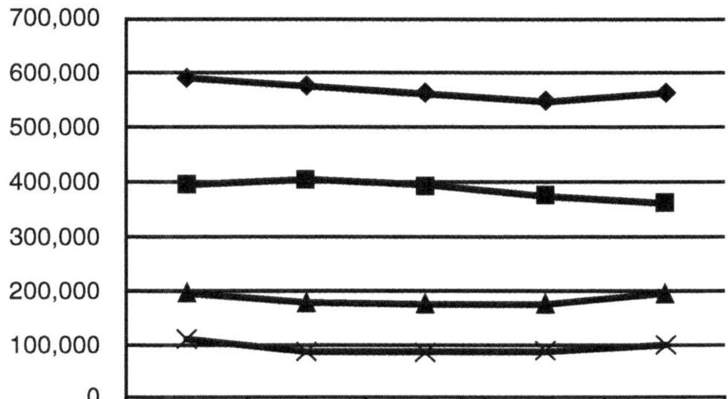

	2013	2014	2015	2016	2017
Total Homeless	590,634	576,450	564,708	549,928	563,742
Sheltered	394,698	401,051	391,440	373,571	360,867
Unsheltered	195,666	175,399	173,268	176,357	192,875
Chronic Homeless	109,132	84,291	83,170	86,132	95,419

Fig. 1.1 HUD PIT count data trends (HUD 2016b, 2017a)

in January, which may create challenges in easily finding people in communities that experience cold winter weather. Because of these identified limitations in the available data, many communities conduct additional counts throughout the year. They are also working to collect better data on unsheltered individuals by developing more assertive community count strategies.

Homeless Populations

There are several vulnerable groups that are frequently found within any given community's homeless population. Some of these groups may not be surprising, such as adults who face serious mental illness, substance use challenges, and/or chronic homelessness. However, it may be surprising to find out about other vulnerable groups that experience high rates of homelessness, such as families, people with high rates of trauma, youth and young adults, individuals fleeing domestic violence, veterans, immigrants, students, and LGBTQ+ individuals. This section of the chapter describes these related impacts and the groups that often intersect to comprise homeless populations, their unique characteristics, and needs.

Health, Mental Health, Trauma, and Substance Use

The homeless population is diverse. However, many homeless individuals and families hold in common the fact that they experience significant, disproportionate, and intersecting health, mental health, trauma, and substance use disparities and resulting disorders at rates higher than their housed counterparts. These disparities are described in this next section.

Health

Considering the potential impacts of such challenges, it is not surprising that people who are homeless are especially susceptible to health problems, including infectious diseases like influenza, tuberculosis, Hepatitis C, and HIV/AIDS, all of which have been documented at disproportionately high rates, as well as medication non-adherence that may contribute to higher rates of disease (Beijer et al. 2012). The prevalence of HIV/AIDS among people experiencing homelessness is especially concerning. Older mortality studies identified HIV/AIDS as a leading cause of death in persons who experience homelessness, especially homeless women (Cheung and Hwang 2004). More recent research suggests that adults experiencing homelessness are three to nine times more likely to be infected with HIV/AIDS than those with stable housing (Riley et al. 2012; Wenzel et al. 2012), and unstably housed youths are at two to ten times greater risk of contracting HIV than stably housed youth (Young and Rice 2011).

Mental Illness

Despite a great deal of variation in the documented prevalence rates of mental illness among homeless adults, it is clear that individuals who experience homelessness also have disproportionally high rates of mental illness. According to HUD's (2017a) PIT count, of the 553,742 counted individuals, 111,902 (20.2%) reported having a severe mental illness (i.e., schizophrenia, bipolar disorder, or major depression). Since other sources report that homeless people experience serious mental illness at rates ranging from 33 to 46% of the population (National Alliance on Mental illness 2017; Treatment Advocacy Center 2014), the current PIT data are likely undercounts. The negative impacts that serious mental illness can have on functioning in work, daily life, and relationships may make this population particularly vulnerable to homelessness (National Coalition for the Homeless 2009).

Trauma and Trauma-Related Disorders

Research suggests that youths who experience homelessness also have disproportionately higher rates of trauma both before and during homelessness. For example, a study of 400 homeless Los Angeles youths found that prior to homelessness, 33% had experienced sexual assault, 51% had experienced physical abuse, and almost three quarters (71%) of the youth reported that they came from homes that included domestic violence and/or substance abuse (Wong et al. 2016). Stewart et al. (2004) found that up to 83% of homeless youth had been physically or sexually abused after becoming homeless. The impacts of this trauma have been found to be serious as Bender et al.'s (2014) research showed that homeless youths who have experienced trauma or witnessed traumatic events were at significantly increased risk of developing post-traumatic stress disorder when compared to their non-homeless counterparts. Researchers have also examined prior adverse childhood experiences (ACEs) in studies with adult homeless populations, finding that 87% reported at least one ACE before age 18 and more than half (53%) reported four or more ACEs (Larkin and Park 2012).

Complex trauma and its health and mental health-related impacts also appear to be highly related to other disparities experienced by individuals and families experiencing homelessness. Not only do homeless populations have high rates of health issues, serious mental illness, and substance-related disorders, they also experience high rates of post-traumatic stress disorder (PTSD) related to prior trauma and victimization, including the trauma of experiencing homelessness itself. However, high prevalence rates of trauma and resulting PTSD among individuals and families experiencing homelessness are difficult to estimate, as individual trauma histories and its impacts are not data points collected during annual community PIT counts. However, some individual studies have indicated rates of PTSD among homeless people ranging as high as 50 to 100% (Christensen et al. 2005; Kim et al. 2010; Schuster et al. 2011; Stewart et al. 2004).

Substance Use

While not all homeless individuals have substance use disorders, substance use commonly co-occurs with mental health conditions and is highly associated with initially becoming homeless (Thompson et al. 2013) and lengthier homeless experiences, including chronic homelessness (Johnson and Chamberlain 2008). Additionally, national estimates from the 2017 PIT count suggest that approximately 46,862 sheltered and 42,471 unsheltered homeless individuals, or 16.1% of the total count, self-reported having a chronic substance use issue (HUD 2017a), which is likely an undercount.

Addressing substance use while an individual remains homeless can be particularly challenging. Arguments have been made that reducing problematic substance use and associated risk behaviors is maximized only after an individual is housed, and basic needs are met (Tsemberis et al. 2004). Research has indicated that individuals with substance use challenges can attain long-term retention in supportive housing (Collins et al. 2013); other research, however, has indicated that substance use is also a risk factor for returning to homelessness among supportive housing residents (O'Connell et al. 2008).

Chronic Homelessness

The most recent data shows that almost one in five individuals experiencing homelessness exhibited chronic patterns of homelessness (HUD 2017a). For people who experience chronic homelessness, they typically also experience other long-standing and intersecting issues such as trauma, mental illness, substance use disorders, disabilities, and/or other health and medical conditions (National Alliance to End Homelessness 2018). Most individuals experiencing chronic homelessness are currently unsheltered and living in places not meant for human habitation. In fact, this is the only subpopulation of homeless individuals for whom this is the case, greatly increasing the vulnerability to certain health impairments as well as threats to physical safety. According to the National Alliance to End Homelessness (2018), it is difficult to obtain housing for this group due to complex needs and barriers.

Homeless Families with Children

Family homelessness is widespread. The National Center on Family Homelessness ([NCFH] 2016) reports that over the course of a year, nearly 500,000 people in families stay in a homeless shelter, more than half of which are children. Homelessness, as well as the factors that can lead to it (e.g., mental illness, substance abuse, domestic violence), can also disrupt family units, resulting in parents and children becoming separated. Roughly 60% of homeless women have children under the age of 18, but only 65% of them are living with at least one of their children. There is an even greater disparity among homeless men, with 41% of homeless men having children under the age of 18 and only 7% of them living with one of their children (NCFH 2011). Certainly, the issue of homelessness has a profound impact on the health and development of these family systems and the individuals who are a part of them.

The statistics above strongly suggest that women are more frequently caring for their minor children when experiencing homelessness, as might be expected given common conceptions regarding caregiver roles. Existing data supports this notion, with an estimated 80% of homeless adult women leading or co-leading a family unit and 71% of single-parent families led by women (NCFH 2011). This dynamic informs our understanding of the characteristics likely displayed by those families experiencing homelessness. For example, mothers who are homeless have more frequently experienced traumatic stress, interpersonal violence, psychiatric health impairments, and problematic drug and alcohol use as compared to other women (Hayes et al. 2013). This lifetime experience of adversity likely leads to decreased coping capacity, which makes issues such as lack of affordable housing and inadequate wages even more difficult to navigate. Further, there are very similar profiles between women who utilize services at domestic violence shelters and those at homeless shelters, including comparable rates of psychiatric illness, problematic substance use, and rates of trauma and victimization (Stainbrook 2006). This suggests that the number of women and families experiencing homelessness is not measured in full, due to the use of domestic violence services rather than services explicitly for homeless families.

These issues experienced by women who are homeless undoubtedly have a profound impact on their children. As might be expected given the higher rates of violence, mental health impairment, and substance use issues experienced by mothers in homelessness, children in homeless families are more likely to have witnessed acts of violence than the general population and are more frequently the subject of Child Protective Services investigations (Guarino and Bassuk 2010). Even in the absence of childhood traumatic experiences while experiencing homelessness, the role of parenting in this environment is noteworthy. Research has shown that disrupted family processes—like those that a family is likely to experience on a trajectory toward homelessness—can intensify any conflict or other negative dynamics within the family system, reducing the quality of parenting and increasing the likelihood of attachment and behavioral issues in children (Gerwitz et al. 2009). Further, homelessness has been associated with children's increased risk of serious emotional, behavioral, and health problems, a higher likelihood of separation from their family, and lower academic achievement (NCFH 2016).

Homeless Youth and Transitional Age Youth

Unaccompanied homeless youth and transitional age youth represent almost 8% of the total population of homeless individuals, with most of these youth ranging between ages 18 and 24, a subpopulation somewhat less likely to be sheltered than their younger counterparts (HUD 2017a). Research strongly suggests that most youths who become homeless do so to escape untenable living situations, particularly those characterized by abuse and trauma (Thompson et al. 2010). There are also youths who are forced out of their homes by parents or other caregivers, young people termed throwaway youth. Family conflict and family breakdown in general are identified by homeless youth as a key factor in their homelessness, with strained family relationships, conflict, poor communication, and parental mental health impairments and/or substance abuse creating a set of circumstances that dramatically increases the risk for youth homelessness (Nooe and Patterson 2010).

Like homeless adults, a strong relationship between homelessness and mental health challenges, even when mental health problems were not the cause of their homelessness, has been documented among homeless youth. Researchers report that youth and young adults who experience homelessness have high rates of mental health disorders, with over two-thirds meeting the criteria for a mental disorder (Hodge et al. 2017; Quimby et al. 2012; Whitbeck et al. 2007). Studies have shown homeless youths exhibit higher rates of conduct problems and delinquency and crime, which are understood as resulting in part from family, peer, and street factors (Chen et al. 2007). Unaccompanied homeless youths exhibit higher rates of anxiety, attention deficit hyperactivity disorder, depression, and developmental delays, and those with trauma histories are more likely to meet the diagnostic criteria for depression and to attempt suicide (Thompson et al. 2010). Further, once a youth becomes homeless, limited social and individual resources, legal status if under the age of 18, and developmental considerations create a unique profile of risk and vulnerability. Indeed, youth and transitional age youth are disproportionately at higher risk of exposure to violence, victimization, exploitation, and substance abuse (Hayashi et al. 2016).

LGBTQ+ Youth

According to researchers, of the 1.6 million American youths who experience homelessness, up to 40% are identified as LGBTQ+ (Durso and Gates 2012; National Coalition for the Homeless 2017b; True Colors Fund 2017). Given the fact that only 12% of the general population and 20% of 18- to 34-year-olds identified as LGBTQ (Harris Poll 2017), this disparity illustrates a large overrepresentation within the homeless population and highlights the fact that LGBTQ+ youths become homeless at rates higher than their non-LBGTQ+ counterparts. Further, given the likelihood that youth may underreport a LGBTQ+ sexual orientation and/or alternative gender identity (Cray et al. 2013), this disparity may be even starker.

LGBTQ+ homeless youths also face additional adversity and risks from their heterosexual or cisgender homeless peers. Choi et al. (2015) report that LGBTQ+ homeless youths have considerably higher rates of substance abuse, violence, victimization, discrimination, and family rejection. Additionally, these researchers found that LGBTQ+ youths experience homelessness for longer periods of time, have more health and mental health problems, and have specific needs for acceptance and support. It is not surprising that given the complexity of needs, vulnerabilities, and marginalization of LGBTQ+ youth, services tailored to support this subpopulation are critically needed. However, a recent study by Maccio and Ferguson (2016) found significant gaps in housing, education, employment, family, and LGBTQ+ affirming homeless services for LGBTQ+ homeless youth.

Students/College Students

When families with children and youth flee from violent homes and seek shelter, not only do those youth lose their home and housing, they often experience disruption of their education. Shelters or other emergency housing may not be located near a student's school, and transportation can be a key barrier to maintaining educational stability. The McKinney-Vento Homeless Education Assistance Act requires school districts to provide transportation to the homeless student's school they attended when they were permanently housed or were last enrolled in. Every state is required to have a State Coordinator for Homeless Education, and every school district is required to have a local homeless education liaison. Homeless education liaisons are tasked with identifying students experiencing homelessness and facilitating enrollment, attendance, immunizations, referrals to other needed services and other opportunities related to student retention and success (National Center for Homeless Education n.d.).

School-aged children and youth are not the only students who experience educational challenges related to homelessness. Recently, researchers have started to consider the prevalence of food and housing insecurity and homelessness among America's college students and its impacts on academic achievement and student well-being (see Chap. 17 for more about homelessness and housing insecurity among students in higher education). Homeless college students have long been able to qualify as independent for purposes of federal financial aid thanks to the College Cost Reduction and Access Act of 2007, and the Higher Education Opportunity Act: Homeless and Foster Youth of 2008 increased access to postsecondary education for homeless and former foster care youth. More recently, the Every Student Succeeds Act of 2015 includes provisions to assist homeless students' transition from high school to higher education. However, even with the aforementioned provisions, homeless college students remain a largely invisible group. Students' Federal Application for Student Aid (FAFSA) applications have been the only available means for identifying homelessness among postsecondary students. The 2015/2016 FAFSA data identified 31,948 homeless students, which represents less than 1% of applicants (NCHE 2017b). It should be noted that the information that can be drawn from FAFSA is not intended to be an accurate count of homelessness and only points to the need for better data.

Only recently have researchers begun to look beyond FAFSA numbers to more fully understand homelessness in higher education. A groundbreaking 2015 survey of about 4000 community college students at 10 community colleges found that approximately one-half of surveyed students were food insecure, about one-half housing insecure, and between 13 and 14% were homeless (Goldrick-Rab et al. 2015). A more recent survey of 22,000 students at 70 community colleges across 24 states found that approximately one-half of surveyed students were living in insecure housing and almost 14% were homeless. Homeless students who had previously lived in foster care and those who had children experienced disproportionately higher rates of homelessness than the other homeless students (Goldrick-Rab et al. 2017).

Recently, California State University (CSU) supported a large study to assess how their campuses were meeting the needs of students who were displaced and/or food insecure. As part of the study, researchers surveyed, interviewed, and conducted focus groups with CSU students across several campuses, finding that up to 12% were homeless and up to 24% were food insecure (Crutchfield et al. 2016).

These findings are similar to a 2017 pilot study in Alaska (Trawver and Hedwig 2017) that surveyed a sample of 193 students attending an open enrollment university in which researchers found that between 19 and 23% of responding students had lived in temporary shelter or as unsheltered and homeless during the prior 12 months. Roughly 11% reported living in unstable housing where they could not continue to stay, and 25% agreed that their housing negatively impacted their education. Finally, 8.3% of the responding students reported having experienced homelessness since beginning college.

K-12 schools, colleges, and universities can continue to find ways to better identify struggling students and link them with university and/or community resources. Further research is needed to more fully understand how food and housing insecurity impacts students and academic success, as well as how to better meet their needs.

Individuals and Families Fleeing Domestic Violence

There is a well-established link between domestic violence and homelessness. Research estimates that more than 80% of homeless women previously have experienced domestic violence (Artani 2009). Domestic violence, also known as intimate partner violence, has been identified as a primary cause of homelessness among women and their children. In the 2017 homeless PIT count, 49,077 of sheltered individuals and 38,252 of unsheltered individuals, or 15.8% of all individuals who were counted, reported that they were currently homeless due to fleeing a domestic violence situation (HUD 2017a).

Abusive home conditions often force victims to leave their home, with their only housing options being shelters or other temporary and insecure locations. Clough et al. (2014) report that a need to find and afford safe and stable housing are two of the principal concerns of women as they leave or consider leaving abusive partners. In fact, in a study of 3410 female shelter residents of 215 domestic violence shelters across 8 states, 83% reported a need for affordable housing (Lyon et al. 2008).

While we know that men experience domestic violence, the prevalence among women is far greater. Knowing the strong relationship between trauma histories and homeless women points to the need for gender-specific services and interventions that are tailored and responsive to their unique needs, including trauma-informed care and protection from further violence while staying in shelters and other temporary housing.

Older Adults

The homeless population in the United States is aging at a rapid rate. Data from New York City suggests that the age cohort at highest risk for homelessness went from 34 through 36 in 1990 to 49 through 51 in 2010, with one-third of homeless adults being over the age of 50 (Culhane et al. 2013). This population experiences the consequences of aging far earlier than their housed counterparts; a homeless person at age 50 years is likely to experience conditions associated with old age that are typically seen in the general population 20 years later. Some of these conditions include functional impairments, cognitive impairments, falls, and urinary incontinence (Brown et al. 2012). Further, homeless older adults face significant medical vulnerabilities due to the compounded effects of acute and chronic stress associated with homelessness, chronic health and behavioral health conditions (e.g., diabetes, HIV/AIDS, mental illness, substance use), and geriatric syndromes, such as mobility problems, vision and hearing impairment, weight loss and malnutrition, Dementia, and Alzheimer's. As a result, homeless people are at three to four times higher risk for dying prematurely than non-homeless people (Brown et al. 2013).

Veterans

Even though the number of homeless veterans has dropped considerably in recent years, veterans continue to represent a disproportionate percentage of the homeless population in the United States (Hamilton et al. 2012). While active duty service is widely understood as containing several risk factors pertaining to trauma and difficulty with assimilation to nonmilitary culture, it is also understood as having the capacity to be protective and to serve as a positive, life-changing event for many young men and women, and so disseminating how military service increases the likelihood of homelessness is crucial. Metraux et al. (2017) found that veterans reported becoming homeless due to transitioning from military to civilian life, relationships and employment, mental and behavioral health, lifetime and adverse events, and use of veteran-specific services. Further Metraux and others (2013) found that while posttraumatic stress presents a moderate risk factor for homelessness, socioeconomic, behavioral health, and traumatic brain injury were found to be higher risk factors for veteran homelessness.

Montgomery et al. (2013) found that individuals who served in the military were slightly more likely to have experienced childhood adversity than the general population, and that this adversity predicted homelessness more than military service itself. In fact, military service seemed to reduce the homelessness risk in these individuals, due in part to greater service access as veterans. However, military service drastically increased the risk for mental health impairment in adulthood.

There are cohort factors that provide some insight pertaining to the characteristics of homeless veterans. For example, while homeless veterans are on average younger than the total veteran population, approximately one-half of all homeless veterans are over the age of 50, most of whom served during the Vietnam era. This is not the case with female veterans, whose homelessness is experienced far more acutely in younger cohorts, perhaps due to the additional stress pertaining to heading families with young children following their service (Fargo et al. 2012). In fact, veteran women are approximately four times more likely to be homeless than non-veteran women (Hamilton et al. 2012). This dynamic is commonly attributed to the increased likelihood of experiencing trauma while enlisted as well as the unique difficulties experienced by women readjusting to life at home following their tour. Further, veteran women experiencing homelessness identify premilitary adversity along with military trauma, substance abuse during their enlistment, post-military violence and abuse, post-military unemployment, and criminal justice involvement as issues also worthy of consideration in this population (Hamilton et al. 2012).

Immigrants and Refugees

The process of immigrating from one country to another is full of unique stressors and can result in immigrants leaving behind key aspects of their existing support network, including friends, family, and familiar surroundings, which is a loss at a moment where these individuals are attempting to navigate the unenviable task of assimilating into a new culture while also hoping to retain a part of their own cultural identities (National Center for Homeless Education [NCHE] 2017a). Even immigrants with extensive professional experience in their country of origin may experience an initial decrease in status and earnings while improving their language skills, pursuing needed education, and passing relevant licensing exams. During this transition, these challenges often lead to decreased incomes, lower quality housing, and even housing instability (NCHE 2017a). The high levels of stress created by these circumstances can significantly compromise the ability of these individuals to successfully adjust in their new country (Levitt et al. 2005) and therefore create social and economic instabilities that may increase risk for homelessness.

Individuals designated as refugees may be particularly vulnerable to homelessness during the immigration process. US Citizenship and Immigration Services (2015) define refugees as individuals outside their country of origin who are unable or unwilling to return due to fear of serious harm. This presents risk for trauma as a result of war or persecution, an increased likelihood of separation from important support systems, and a potential for a lengthy displacement prior to arriving in a new home country (NCHE 2017a). The high rate of child refugees increases the vulnerability of this group, with nearly half of the world's refugee population and one-third of children living outside their country of birth (UNICEF 2015). Refugee children encounter lost social stability, much like their adult counterparts, but also are likely to be affected educationally and developmentally in ways unique to this demographic. They are also less likely than their adult counterparts to experience improved adjustment as a result of social supports in their new home country (Levitt et al. 2005).

The way an individual enters their new home country and their immigration status appears relevant in terms of safety and security generally and housing in particular. Paradis et al. (2009) found that while Toronto immigrant women with permanent resident status were more likely to live in overcrowded conditions, in almost all other measures they were better off than their non-status counterparts. For example, they moved less frequently, their living situations tended to be more secure and less vulnerable to sudden eviction or violations of privacy, and they were more likely to be residing with a dependent child and less likely to be evicted due to pregnancy. It should be noted that nonpermanent status might be restrictive in terms of employment options and access to benefits, potentially further increasing risk for not only homelessness but also extreme poverty and exploitation.

DeVerteuil (2011) theorizes that some immigrant communities have developed survival strategies that reduce incidents of "absolute" homelessness. One such strategy is overcrowding, wherein housing instability is resolved not by accessing public services but rather by moving in with family or friends from the same immigrant group, regardless of available space. This has the benefit of creating an environment of shared faith, language, ethnicity, place of origin, and perhaps time of arrival, potentially increasing trust and mutual understanding in a manner that supports healthy adjustment. While this process is also believed to restrict upward mobility and increase segregation and exclusion from services, these problematic outcomes are more reasonably attributed to broader social circumstances—including implicit and explicit bias toward immigrant populations. Further, overcrowding lends itself to a degree of housing instability, household stress, and potential vulnerability.

Race

People of color are overrepresented within the US homeless population, driven by poverty and historical and systemic racism. According to the 2016 Annual Homelessness Assessment Report, 39% of the homeless population was Black or African American (2016b). A recent study conducted by the Center for Social Innovation (2018) assessing race and homelessness in six communities (Atlanta, San Francisco, Columbus, Dallas, Syracuse, and Pierce County, Washington) found that over 78% of individuals experiencing homelessness were people of color. Further, the study found a racial disparity for Black people. While African Americans represented 18% of the general population within the study communities, 65% of the homeless population within those communities was Black. Racial disparities have also been found among homeless young adults. The Voices of Youth Count study found that, compared to non-Hispanic white youth, Black or African American youth had an 83% higher risk of experiencing homelessness and Hispanic youth had a 33% higher risk (Morton et al. 2017).

Consequences of Homelessness

Homelessness remains wrought with consequences for the individuals and families who experience it. This section discusses the impacts of stigma and experienced disparities in health, safety, stability, and daily living, as well as criminalization associated with homelessness.

Stigma

People who experience homelessness often face social stigma and discrimination largely resulting from negative stereotypes held by society. These stereotypes often stem from a high sense of individualism, which tends to blame the individual for their status rather than focusing on systemic issues that contribute to homelessness, such as high unemployment rates, insufficient units of affordable housing, and poverty (Belcher and DeForge 2012; Clapham 2003). Despite waves of support from the public to end homelessness, individuals facing homelessness continue to be largely viewed negatively, devalued, and seen as unworthy of equal rights and resources (Link et al. 1995). This public perception results in the societal belief that it is the individual's responsibility to attain housing rather than a shared, public concern.

The FrameWorks Institute (2016) found that many people hold negative views of people who are homeless, including the belief that those struggling for housing were lazy and unwilling to accept responsibility for their own problems, have made bad decisions, and are managing their money poorly. The research further found that when issues of racial and economic segregation within the context of housing are raised, the public falls back on a "we already have solved racial issues" narrative, seeing discrimination as a thing of the past or believing that racial and economic segregation are natural and inevitable. These views create many barriers for homeless people in attaining social inclusion and in accessing resources, such as safe, affordable housing.

Health and Safety Impacts

Health Disparities

It is well established that people experiencing homelessness have significantly worse health and health outcomes than people who have housing. Life expectancy is shorter, and mortality rates among people who are homeless are up to four times higher than in the general population (Geddes and Fazel 2011). Life on the streets and in shelters is both physically and mentally stressful and is associated with higher rates of negative health conditions than are found in the general population

(Fazel et al. 2014; Morrison 2009). The rates of tuberculosis, respiratory illnesses, and HIV are particularly high. Noncommunicable diseases, such as high blood pressure, diabetes, and asthma, are exacerbated by homelessness because it is difficult to store medications properly. Even minor injuries or common colds are harder to manage because bathing, access to clean bandages, and a good night sleep are difficult to obtain on the streets or in a shelter (Beijer et al. 2012; Singer 2003). Maintaining a healthy diet to prevent or manage these diseases also becomes a difficult task as soup kitchens and shelters often serve food that is high in starch, salt, and sugar, ingredients for an economical meal but with little to no nutritional benefit (Davis et al. 2008).

Exposure to adverse conditions often leads to higher stress levels, which in turn lead to higher rates of behavioral health issues. The prevalence of psychiatric diagnoses is consistently higher in homeless people than in the general population, particularly for drug and alcohol dependence. The prevalence of psychosis and depression is also higher when compared to the general population (Fazel et al. 2008).

Individuals who experience homelessness often lack health insurance to cover physical or mental health appointments and report that finding food or shelter often competes for priority with obtaining medical care (Gelberg et al. 1997; Kushel et al. 2001). As a result, people experiencing homelessness are frequent visitors of emergency departments (EDs), only seeking medical care when it cannot be avoided and a condition is too severe to ignore. One study found that they were twice as likely to have unmet medical needs and were twice as likely to have an ED visit (Lebrun-Harris et al. 2013). Emergency care is much more costly than non-emergency care, and this reliance on high cost of emergency services contributes to the overall rising cost of healthcare (Mitchell et al. 2017).

Increased risk of violence and victimization is also exceedingly common for homeless individuals. Meinbresse et al. (2014) found that nearly one-half of homeless individuals included in a five-city study across the United States were victims of violence. Rates increased further for older individuals and those who had been homeless more than 2 years. Women and sexual minorities are more likely to experience sexual violence than their heterosexual and male counterparts (Meinbresse et al. 2014; Tyler 2008).

These adverse physical health, mental health, and environmental conditions seem to accelerate the aging process and increased mortality rates among individuals who experience homelessness. A homeless person aged 50 years or older is more likely to experience conditions associated with old age that are typically seen in the general population 20 years later, such as functional and cognitive impairments, falls, and urinary incontinence (Brown et al. 2012). As a result, research has shown that people who are homeless are three to four times at higher risk for dying prematurely than the non-homeless (Morrison 2009), with some research showing homeless women at higher risk of premature death compared to homeless men (Nusselder et al. 2013).

Stability and Daily Living Impacts

Daily routines and rituals can be a protective factor for individuals, particularly when they experience the extreme stress of homelessness (Weisner 2010). When forced to move through different housing systems or living on the streets, people experiencing homelessness are denied the opportunity to adhere to a fixed and predictable schedule. For example, when they attempt to develop stability and routine through employment, they face a variety of barriers, including a lack of access to utilities for personal hygiene, limitations due to mental and physical disabilities, a lack of jobs that align with shelter hours, and lack of transportation (Barber et al. 2005; Long et al. 2007; McGurk et al. 2003; Taylor 2001; Zuvekas and Hill 2001).

For families and children, the impact of homelessness-related instability can be significant. Mayberry et al. (2014) interviewed parents with unstable housing and found that they struggled to maintain family processes and routines across different housing programs. Some shelters and traditional housing programs have strict rules that can cause family processes to be interrupted and can cause parents to feel judged for differing parenting styles or to fear being threatened by child protective service involvement (Mayberry et al. 2014).

Instability also affects children's educational outcomes. When children are homeless, they may change schools frequently, lack access to transportation to and from school, and live in a setting not ideal to complete homework, and some may have complicated physical and mental health problems, making it difficult to perform at school in educational tasks and social interactions (Cunningham et al. 2010; Dworsky 2008; Fantuzzo et al. 2012; Huntington et al. 2008; Obradović et al. 2009). These poor academic and social outcomes for children have strong negative effects on future academic and social development (Children's Defense Fund 2007).

Conclusion

Homelessness has been a long-standing condition in the United States, significantly intersecting with poverty and racial disparities, health and behavioral health disparities, criminal justice contact, and general life instability. Historically, a broad variety of populations have experienced homelessness; however, its significant impacts of marginalization and stigmatization span across both time and people. Social work as a profession is especially well positioned to lead efforts to end homelessness, both through continuing to define homelessness as an issue of social justice and through goal-directed professional practice and advocacy.

References

Artani, Y. (2009). *Homeless children and youth: Causes and consequences*. New York, NY: National Center for Children in Poverty, Mailman School of Public Health, Columbia University.

Barber, C. C., Fonagy, P., Fultz, J., Simulinas, M., & Yates, M. (2005). Homeless near a thousand homes: Outcomes of homeless youth in a crisis shelter. *American Journal of Orthopsychiatry, 75*(3), 347–355.

Belcher, J. R., & DeForge, B. R. (2012). Social stigma and homelessness: The limits of social change. *Journal of Human Behavior in the Social Environment, 22*(8), 929–946.

Beijer, U., Wolf, A., & Fazel, S. (2012). Prevalence of tuberculosis, hepatitis C virus, and HIV in homeless people: A systematic review and meta-analysis. *The Lancet Infectious Diseases, 12*(11), 859–870.

Bender, K. A., Thompson, S. J., Ferguson, K. M., Yoder, J. R., & Kern, L. (2014). Trauma among street-involved youth. *Journal of Emotional and Behavioral Disorders, 22*(1), 53–64.

Brown, R. T., Kiely, D. K., Bharel, M., & Mitchell, S. L. (2012). Geriatric syndromes in older homeless adults. *Journal of General Internal Medicine, 27*(1), 16–22.

Brown, R. T., Kiely, D. K., Bharel, M., & Mitchell, S. L. (2013). Factors associated with geriatric syndromes in older homeless adults. *Journal of Health Care for the Poor and Underserved, 24*(2), 456–468.

Byrne, T., Fargo, J. D., Montgomery, A. E., Munley, E., & Culhane, D. (2014). The relationship between community investment in permanent supportive housing and chronic homelessness. *Social Service Review, 88*(2), 234–263.

Canfield, J. P., Harley, D., Teasley, M. L., & Nolan, J. (2017). Validating the McKinney-Vento Act Implementation Scale: Examining the factor structure and reliability. *Children & Schools, 39*(1), 53–60.

Center on Budget and Policy Priorities. (2017). National and state housing fact sheets and data. Author. https://www.cbpp.org/research/housing/national-and-state-housing-fact-sheets-data. Accessed 30 June 2018.

Center for Social Innovation. (2018). Supporting partnerships for anti-racist communities: Phase one study findings. Author. http://center4si.com/wp-content/uploads/2018/03/SPARC-Phase-1-Findings-March-20181.pdf. Accessed 30 June 2018.

Chen, X., Thrane, L., Whitbeck, L. B., Johnson, K. D., & Hoyt, D. R. (2007). Onset of conduct disorder, use of delinquent subsistence strategies, and street victimization among homeless and runaway adolescents in the Midwest. *Journal of Interpersonal Violence, 22*(9), 1156–1183.

Cheung, A. M., & Hwang, S. W. (2004). Risk of death among homeless women: A cohort study and review of the literature. *Canadian Medical Association Journal, 170*(8), 1243–1247.

Cheyne, G. C. (2009). Facially discriminatory admissions policies in homeless shelters and the Fair Housing Act. University of Chicago Legal Forum. http://chicagounbound.uchicago.edu/uclf/vol2009/iss1/13. Accessed 30 June 2018.

Children's Defense Fund. (2007). *America's cradle to prison pipeline*. Washington, D.C.: Author.

Choi, S. K., Wilson, B. D. M., Shelton, J., & Gates, G. (2015). Serving our youth 2015: The needs and experiences of lesbian, gay, bisexual, transgender, and questioning youth experiencing homelessness. *The Williams Institute*. https://escholarship.org/uc/item/1pd9886n. Accessed 30 June 2018.

Christensen, R. C., Hodgkins, C. C., Garces, L., Estlund, K. L., Miller, M. D., & Touchton, R. (2005). Homeless, mentally ill and addicted: The need for abuse and trauma services. *Journal of Health Care for the Poor and Underserved, 16*(4), 615–622.

Clapham, D. (2003). Pathways approaches to homelessness research. *Journal of Community and Applied Social Psychology, 13*(2), 119–127.

Clough, A., Draughon, J. E., Njie-Carr, V., Rollins, C., & Glass, N. (2014). "Having housing made everything else possible": Affordable, safe and stable housing for women survivors of violence. *Qualitative Social Work, 13*(5), 671–688.

Collins, S. E., Malone, D. K., & Clifasefi, S. L. (2013). Housing retention in single-site housing first for chronically homeless individuals with severe alcohol problems. *American Journal of Public Health, 103*(S2), S269–S274.

Cray, A., Miller, K., & Durso L. E. (2013). Seeking shelter: The experiences and unmet needs of LGBT homeless youth. Center for American Progress. https://www.americanprogress.org/wp-content/uploads/2013/09/LGBTHomelessYouth.pdf. Accessed 30 June 2018.

Crutchfield, R., Clark, K., Gamez, S., Green, A., Munson, D., & Stribling, H. (2016). Serving displaced and food insecure students in the CSU. California State University. https://www2.calstate.edu/impact-of-the-csu/student-success/basic-needs-initiative/Documents/ServingDisplacedandFoodInsecureStudetnsintheCSUJanuary20163.8.16.pdf. Accessed 30 June 2018.

Culhane, D. P., Metraux, S., Byrne, T., Stino, M., & Bainbridge, J. (2013). The age structure of contemporary homelessness: Evidence and implications for public policy. *Analyses of Social Issues and Public Policy, 13*(1), 228–244.

Cunningham, M., Harwood, R., & Hall, S. (2010). Residential instability and the McKinney-Vento Homeless Children and Education Program: What we know, plus gaps in research. *Urban Institute*. https://eric.ed.gov/?id=ED510555. Accessed 30 June 2018.

Davis, L. R., Weller, N. F., Jadhav, M., & Holleman, W. L. (2008). Dietary intake of homeless women residing at a transitional living center. *Journal of Health Care for the Poor and Underserved, 19*(3), 952–962.

DePastino, T. (2004). Great depression. In D. Levinson (Ed.), *Encyclopedia of homelessness* (pp. 184–188). Thousand Oaks, CA: Sage Publications.

DeVerteuil, G. (2011). Survive but not thrive? Geographical strategies for avoiding absolute homelessness among immigrant communities. *Social & Cultural Geography, 12*(8), 929–945.

Durso, L. E., & Gates, G. J. (2012). *Serving our youth: Findings from a national survey of service providers working with lesbian, gay, bisexual, and transgender youth who are homeless or at risk of becoming homeless*. Los Angeles, CA: The Williams Institute with True Colors Fund and the Palette Fund.

Dworsky, A. (2008). *Educating homeless children in Chicago: A case study of children in the family regeneration program*. Chicago, IL: Chapin Hall at the University of Chicago.

Fantuzzo, J. W., LeBoeuf, W. A., Chen, C. C., Rouse, H. L., & Culhane, D. P. (2012). The unique and combined effects of homelessness and school mobility on the educational outcomes of young children. *Educational Researcher, 41*(9), 393–402.

Fargo, J., Metraux, S., Byrne, T., Munley, E., Montgomery, A. E., & Jones…Culhane, D. (2012). Prevalence and risk of homelessness among US veterans. *Preventing Chronic Disease, 9*, 110–112.

Fausset, R., & Robertson, C. (September 11, 2017). Houstonians adrift in their city, trying to call somewhere home. *New York Times*. https://www.nytimes.com/2017/09/11/us/houston-harvey-home-displaced.html. Accessed 30 June 2018.

Fazel, S., Geddes, J. R., & Kushel, M. (2014). The health of homeless people in high-income countries: Descriptive epidemiology, health consequences, and clinical and policy recommendations. *The Lancet, 384*(9953), 1529–1540.

Fazel, S., Khosla, V., Doll, H., & Geddes, J. (2008). The prevalence of mental disorders among the homeless in western countries: Systematic review and meta-regression analysis. *PLoS Medicine, 5*(12), e225.

FrameWorks Institute. (2016). *You don't have to live here:' Why housing messages are backfiring and 10 things we can do about it*. [Research Report]. Washington, D.C.: Author.

Geddes, J. R., & Fazel, S. (2011). Extreme health inequalities: Mortality in homeless people. *Lancet, 377*, 2156–2157.

Gelberg, L., Gallagher, T. C., Andersen, R. M., & Koegel, P. (1997). Competing priorities as a barrier to medical care among homeless adults in Los Angeles. *American Journal of Public Health, 87*(2), 217–220.

Gerwitz, A. H., DeGarmo, D. S., Plowman, E. J., August, G., & Realmuto, G. (2009). Parenting, parental mental health, and child functioning in families residing in supportive housing. *American Journal of Orthopsychiatry, 79*(3), 336–347.

Goldrick-Rab, S., Broton, K., & Eisenberg, D. (2015). *Hungry to learn: Addressing food and housing insecurity among undergraduates*. Madison, WI: Wisconsin HOPE Lab.

Goldrick-Rab, S., Richardson, J., & Hernandez, A. (2017). *Hungry and homeless in college: Results from a national study of basic needs insecurity in higher education*. Madison, WI: Wisconsin HOPE Lab.

Guarino, K., & Bassuk, E. (2010). Working with families experiencing homelessness: Understanding trauma and its impact. *Zero to Three, 30*(3), 11–20.

Hamilton, A., Poza, I., Hines, V., & Washington, D. (2012). Barriers to psychosocial services among homeless women veterans. *Journal of Social Work Practice in the Addictions, 12*(1), 52–68. https://doi.org/10.1080/1533256X.2012.647584.

Harris Poll. (2017). Accelerating acceptance 2017: A Harris Poll survey of Americans' acceptance of LGBTQ people. GLAAD. http://www.glaad.org/files/aa/2017_GLAAD_Accelerating_Acceptance.pdf. Accessed 30 June 2018.

Hayashi, K., Daly-Grafstein, B., Dong, H., Wood, E., & Kerr, T. (2016). The relationship between violence and engagement in drug dealing and sex work among street-involved youth. *Canadian Journal of Public Health, 107*(1), 88–93.

Hayes, M., Zonneville, M., & Bassuk, E. (2013). *The SHIFT study: Final report*. Needham, MA: The National Center on Family Homelessness.

Henwood, B. F., Wenzel, S. L., Mangana, P. F., Hombs, M., Padgett, D. K., Byrne, T., et al. (2015). *The grand challenge of ending homelessness [working paper #9]*. Columbia, SC: American Academy of Social Work and Social Welfare.

Hoch, C. (2004). Chicago skid row. In D. Levinson (Ed.), *Encyclopedia of homelessness* (pp. 59–62). Thousand Oaks, CA: Sage Publications.

Hodge, J. G., Jr., DiPietro, B., & Horton-Newell, A. E. (2017). Homelessness and the public's health: Legal responses. *Journal of Law, Medicine & Ethics, 45*, 28–32.

Homeless Assistance and Rapid Transition to Housing (HEARTH) Act. §896.

Huntington, N., Buckner, J. C., & Bassuk, E. L. (2008). Adaptation in homeless children: An empirical examination using cluster analysis. *American Behavioral Scientist, 51*(6), 737–755.

Johnson, G., & Chamberlain, C. (2008). Homelessness and substance abuse: Which comes first? *Australian Social Work, 61*(4), 342–356.

Kim, M. M., Ford, J. D., Howard, D. L., & Bradford, D. W. (2010). Assessing trauma, substance abuse, and mental health in a sample of homeless men. *Health & Social Work, 35*(1), 39–48.

Kingsley, G. T. (2017). *Trends in housing problems and federal housing assistance*. Washington, D.C.: The Urban Institute.

Kushel, M. B., Vittinghoff, E., & Haas, J. S. (2001). Factors associated with the health care utilization of homeless persons. *Journal of the American Medical Association, 285*(2), 200–206.

Kusmer, K. L. (2002). *Down and out, on the road: The homeless in American history*. New York, NY: Oxford University Press.

Landis, J. D., & McClure, K. (2010). Rethinking federal housing policy. *Journal of the American Planning Association, 76*(3), 319–348.

Larkin, H., Henwood, B., Fogel, S. J., Aykanian, A., Briar-Lawson, K. H., Donaldson, L. P., Herman, D., Little, S., Meyer-Adams, N., Padgett, D., Patchner, M., & Streeter, C. L. (2016). Responding to the grand challenge to end homelessness: The National Homelessness Social Work Initiative. *Families in Society, 97*(3), 153–159.

Larkin, H., & Park, J. (2012). Adverse childhood experiences (ACEs), service use, and service helpfulness among people experiencing homelessness. *Families in Society: The Journal of Contemporary Social Services, 93*(2), 85–93.

Lebrun-Harris, L. A., Baggett, T. P., Jenkins, D. M., Sripipatana, A., Sharma, R., Hayashi, A. S., & Ngo-Metzger, Q. (2013). Health status and health care experiences among homeless patients in federally supported health centers: Findings from the 2009 patient survey. *Health Services Research, 48*(3), 992–1017.

Levitt, M. J., Lane, J. D., & Levitt, J. (2005). Immigration stress, social support, and adjustment in the first postmigration year: An intergenerational analysis. *Research in Human Development, 2*(4), 159–177.

Link, B. G., Schwartz, S., Moore, R., Phelan, J., Struening, E., Stueve, A., & Colten, M. E. (1995). Public knowledge, attitudes, and beliefs about homeless people: Evidence for compassion fatigue? *American Journal of Community Psychology, 23*(4), 533–555.

Long, D., Rio, J., & Rosen, J. (2007). *Employment and income supports for homeless people*. Washington, D.C.: Office of the Assistant Secretary for Planning and Evaluation, U.S. Department of Health and Human Services.

Losinski, M., Katsiyannis, A., & Ryan, J. B. (2013). The McKinney-Vento Education for Homeless Children and Youth Program: Implications for Special Educators. *Intervention in School and Clinic, 49*(2), 92–98.

Lyon, E., Lane, S., & Menard, A. (2008). *Meeting survivors needs: A multi-state study of domestic violence shelter experiences, final report*. Washington, D.C.: National Institute of Justice.

Maccio, E. M., & Ferguson, K. M. (2016). Services to LGBTQ runaway and homeless youth: Gaps and recommendations. *Children and Youth Services Review, 63*, 47–57.

Mayberry, L. S., Shinn, M., Benton, J. G., & Wise, J. (2014). Families experiencing housing instability: The effects of housing programs on family routines and rituals. *American Journal of Orthopsychiatry, 84*(1), 95–109.

McGurk, S., Mueser, K., Harvey, P., LaPuglia, R., & Marder, J. (2003). Cognitive and symptom predictors of work outcomes for clients with schizophrenia in supported employment. *Psychiatric Services, 54*(8), 1129–1135.

Meinbresse, M., Brinkley-Rubinstein, L., Grassette, A., Benson, J., Hamilton, R., Mallot, M., & Jenkins, D. (2014). Exploring the experiences of violence among individuals who are homeless using a consumer-led approach. *Violence and Victims, 29*(1), 122–136.

Metraux, S., Glegg, L. X., Daighe, J. D., Chuhane, D. P., & Kane, V. (2013). Risk factors for becoming homeless among a cohort of veterans who served in the era of the Iraq and Afghanistan conflicts. *Journal of Public Health, 102*(Supplement 2), S255–S262.

Metraux, S., Cusack, M., Byrned, T. H., Hunt-Johnson, N., & True, G. (2017). Pathways into homelessness among post-9/11-era veterans. *Psychological Services, 14*(2), 229–223.

Mitchell, M. S., León, K. L., Byrne, T. H., Lin, W. C., & Bharel, M. (2017). Cost of health care utilization among homeless frequent emergency department users. *Psychological Services, 14*(2), 193–202.

Montgomery, A. E., Hill, L. L., Kane, V., & Culhane, D. P. (2013). Housing chronically homeless veterans: Evaluation the efficacy of a housing first approach to HUD-VASH. *Journal of Community Psychology, 41*(4), 505–514.

Morrison, D. S. (2009). Homelessness as an independent risk factor for mortality: Results from a retrospective cohort study. *International Journal of Epidemiology, 38*(3), 877–883.

Morton, M. H., Dworsky, A., & Samuels, G. M. (2017). *Missed opportunities: Youth homelessness in America. National estimates*. Chicago, IL: Chapin Hall at the University of Chicago.

National Alliance on Mental Illness. (2017). Mental health by the numbers. https://www.nami.org/Learn-More/Mental-Health-By-the-Numbers. Accessed 30 June 2018.

National Alliance to End Homelessness. (2016). The state of homelessness in America. http://endhomelessness.org/wp-content/uploads/2016/10/2016-soh.pdf. Accessed 30 June 2018.

National Alliance to End Homelessness. (2018). Chronically homeless. https://endhomelessness.org/homelessness-in-america/who-experiences-homelessness/chronically-homeless/. Accessed 30 June 2018.

National Center for Homeless Education. (n.d.). Local homeless education liaisons: McKinney-Vento – Law into practice. https://nche.ed.gov/downloads/briefs/liaisons.pdf. Accessed 30 June 2018.

National Center for Homeless Education. (2017a). FAFSA data on unaccompanied homeless youth. https://nche.ed.gov/ibt/fafsa.php. Accessed 30 June 2018.

National Center for Homeless Education. (2017b). Best practices in homeless education series: Supporting the education of immigrant students experiencing homelessness. https://nche.ed.gov/downloads/briefs/imm_lia.pdf. Accessed 30 June 2018.

National Coalition for the Homeless. (2009). Mental illness and homelessness. http://www.nationalhomeless.org/factsheets/Mental_Illness.pdf. Accessed 30 June 2018.

National Coalition for the Homeless. (2017a). Homelessness in America: Reasons people become homeless. http://nationalhomeless.org/tag/history/. Accessed 30 June 2018.

National Coalition for the Homeless. (2017b). LGBTQ homelessness. http://nationalhomeless.org/wp-content/uploads/2017/06/LGBTQ-Homelessness.pdf. Accessed 30 June 2018.

National Center on Family Homelessness (NCFH). (2011). The characteristics and needs of families experiencing homelessness. http://files.eric.ed.gov/fulltext/ED535499.pdf. Accessed 30 June 2018.

National Center on Family Homelessness (NCFH). (2016). How many children and families experience homelessness? https://endhomelessness.org/homelessness-in-america/who-experiences-homelessness/children-and-families/. Accessed 30 June 2018.

National Health Care for the Homeless Council. (2017). What is the official definition of homelessness? https://www.nhchc.org/faq/official-definition-homelessness/. Accessed 30 June 2018.

National Law Center on Homelessness and Poverty. (2015). Homelessness in America: Overview of data and causes. https://www.nlchp.org/documents/Homeless_Stats_Fact_Sheet. Accessed 30 June 2018.

National Law Center on Homelessness & Poverty. (2016). *Housing not handcuffs: Ending the criminalization of homelessness in U.S. cities*. Washington, D.C.: Author.

Nooe, R. M., & Patterson, D. A. (2010). The ecology of homelessness. *Journal of Human Behavior in the Social Environment, 20*(2), 105–152.

Nusselder, W. J., Slockers, M. T., Krol, L., Slockers, C. T., Looman, C. W. N., & van Beeck, E. F. (2013). Mortality and life expectancy in homeless men and women in Rotterdam: 2001–2010. *PLoS One, 8*(10), e73979.

O'Connell, M. J., Kasprow, W., & Rosenheck, R. A. (2008). Rates and risk factors for homelessness after successful housing in a sample of formerly homeless veterans. *Psychiatric Services, 59*(3), 268–275.

Obradović, J., Long, J. D., Cutuli, J. J., Chan, C. K., Hinz, E., Heistad, D., & Masten, A. S. (2009). Academic achievement of homeless and highly mobile children in an urban school district: Longitudinal evidence on risk, growth, and resilience. *Development and Psychopathology, 21*(2), 493–518.

Quimby, E. G., Edidin, J. P., Ganim, Z., Gustafson, E., Hunter, S. J., & Karnik, N. S. (2012). Psychiatric disorders and substance use in homeless youth: A preliminary comparison of San Francisco and Chicago. *Behavioral Science, 2*(3), 186–194.

Paradis, E., Novac, S., Sarty, M., & Hulchanski, J. D. (2009). Better off in a shelter? A year of homelessness and housing among status immigrant, non-status migrant, and Canadian-born families. In J. D. Hulchanski, P. Campsie, S. Chau, S. Hwang, & E. Paradis (Eds.), *Finding home: Policy options for addressing homelessness in Canada*. Toronto, ON: Cities Centre, University of Toronto.

Primeau, A., Bowers, T. G., & Harrison, M. A. (2013). Deinstitutionalization of the mentally ill: Evidence for transinstitutionalization from psychiatric hospitals to penal institutions. *Comprehensive Psychology, 2*(2), 1–10.

Riley, E. D., Torsten, B. N., Moore, K., Cohen, J., Bangsber, D. R., & Havlir, D. (2012). Social, structural and behavioral determinants of overall health status in a cohort of homeless and unstably housed HIV-infected men. *PLoS One, 7*(4), e35207.

Rog, D. J., Marshall, T., Dougherty, R. H., George, P., Daniels, A. S., Ghose, S. S., & Delphin-Rittmon, M. E. (2014). Permanent supportive housing: Assessing the evidence. *Psychiatric Services, 65*(3), 287–294.

Schuster, J., Park, C. L., & Frisman, L. K. (2011). Trauma exposure and PTSD symptoms among homeless mothers: Predicting coping and mental health outcomes. *Journal of Social and Clinical Psychology, 30*(8), 887–904.

Singer, J. (2003). Taking it to the streets: Homelessness, health, and health care in the United States. *Journal of General Internal Medicine, 18*(11), 964–965.

Stainbrook, K. (2006). Similarities in the characteristics and needs of women with children in homeless family and domestic violence shelters. *Families in Society, 87*(1), 3–62.

Stewart, A. J., Steiman, M., Cauce, A. M., Cochran, B. N., Whitbeck, L. B., & Hoyt, D. R. (2004). Victimization and posttraumatic stress disorder among homeless adolescents. *Journal of the American Academy of Child & Adolescent Psychiatry, 43*(3), 325–331.

Taylor, L. C. (2001). Work attitudes, employment barriers, and mental health symptoms in a sample of rural welfare recipients. *American Journal of Community Psychology, 29*(3), 443–463.

Thompson, R. G., Wall, M. M., Greenstein, E., Grant, B. F., & Hasin, D. S. (2013). Substance-use disorders and poverty as prospective predictors of first-time homelessness in the United States. *American Journal of Public Health, 103*(Suppl 2), S282–S288.

Thompson, S. J., Bender, K., Windsor, L., Cook, M. J., & Williams, T. (2010). Homeless youth: Characteristics, contributing factors, and service options. *Journal of Human Behavior in the Social Environment, 20*(2), 193–217.

Trawver, K. R., & Hedwig, T. (2017). Food and housing insecurity and homelessness among students attending an open-enrollment university.. Unpublished manuscript.

Treatment Advocacy Center. (2014). How many people with serious mental illness are homeless? http://www.treatmentadvocacycenter.org/fixing-the-system/features-and-news/2596-how-many-people-with-serious-mental-illness-are-homeless. Accessed 30 June 2018.

True Colors Fund. (2017). Our issue. https://truecolorsfund.org/our-issue/. Accessed 30 June 2018.

Tsemberis, S., Gulcur, L., & Nakae, B. A. (2004). Housing First, consumer choice, and harm reduction for homeless individuals with a dual diagnosis. *American Journal of Public Health, 94*(4), 651–656.

Tyler, K. A. (2008). A comparison of risk factors for sexual victimization among gay, lesbian, bisexual, and heterosexual homeless young adults. *Violence and Victims, 23*(5), 586–602.

UNICEF. (2015). Uprooted: The growing crisis for refugee and migrant children. https://www.unicef.org/publications/index_92710.html. Accessed 30 June 2018.

United States Citizenship and Immigration Services. (2015). Refugees and asylum. https://www.uscis.gov/humanitarian/refugees-asylum. Accessed 30 June 2018.

United States Code of Federal Regulations. (2006a). The Public Health and Welfare: Fair Housing. 42 USC § 3604(a).

United States Code of Federal Regulations. (2006b). The Public Health and Welfare: Fair Housing. 42 USC § 3604(f)(1).

United States Code of Federal Regulations. (2006c). The Public Health and Welfare: 42 USC § 11302.

United States Code of Federal Regulations. (2006d). The Public Health and Welfare: 42 USC § 42 U.S.C § 11431(1) & (3).

United States Code of Federal Regulations. (2006e). The Public Health and Welfare: 42 USC § (42 U.S.C. § 11431.723(d)).

United States Code of Federal Regulations. (2006f). The Public Health and Welfare: 42 USC § 11432(3)(C)(i)(I)-(III).

United States Code of Federal Regulations. (2006g). The Public Health and Welfare: 42 USC § 42 U.S.C. § 11434a(2)(A-B).

United States Department of Education. (2004). Education for homeless children and youth program. https://www2.ed.gov/programs/homeless/guidance.pdf. Accessed 30 June 2018.

United States Department of Housing and Urban Development. (n.d.) Continuum of Care (COC) program eligibility requirements. https://www.hudexchange.info/programs/coc/coc-program-eligibility-requirements/. Accessed 30 June 2018.

United States Department of Housing and Urban Development. (2012). Criteria for definition of at risk of homelessness. https://www.hudexchange.info/resource/1975/criteria-for-definition-of-at-risk-of-homelessness/. Accessed 30 June 2018.

United States Department of Housing and Urban Development. (2015a). Rapid re-housing. https://www.hudexchange.info/resources/documents/Rapid-Re-Housing-Brief.pdf. Accessed 30 June 2018.

United States Department of Housing and Urban Development. (2015b). Federal Register: Rules and Regulations, (80)233, 75792. https://www.hudexchange.info/resources/documents/Defining-Chronically-Homeless-Final-Rule.pdf. Accessed 30 June 2018.

United States Department of Housing and Urban Development. (2016a). HUD 2016 continuum of care homeless assistance programs homeless populations and subpopulations. https://www.hudexchange.info/resource/reportmanagement/published/CoC_PopSub_NatlTerrDC_2016.pdf. Accessed 30 June 2018.

United States Department of Housing and Urban Development. (2016b). *The 2016 Annual Homeless Assessment Report (AHAR) to Congress*. Washington, D.C.: Author.

United States Department of Housing and Urban Development. (2017a). HUD 2017 continuum of care homeless assistance programs homeless populations and subpopulations. https://www.hudexchange.info/resource/reportmanagement/published/CoC_PopSub_NatTerrDC_2017.pdf. Accessed 30 June 2018.

United States Department of Housing and Urban Development. (2017b). *Mission*. https://portal.hud.gov/hudportal/HUD?src=/about/mission. Accessed 30 June 2018.

United States Department of Housing and Urban Development. (2017c). Community Planning and Development Homeless Assistance Grants: 2018 summary statement and initiatives. https://portal.hud.gov/hudportal/documents/huddoc?id=22-HomelessAGrants.pdf. Accessed 30 June 2018.

United States Department of Housing and Urban Development. (2017d). Continuum of Care (COC) program eligibility requirements. https://www.hudexchange.info/programs/coc/coc-program-eligibility-requirements/. Accessed 30 June 2018.

United States Department of Housing and Urban Development. (2018). AHAR reports, guides, tools, and webinars. https://www.hudexchange.info/programs/hdx/guides/ahar/#reports. Accessed 30 June 2018.

United States Interagency on Homelessness. (2018). Key Federal terms and definitions of homelessness among youth. https://www.usich.gov/resources/uploads/asset_library/Federal-Definitions-of-YouthHomelessness.pdf. Accessed 30 June 2018.

Weisner, T. S. (2010). Well-being, chaos, and culture: Sustaining a meaningful daily routine. In G. W. Evans & T. D. Wachs (Eds.), *Chaos and its influence on children's development: An ecological perspective* (pp. 211–224). Washington, D.C.: American Psychological Association.

Wenzel, S. L., Rhoades, H., Tucker, J. S., Golinelli, D., Kennedy, D. P., Zhou, A., & Ewing, B. (2012). HIV risk behavior and access to services: What predicts HIV testing among heterosexually active homeless men? *AIDS Education and Prevention, 24*(3), 270–279.

Whitbeck, L. B., Hoyt, D. R., Johnson, K., & Chen, X. (2007). Victimization and posttraumatic stress disorder among runaway and homeless adolescents. *Violence and Victimization, 22*(6), 721–734.

Whoriskey, P. (2006). Katrina displaced 400,000, study says. *Washington Post*. http://www.washingtonpost.com/wp-dyn/content/article/2006/06/06/AR2006060601729.html. Accessed 30 June 2018.

Wilkins, B. T., Mullins, M. H., Mahan, A., & Canfield, J. (2016). Homeless liaisons' awareness about the implementation of the McKinney-Vento Act. *Children & Schools, 38*(1), 57–64.

Wong, K. (2009). Narrowing the definition of "dwelling" under the Fair Housing Act. *UCLA Law Review, 56*(6), 1867–1898.

Wong, C. F., Clark, L. F., & Marlotte, L. (2016). The impact of specific and complex trauma on the mental health of homeless youth. *Journal of Interpersonal Violence, 31*(5), 831–854.

Young, S. D., & Rice, E. (2011). Online social networking technologies, HIV knowledge, and sexual risk and testing behaviors among homeless youth. *AIDS Behavior, 15*(2), 253–260.

Zuvekas, S. H., & Hill, S. C. (2001). Income and employment among homeless people: The role of mental health, health and substance abuse. *The Journal of Mental Health Policy and Economics, 3*(3), 153–163.

Chapter 2
Trauma and Adversity in the Lives of People Experiencing Homelessness

Stephanie Duncan, Stephen Oby, and Heather Larkin

Who Is Homeless and Why

Homelessness is a profoundly devastating experience that negatively affects the health and well-being of those who experience it. Several issues explicitly contribute to homelessness, including a lack of affordable housing, unemployment, lack of access to needed resources and supports, physical and psychiatric health impairments, and physical violence. What appears to also contribute to experiences of homelessness, albeit perhaps less explicitly, is the presence of trauma.

The prevalence of trauma in individuals and families experiencing homelessness is remarkably high, both as victims of and witnesses to singular and repeated traumatic events, such as acts of violence, lack of safety and security, and loss of home. These experiences with trauma can significantly impact individuals, altering how they experience their world, relate to others, manage their own needs, and think and behave generally (Guarino and Bassuk 2010). The combination of trauma and homelessness, not only in how one contributes to the other but how they interact over the lifespan, warrants careful consideration and examination by service providers.

Electronic supplementary material: The online version of this chapter (https://doi.org/10.1007/978-3-030-03727-7_2) contains supplementary material, which is available to authorized users.

S. Duncan
University of Texas at Austin, Austin, TX, USA
e-mail: stephanie.duncan@utexas.edu

S. Oby
University at Albany, Albany, NY, USA
e-mail: soby@albany.edu

H. Larkin (✉)
School of Social Welfare, University at Albany, Albany, NY, USA
e-mail: hlarkin@albany.edu

H. Larkin et al. (eds.), *Homelessness Prevention and Intervention in Social Work*, https://doi.org/10.1007/978-3-030-03727-7_2

The interaction between trauma and homelessness manifests in several ways. For example, research shows that adults experiencing homelessness exhibit not only high rates of trauma (Guarino and Bassuk 2010) but also high rates of chronic health issues, mental health impairments, and substance use issues, and they are more likely than the general population to experience multiple problems at once (Zlotnick and Zerger 2008). Substance abuse is understood as a key impediment to successful management of a psychiatric health disorder, an interaction that increases vulnerability to additional health problems, victimization, incarceration, and indeed homelessness, with no fewer than half of all homeless individuals with a psychiatric illness also abusing substances (Padgett et al. 2011). With high rates of trauma and co-occurring disorders among this population, homeless individuals are uniquely vulnerable to a particularly troublesome dynamic in which recovery is less likely.

The unique experiences of homeless women further highlight the interplay between trauma, homelessness, and related impairments, such as mental illness and substance abuse. Women who had experienced co-occurring homelessness and psychiatric illness revealed in interviews that they encountered horrific incidents of trauma in their lives, as well as betrayals of trust, anxiety around interacting with the world, and loss of status as homeless women (Padgett et al. 2006), factors specific to a population simultaneously navigating trauma and homelessness. This is particularly important when considering families experiencing homelessness, given how commonly women are single heads of household in these circumstances and the degree to which a child's health and well-being are tied to that of their parent (Guarino and Bassuk 2010). Children experiencing homelessness often live in unsafe environments and are exposed to greater trauma and adversity than their peers who have not experienced homelessness, including witnessing or experiencing violence. Further, children who are experiencing homelessness are more likely to have health issues, developmental delays, mental health impairments, and academic difficulties than their housed peers (Hayes et al. 2013).

Another population navigating unique interactions between trauma and homelessness are veterans of the military. While the number of homeless veterans has dropped considerably in recent years, veterans continue to represent a disproportionate percentage of the homeless population in the USA (Henry et al. 2017). Active service is widely understood as containing several risk factors pertaining to trauma and difficulty with assimilation to nonmilitary culture; military service, however, is also understood as having the capacity to be protective and can be a positive, life-changing event for many. Thus, discerning how military service increases the likelihood of homelessness is crucial. Montgomery et al. (2013) found that individuals who served in the military were slightly more likely to have experienced childhood adversity than the general population and that this adversity predicted homelessness more than military service itself. In fact, military service was associated with a reduced homelessness risk in these individuals, due in part to access to services for veterans to which nonveterans do not have access. Yet, military service drastically increased the risk for mental health impairment in adulthood, and a qualitative inquiry with women veterans revealed increased vulnerability following service including: post-military violence, abuse, and relationship termination; post-military substance abuse and medical conditions; and unemployment (Hamilton et al. 2011).

The consequences of childhood adversity for veterans who experience homelessness appear to differ from those described by homeless women with psychiatric illness. This is highlighted by findings in Kim et al. (2010), which showed a lack of relationship between childhood trauma and certain outcomes known to be associated with trauma, such as substance abuse and physical health impairments. The lack of relationship between childhood adversity and later-in-life problems may be due to the narrow definition of trauma used in the study. It may also reflect the need to conceive of trauma not only as single, significant events but as lower-level difficulties that can similarly affect individual functioning.

The Role of Trauma and Adversity in Homelessness

Understanding the impact that trauma can have on the daily functioning of individuals and families is crucial to understanding how it contributes to an issue such as homelessness. Guarino and Bassuk (2010) describe a "natural alarm system" within the brain that is used to detect and respond to danger. When a threat cannot be successfully addressed with one of the three responses—an active response to address the threat, avoiding the threat, or simply freezing—it can become traumatic, creating feelings of hopelessness and anger as well as a lack of control. Complex trauma can leave individuals in a state of almost constant arousal as they look to identify and address potential dangers, affecting their ability to think, plan, solve problems, manage their emotions, and pursue and maintain meaningful relationships (van der Kolk et al. 2005). Certainly, attempting to navigate experiences of complex trauma is demanding enough that to manage a lack of adequate housing or well-paying jobs, not to mention a loss of housing and the experience of homelessness, is an almost insurmountable challenge.

The debilitating effects of trauma may be particularly influential in early childhood. Early childhood trauma has been conceived of as resulting in a series of neurobiological responses related to the brain's ability to manage stress, with early adverse experiences manifesting biologically and in lived experiences accumulating over the lifespan, overwhelming the brain and body in what is described as allostatic overload (McEwen 2012). The implication appears to be that early childhood trauma has the potential to put an affected individual on a trajectory in which more difficulties are encountered because of that trauma, further challenging the individual's capacity to cope and yielding additional negative outcomes.

Appreciating the interplay between trauma, related social and emotional challenges, and homelessness warrants a certain conception of the issue. Moving beyond understandings of the causes and consequences of homelessness that focus on the individual—which might see trauma as explicitly causing homelessness—or on systems, which might interrogate the failure of society to adequately support traumatized individuals or resolve housing shortages, to a biopsychosocial approach is a significant step in more meaningfully explaining an otherwise elusive phenomenon. This perspective attributes disease and other negative health outcomes to complex and highly variable interactions between biological, psychological, and social factors (Santrock 2012). By examining the intricate components that lead to homelessness, including trauma, and by understanding their interplay as unpredictable and dynamic, we are well-positioned to more meaningfully understand the phenomenon.

This interplay is exemplified in the role of not just trauma but adversity. Research now tells us that adversity early in life has greater long-term impacts on an individual's functioning than were previously understood. It not only has the potential to impact factors relevant to housing, including educational attainment (Dupre 2008) and experiences of unemployment and poverty (Zielinski 2009), but also increases the likelihood of further adversity into adulthood. This evolving and accumulating adversity affects individuals' ability to cope, exposes them to experiences that increase their risk for homelessness (e.g., domestic violence), and makes the risk of victimization greater (Hopper et al. 2010). It appears that trauma and adversity each can play a role in experiences of homelessness.

Homelessness as Trauma

The disruptive nature of trauma and its potential role in creating or contributing to pathways toward homelessness do not entirely account for the degree to which homelessness itself serves as trauma, likely as part of an accumulation of adversity and a larger pattern of disturbance of healthy development. Oppenheimer et al. (2016) demonstrate the degree to which health and mental health impairment is amplified in populations of individuals who have experienced homelessness, conceiving of these issues as part of a broader trend that may have begun prior to experiences of homelessness but were exacerbated during that time. Further, these authors point to greater health-risk behaviors and diminished access to social support in this population, factors that almost certainly were worsened during stretches of homelessness. It is not enough to hypothesize that homelessness caused these impairments, or vice versa, but rather it is likely that the conditions of homelessness served to worsen their effect and therefore made the experience of homelessness itself problematic and potentially traumatic.

The experience of homelessness can be particularly hard on minor children, who are already at higher risk for adverse childhood experiences due to higher rates of witnessing and experiencing violence as well as psychiatric illness and drug and alcohol use among caregivers (Guarino and Bassuk 2010). This is further complicated by the volatile behaviors and responses that might be exhibited by caregivers, as well as the turmoil that accompanies frequent relocation, including an increased likelihood among homeless children of being separated from their families and potentially placed in foster care. These disruptions create a general sense of instability that can be felt in practical ways too; for example, multiple relocations can result in having to change schools numerous times even within a given year, disrupting academic achievement as well as peer and adult connections. Trauma becomes complex trauma when it is persistent and sustained over a length of time and particularly when it is facilitated or enabled by caregivers during formative years. This can create a dynamic in which individuals who have experienced homelessness, or who may be currently experiencing homelessness, are at considerably greater risk for the effects of complex trauma (Guarino and Bassuk 2010).

Homeless youth experience increased risk for victimization, which is associated with a range of negative health outcomes, including substance abuse, self-harm, depression, and posttraumatic stress disorder (Bender et al. 2016). Young people experiencing homelessness lack emotional support, and the ensuing distress serves to produce mental health issues or exacerbate existing issues, with youth reporting increased symptoms of depression affecting daily functioning and self-esteem (Thompson et al. 2010). Young people are often in a stage of development where their coping skills are limited. Limited coping skills combined with the risk of previous trauma and family stress create a set of circumstances where youth are unable to navigate the demands that accompany homelessness, increasing the risk for vulnerability, which is associated with increased rates of suicidal ideation and suicide attempts (Thompson et al. 2010). This is another example not only of the detrimental effects of homelessness but the complicated back-and-forth relationship between precursors to homelessness, such as trauma and adversity, negative health outcomes, and homelessness itself.

The Adverse Childhood Experiences (ACE) Study

Adverse childhood experiences (ACEs) is a term that grew out of a study by medical researchers at Kaiser Permanente and the Centers for Disease Control and Prevention (Felitti et al. 1998). The goal of the study was to develop a sense of how the exposure to adverse experiences as a child might affect long-term health in adulthood. ACEs do not describe numbers of incidents but rather categories of events experienced prior to the age of 18 that were conceived of as potentially contributing to negative health outcomes later in life. The original ACE study consisted of approximately 17,000 patients from a notably middle-class, Caucasian population in San Diego, California. Researchers asked patients to report retrospectively on their experience with ten ACE categories, including sexual, physical, or emotional abuse; physical or emotional neglect; loss of a parent due to death, divorce, or incarceration; mental illness in a parent; and drug or alcohol abuse by a parent. The number of "yes" responses is summed to create an ACE score that ranges from 0 to 10, which was hypothesized to be correlated with negative health outcomes in adulthood. Indeed, the ACE study revealed powerful relationships between higher ACE scores and emotional and physical health problems later in life, and ACEs are now implicated in many of the leading causes of death in the USA. The ACE study has been extended by several researchers, and departments of health in a number of states have included the ACE questions on the Behavioral Risk Factor Surveillance

System (BRFSS), making it one of the most influential studies ever conducted (Centers for Disease Control and Prevention 2018a, b).

ACEs and Health Disparities

As noted above, ACEs are implicated in many of the leading causes of death in the USA. To understand how early childhood adversity would ultimately result in early death, researchers have examined how accumulated early adversity can lead to social, emotional, and cognitive impairment, which then increases the likelihood of individuals adopting health-risk behaviors. The connection between higher ACE scores and an increase in social, emotional, and cognitive impairment has been explained by neurobiological factors that impact early brain development, the immune system, and the endocrine system (Metzler et al. 2017; McCrory et al. 2011; Shonkoff et al. 2009, 2012; Danese et al. 2008). The devastating outcomes often experienced by individuals with high ACE scores imply the need to incorporate the ACE questionnaire into routine services. This would support the ability to provide preventive services and address the negative health outcomes of those who have high ACE scores (Larkin et al. 2014).

It has become clear that adverse experiences during childhood can deeply affect a young person and profoundly influence emotional and physical health. The conceptual framework developed by the original ACE study authors is an attempt to explain why the accumulation of adversity would be associated with later-in-life health problems and even early death, a correlation that is not self-evident. The pyramid model (Fig. 2.1) depicts a trajectory of adverse childhood experiences contributing to but not guaranteeing disrupted neurodevelopment, which then creates risk for social, emotional, and cognitive impairment and potential subsequent adoption of health-risk behaviors. These behaviors increase the odds of disease, disability, and social problems, which may then contribute to death. Individuals experiencing early adversity do not always experience early death as a result, of course, but rather this is a potential outcome mitigated by an individual's supports and degree of resilience. However, as the pyramid illustrates, each outcome may potentially lead to the next, and as the pyramid narrows, fewer individuals may be affected; yet, the potential sequence is clear. This interpretation points to opportunities for prevention and intervention activities across the lifespan. Furthermore, viewing individuals within a biopsychosocial context could support our ability to improve the health of more people who have experienced adversity, reducing negative health outcomes or even premature death (Larkin et al. 2014).

ACEs and Homelessness

Homelessness is by now well established as not strictly a structural or an individual issue but a combination of the two, and individual factors related to homelessness reflect a long-term trajectory of adversity and hardship that interact and accumulate

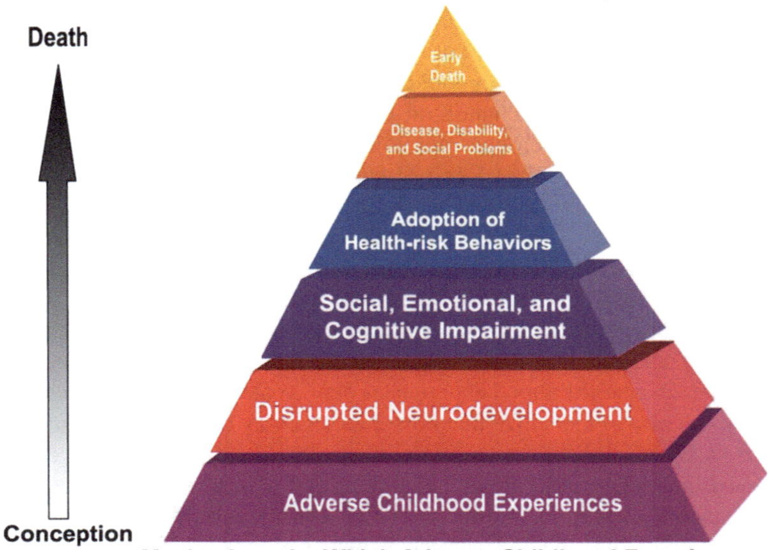

Fig. 2.1 The pyramid model illustrates a potential pathway from early childhood experiences to later-in-life health consequences (Centers for Disease Control and Prevention 2018b)

over time. Life stresses have been consistently linked to depression, substance abuse, poor health, and premature mortality, including suicide (Felitti et al. 1998; Gould et al. 1994; Horwitz et al. 2001; Thorncroft 2011). Recent research indicates that ACE scores are considerably higher among homeless populations than the general population (Larkin and Park 2012; Roos et al. 2013). Larkin and Park (2012) found that 87% of a convenience sample of homeless adults reported at least one ACE and more than half reported four or more. This is in stark contrast to the original ACE study, which found approximately half of all respondents reported one ACE and six percent reported four or more. While this correlation might be expected given what is known about correlates to homelessness, these figures are nonetheless striking. Further, ACE categories are interrelated, meaning that having experienced one ACE increases the likelihood of experiencing another (Larkin and Park 2012; Dong et al. 2004). These findings support the notion of a complex interplay between trauma, adversity, and homelessness. Adults experiencing homelessness exhibit high rates of chronic health issues, as well as mental health and substance use disorders, and are more likely than the general population to be experiencing co-occurring problems (Zlotnick and Zerger 2008), factors that may be indicative of high ACE scores. It is surmised that higher ACE scores increase individual vulnerability to various societal conditions (e.g., lack of jobs and affordable housing, various types of oppression) that cause homelessness (Larkin and Park 2012).

It may be tempting to see a single instance of homelessness as an event in isolation that can be resolved through short-term crisis intervention to meet basic needs along with improved housing and job opportunities. Yet, this interpretation fails to account for how the additive effect of childhood adversities becomes entwined with ongoing life events, which in turn yield lifelong challenges. A limitation of current ACE research includes its reliance on cross-sectional studies with retrospective reporting. Thus, the research does not define a causal relationship between ACEs and homelessness and can therefore not explain why person X with an ACE score of eight experienced homelessness while person Y who also has an ACE score of eight did not. Yet, even with a lack of causal evidence, the correlational research is compelling (Cutuli et al. 2013). Thus, while certain aspects of retrospective reporting may be called into question, the weight of these correlations puts the relationship between accumulated early adversity, the health-risk factors that contribute to homelessness, and homelessness itself beyond doubt. In addition to understanding the ways that adverse childhood experiences may create a pathway to homelessness, it is also necessary to recognize that homelessness may contribute to a greater incidence of ACEs.

Formerly homeless individuals have identified patterns of social losses, acute traumatic events as well as chronic stressors, and the interrelated and cumulative nature of adversity over the lifespan as key themes of lived adversity (Padgett 2012). Yet, the ACE questionnaire does not include the experience of being homeless as a youth as one of its ten categories. Homeless youth have high rates of past substance abuse, with up to two-thirds of homeless youth reporting a history of childhood physical or sexual abuse (Keeshin and Campbell 2011; Busen and Engebretson 2008; Kral et al. 1997; Ryan et al. 2000). Existing findings have identified homeless youth compared to their non-homeless peers as displaying increased rates of tobacco use, substance abuse, high-risk sexual behavior, victimization, and mental illness (Keeshin and Campbell 2011; McCaskill et al. 1998). Homeless youth often experience several stressors because of the fear developed around not having a safe place to live or separation from family. Research also reveals that many homeless youth score higher on the ACE questionnaire than youth in a family home (Thompson et al. 2010). Those who have a lifetime of homelessness have higher rates of childhood adversities compared to those who have not experienced homelessness (Roos et al. 2013).

The research also suggests that many youth who are homeless experienced a multitude of risk factors leading to homelessness. For example, a reason frequently cited for leaving home is parental drug and alcohol use, which is often associated with parental abandonment, family violence, and neglect, as well as sexual, physical, and psychological abuse (Edidin et al. 2012; Merscham et al. 2009). These factors may also contribute to an increased likelihood of out of home placements or foster care, which may also lead to youth homelessness (Merscham et al. 2009). Although there are limitations, the handful of studies available suggest that adverse experiences and being homeless before the age of 18 can have a profound effect on young people, including diagnoses of posttraumatic stress disorder or other mental illnesses, which can also be tied to substance abuse, incarceration, and suicide. Homeless youth may feel powerless and take part in illicit practices, often because they see themselves as having little value and opportunity and few economic resources (Yoder et al. 2014; Baron and Hartnagel 1998). Homeless youth often rely on survival behaviors, such as drug dealing, prostitution, and theft, rather than gaining traditional employment because they are able to generate immediate income. However, while youth engage in these activities to survive and earn income, it often positions them to enter the criminal justice system (Yoder et al. 2014). Future interventions could focus on treating the trauma and adversity youth have experienced rather than attending exclusively to the illegal behaviors that led to incarceration (Yoder et al. 2014).

Moreover, homeless youth may experience further adversities once homeless and need proper services and supports as well as interventions that are tailored to their needs. Factors such as impaired attachment or inadequate social support contribute to poor outcomes for people who experience ACEs (Roos et al. 2013). Homeless individuals who have high ACE scores may have poor attachment and underdeveloped trust skills, which may compromise their functionality in the community. For example, youth who have run away and become homeless often lack trust because their caregiver was inaccessible emotionally; this may be generalizable to their new social environment, thereby preventing them from having trusting relationships with service providers (Travecchio et al. 1999). High ACE scores are more common among people experiencing homelessness as compared to the sample in the original ACE study, and it is clear that ACEs are powerfully connected to many of the health-risk behaviors that contribute to homelessness and long-term health and psychosocial problems. In one study, people experiencing homelessness with ACE backgrounds reported using a range of supports and services before becoming homeless, which suggests there is an opportunity for ACE-informed services that could play a role in preventing homelessness (Larkin and Park 2012).

The ACE research suggests the need for a lifespan and intergenerational perspective, recognizing opportunities to partner across sectors to break the trajectory from high ACE scores to later-in-life health and social problems. The Restorative Integral Support (RIS) model was first developed within a homeless service agency to facilitate ACE-informed programming for a whole-person approach to addressing ACEs and trauma by fostering resilience in programs and communities (Larkin and Records 2007; Larkin et al. 2012).

ACE Response: The Restorative Integral Support Model

One of the defining elements of social work practice is an integrative, person-in-environment perspective that incorporates all aspects of an individual within the context of their social environments (Garner 2011; Germain and Gitterman 1980). This is particularly important for addressing the issue of homelessness given the biopsychosocial contributions to this phenomenon, suggesting that a broad range of individual and environmental issues are relevant in addressing homelessness. For this reason, a whole-person approach would include simultaneous attention to biological, psychological, and social concerns. Human service providers might seek to address homelessness by raising awareness around the role of ACEs in relevant health outcomes, building capacity to address negative ACE consequences, supporting ACE-appropriate responses by policy makers and other significant stakeholders, and collaborating throughout communities to move toward meaningful ACE responses across sectors (Larkin and Park 2012; Larkin et al. 2018).

This section presents the Restorative Integral Support (RIS) model and addresses training implications for agency leaders and service providers. Agency leaders bring together a variety of best practices to respond to the needs of clients within the context of local resources. RIS unifies a comprehensive knowledge of adversity and trauma with an understanding of resilience and recovery to inform programs. The RIS model is therefore offered as a flexible guide in attending to leadership, service systems, and culture while integrating a range of prevention and intervention activities for a comprehensive approach. More specifically, in applying integral theory (Wilber 2000) to address ACEs, RIS clarifies the distinction between adversity and trauma and offers a framework for building resilience in programs and communities (Larkin and Records 2007).

RIS can be viewed as a map that points to opportunities for bringing together evidence-supported interventions within intentionally developed restorative contexts, involving leadership capacity development, peer supports, and policy and system redesign (Larkin et al. 2012). RIS application reveals that adversity co-arises with a variety of internal and external resources, with trauma emerging as an "all-quadrant" experience.

The quadrants represent four irreducible perspectives—subjective (first person), intersubjective (second person), objective, and inter-objective (third person)—that must be consulted when attempting to fully understand any issue or aspect of reality. The collective, or community, is made up of individuals. This interrelatedness is conveyed through the concept of the quadrants. The top two quadrants represent the individual, and the bottom quadrants represent the community or collective. The right-hand quadrants represent observable qualities, while the left-hand quadrants are subjective and therefore involve asking questions to understand. The upper-left quadrant is a first-person perspective, also referred to as the "I" quadrant or the interior of the individual. The lower left quadrant represents cultural values, shared meanings, and social networks. This quadrant is identified as the "WE" quadrant or second-person perspective. The right-hand quadrants are third-person perspectives, objective, and inter-objective and thus referred to as the "IT" and "ITS" quadrants. Figure 2.2 illustrates the four quadrants by mapping adversity and trauma to these perspectives.

It is often helpful to point out the observable physical impacts of ACEs in the brain, which can bring about a major shift in how people who have experienced trauma are viewed and treated (including how they treat themselves). In this way, an upper-right (IT) quadrant observable consequence can lead to changes in upper-left (I) quadrant perceptions as well as changes in lower-left (WE) quadrant shared meanings and lower-right (ITS) quadrant observable interactions. In mapping ACEs, each quadrant reflects different dimensions of the adversity, including whether an adverse event is also traumatic. The meanings people make of observable

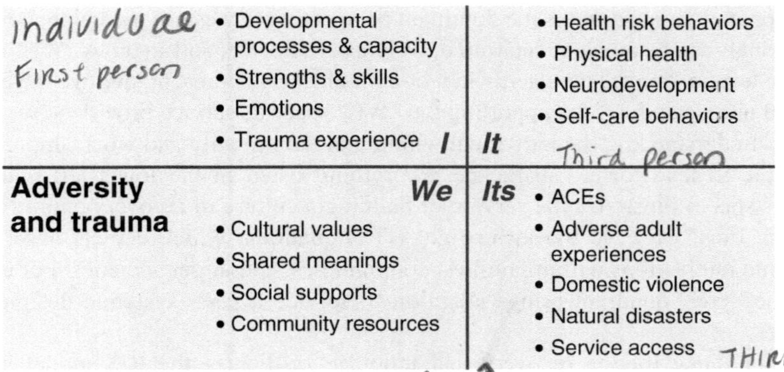

Fig. 2.2 Adversity and trauma: The Restorative Integral Support (RIS) quadrants (Larkin and Records 2011)

adverse interactions (lower-right ITS quadrant) are influenced by lower-left (WE) quadrant culture and upper-left (I) quadrant individual perception. Numerous developmental processes, mapped to the upper-left (I) quadrant, are also taking place within the context of relationships (lower-left WE quadrant). One's developmental capacity is an upper-left resource as are lower-left social supports and lower-right access to services. An adverse event has the potential to derail development, but this can also be counteracted by cultural and systemic supports. Trauma is an upper-left subjective assessment indicating that an adverse event is experienced as overwhelming. Behavioral attempts at coping, including risk behaviors, would be mapped to the upper-right quadrant (Larkin and Records 2007; Larkin and Records 2011).

The RIS model then applies the quadrants for a flexible response that allows one to recognize how leadership, service systems, and culture all work together. Using the RIS model as a guide, resources mapped to each of the quadrants can be mobilized to enhance resilience and fortify development to resume healthy processes. This comprehensive, whole-person response is designed to promote healing (Larkin and Records 2007; Larkin et al. 2012). The key elements of the RIS model are to raise staff and community awareness of ACEs and trauma, integrate resilience and recovery knowledge, engage staff in organizational development activities (including agreement on values and mission), identify and implement best practices, support staff self-care practices, train community leaders in ACEs and resilience, and engage in policy advocacy to advance programs developed in response to client characteristics and needs. Within all of this, leadership capacity development is key (Larkin et al. 2012, 2018).

The upper-left quadrant (the "I" space) represents the interior of the individual: thoughts, feelings, emotions, and beliefs. The interior is very real and present but is not an observable, physical object. It is up to the individual to tell us what they are experiencing for us to develop an understanding. The upper right represents the exterior (the "IT" quadrant). This identifies the physical body and observable behaviors.

The upper-right quadrant is the dominant perspective of western medicine, whereas individuals can be touched, measured, weighed, dissected, and so on. A "WE" space (lower-left quadrant) is created when communication is present, and we develop a mutual understanding. In supporting the "WE" space as service providers, we work toward understanding the individual within their community and what supports are available to lead toward resilience. Everything listed in the lower-left quadrant ("WE" space) illustrates the service of building a culture of recovery and transformation. Last, we have the lower-right (ITS) quadrant, which depicts observable systemic interactions within families, communities, and larger societies. For example, the "ITS" quadrant brings attention to service access, systemic design, and policies.

To facilitate trauma recovery and mobilize resilience, the RIS model brings attention to the interior and exterior of the individual and community, offering a flexible approach to addressing "hot spots" and bringing resources together within the local context. It is important to note that a change in any one quadrant will be reflected in the other quadrants. By using the four quadrants to assess our clients, we can identify the major effects of adversity and work with the community to mobilize resilience and recovery (Larkin and Records 2011). Figure 2.3 illustrates mapping at a community and program level in the "WE" and the "ITS" quadrants.

Self-Care and Leadership Development

We all contribute to the culture of the programs within which we provide services, making our own self-care an important aspect of ACE-informed programming. It is important that we identify self-care practices that nourish each integral part of our whole self, helping us to maintain balance in our personal and professional lives.

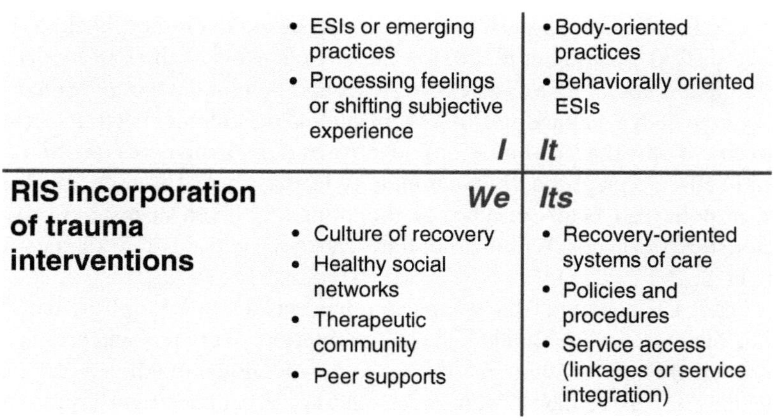

Fig. 2.3 RIS incorporation of trauma interventions (Larkin and Records 2011)

Additionally, it is particularly important to recognize that many providers have their own ACE backgrounds and therefore have an opportunity to role-model resilience as they engage in relationship-building and service delivery (Esaki and Larkin 2013). Agency leaders are encouraged to create a more restorative environment for their workforce. Self-care is a key element for agency leaders to set the tone toward a positive, restorative culture that supports staff members in their own self-care as they provide relationship-building and role-modeling for clients (Esaki and Larkin 2013).

RIS and Human Service Providers

The RIS model was designed to support agencies and service providers working with any high ACE score population and was first applied to assist people experiencing homelessness at the Committee on the Shelterless (COTS) in Petaluma, California. The COTS leadership staff first learned about ACEs through the United Way in 2004. The leadership of COTS engaged staff, shared the ACE study with them, and discussed the implications regarding best practices and responses to these client characteristics. Furthermore, with a mission to break cycles of homelessness, the leadership was interested in what types of programs could support resilience and recovery. The staff looked at the services available within their own agency and in the larger community and worked together to identify the values and principles that pervade programming. The RIS model does not specify values but rather points to the importance of agreeing upon values and principles that pervade the culture, creating the "WE" space of the organization. Program leaders set a tone and example of self-care, building a culture around themselves to support the organizational mission. At COTS, services were integrated within a context of intentionally developed social networks and peer supports to help people move forward and transform their lives (Larkin et al. 2012).

Conclusion

Homelessness is a serious problem throughout the society that is associated with physical and mental illness, social isolation, and exposure to trauma (Roos et al. 2013). The original ACE study revealed powerful relationships between higher ACE scores and emotional and physical health problems later in life, and ACEs are now implicated in many of the leading causes of death in the USA (Centers for Disease Control and Prevention 2018b). It is clear that ACEs are powerfully connected to many of the health-risk behaviors that contribute to homelessness and long-term health and psychosocial problems. This chapter discussed employing strategies, such as the Restorative Integral Support (RIS) model, for a whole-person approach that supports recovery from trauma and builds resilience.

References

Baron, S. W., & Hartnagel, T. F. (1998). Street youth and criminal violence. *Journal of Research in Crime and Delinquency, 35*(2), 166.

Bender, K., Brown, S. M., Begun, S., Barman-Adhikari, A., & Ferguson, K. (2016). Coping styles associated with victimization profiles among homeless youth. *Families in Society: The Journal of Contemporary Social Services, 97*(3), 171–180.

Busen, N. H., & Engebretson, J. C. (2008). Facilitating risk reduction among homeless and street-involved youth. *Journal of the American Academy of Nurse Practitioners, 20*, 567–575.

Centers for Disease Control and Prevention (2018a). Adverse childhood experiences. https://www.cdc.gov/violenceprevention/acestudy/. Accessed 5 August 2018.

Centers for Disease Control and Prevention (2018b). About the CDC-Kaiser ACE study. https://www.cdc.gov/violenceprevention/acestudy/about.html. Accessed 5 August 2018.

Cutuli, J. J., Desjardins, C. D., Herbers, J. E., Long, J. D., Heistad, D., Chan, C. K., & Masten, A. S. (2013). Academic achievement trajectories of homeless and highly mobile students: Resilience in the context of chronic and acute risk. *Child Development, 84*(3), 841–857.

Danese, A., Moffitt, T. E., Pariante, C. M., Ambler, A., Poulton, R., & Caspi, A. (2008). Elevated inflammation levels in depressed adults with a history of childhood maltreatment. *Archives of General Psychiatry, 65*(4), 409–415.

Dong, M., Anda, R. F., Felitti, V. J., Dube, S. R., Williamson, D. F., Thompson, T. J., & Giles, W. H. (2004). The interrelatedness of multiple forms of childhood abuse, neglect, and household dysfunction. *Child Abuse and Neglect, 28*, 771–784.

Dupre, M. (2008). Educational differences in health risks and illness over the life course: A test of cumulative disadvantage theory. *Social Science Research, 37*(4), 1253–1266.

Edidin, J. P., Ganim, Z., Hunter, S. J., & Karnik, N. S. (2012). The mental and physical health of homeless youth: A literature review. *Child Psychiatry and Human Development, 43*(3), 354–375.

Esaki, N., & Larkin, H. (2013). Prevalence of adverse childhood experiences (ACEs) among child service providers. *Families in Society: The Journal of Contemporary Social Services, 94*(1), 31–37.

Felitti, V. J., Anda, R. F., Nordenberg, D., Williamson, D. F., Spitz, A. M., Edwards, V., Koss, M. P., & Marks, J. S. (1998). Relationship of childhood abuse and household dysfunction to many of the leading causes of death in adults: The adverse childhood experiences (ACE) study. *American Journal of Preventative Medicine, 14*(4), 354–364.

Garner, M. D. (2011). Thinking practice: The social work integral model. *Families in Society: The Journal of Contemporary Social Services, 92*(3), 255–261.

Germain, C. B., & Gitterman, A. (1980). *The life model of social work practice: Advances in theory and practice*. New York, NY: Columbia University Press.

Gould D. A., Stevens, N. G., Ward, N. G., Carlin, A. S., Sowell, H. E., Gustafson, B. (1994). Self-reported childhood abuse in an adult population in a primary care setting: Prevalence, correlates, and associated suicide attempts. *Archives of Family Medicine*. (3), 252–256.

Guarino, K., & Bassuk, E. (2010). Working with families experiencing homelessness: Understanding trauma and its impact. *Zero to Three, 30*(3), 11–20.

Hamilton, A., Poza, I., & Washington, D. (2011). "Homelessness and trauma go hand-in-hand": Pathways to homelessness among women veterans. *Women's Health Issues, 21*(4S), S203–S209.

Hayes, M., Zonneville, M., & Bassuk, E. (2013). *The SHIFT study: Final report*. Needham, MA: The National Center on Family Homelessness.

Henry, M., Watt, R., Rosenthal, L., & Azim, S. (2017). The annual homelessness assessment report to Congress. https://www.hudexchange.info/resources/documents/2017-AHAR-Part-1.pdf. Accessed 5 Aug 2018.

Hopper, E., Bassuk, E., & Olivet, J. (2010). Shelter from the storm: Trauma-informed care in homeless service settings. *The Open Health Services and Policy Journal, 3*, 80–100.

Horwitz, A. V., Widom, C. S., McLaughlin, J., White, H. R. (2001). The impact of childhood abuse and neglect on adult mental health: A prospective study. *Journal of Health and Social Behavior*, (42), 184–201.

Keeshin, B. R., & Campbell, K. (2011). Screening homeless youth for histories of abuse: Prevalence, enduring effects, and interest in treatment. *Child Abuse and Neglect, 35*(6), 401–407.

Kim, M. M., Ford, J. D., Howard, D. L., & Bradford, D. W. (2010). Assessing trauma, substance abuse, and mental health in a sample of homeless men. *Health and Social Work, 35*(1), 39–48.

Kral, A. H., Molnar, B. E., Booth, R. E., & Watters, J. K. (1997). Prevalence of sexual risk behaviour and substance use among runaway and homeless adolescents in San Francisco, Denver, and New York City. *International Journal of STD and AIDS, 8*(2), 109–117.

Larkin, H., Felitti, V., & Anda, R. (2014). Social work and adverse childhood experiences (ACE) research: Implications for practice and health policy. *Social Work in Public Health, 29*(1), 1–16.

Larkin, H., Lee, E., Esaki, N., Demasi, M., Trifoso, S., Briar-Lawson, K., et al. (2018). The effects of protective factors and adverse childhood experiences on behavioral health services use: Findings from a population-based sample. *Social Work in Health Care, 57*(7), 548–562.

Larkin, H., & Park, J. (2012). Adverse childhood experiences (ACEs), service use, and service helpfulness among people experiencing homelessness. *Families in Society: The Journal of Contemporary Social Services, 93*(2), 85–93.

Larkin, H., Beckos, B., & Shields, J. (2012). Mobilizing resilience and recovery in response to adverse childhood experiences (ACE): A restorative integral support (RIS) case study. *Journal of Prevention and Intervention in the Community, 40*(4), 335–346.

Larkin, H., & Records, J. (2007). Adverse childhood experiences: Overview, response strategies, and integral theory. *Journal of Integral Theory and Practice, 2*(3), 1–25.

Larkin, H., & Records, J. (2011). Restorative Integral Support (RIS) for trauma wellness. https://web.archive.org/web/20170623125735, http://posttraumawellness.org/. Accessed 25 June 2018.

McCrory, E., De Brito, S. A., & Viding, E. (2011). The impact of childhood maltreatment: A review of neurobiological and genetic factors. *Frontiers in Psychiatry, 2*(48). https://doi.org/10.3389/fpsyt.2011.

McCaskill, P. A., Toro, P. A., & Wolfe, S. M. (1998). Homeless and matched housed adolescents: A comparative study of psychopathology. *Journal of Clinical Child Psychology, 27*(3), 306–319.

McEwen, B. S. (2012). Brain on stress: How the social environment gets under the skin. *Proceedings of the National Academy of Sciences of the United States of America, 109*(Suppl 2), 17180–17185.

Merscham, C., Van Leeuwen, J. M., & McGuire, M. (2009). Mental health and substance abuse indicators among homeless youth in Denver, Colorado. *Child Welfare, 88*, 93–110.

Metzler, M., Merrick, M. T., Klevens, J., Ports, K. A., & Ford, D. C. (2017). Adverse childhood experiences and life opportunities: Shifting the narrative. *Children and Youth Services Review, 72*, 141–149.

Montgomery, A. E., Hill, L. L., Kane, V., & Culhane, D. P. (2013). Housing chronically homeless veterans: Evaluation the efficacy of a housing first approach to HUD-VASH. *Journal of Community Psychology, 41*(4), 505–514. https://www.ncbi.nlm.nih.gov/pmc/articles/PMC3969137/.

Oppenheimer, S., Nurius, P., & Green, S. (2016). Homelessness history impacts on health outcomes and economic and risk behavior intermediaries: New insights from population data. *Families in Society: The Journal of Contemporary Social Services, 97*(3), 230–242.

Padgett, D. (2012). Life course adversity in the lives of formerly homeless persons with serious mental illness: Context and meaning. *American Journal of Orthopsychiatry, 82*(3), 421–430.

Padgett, D., Stanhope, V., Henwood, B., & Stefancic, A. (2011). Substance use outcomes among homeless clients with serious mental illness: Comparing housing first with treatment first programs. *Community Mental Health Journal, 47*, 227–232.

Padgett, D., Hawkins, R., Abrams, C., & Davis, A. (2006). In their own words: Trauma and substance abuse in the lives of formerly homeless women with serious mental illness. *American Journal of Orthopsychiatry, 76*(4), 461–467.

Roos, L. E., Mota, N., Afifi, T. O., Katz, L. Y., Distasio, J., & Sareen, J. (2013). Relationship between adverse childhood experiences and homelessness and the impact of Axis I and II disorders. *American Journal of Public Health, 103*(Suppl 2), S275–S281.

Ryan, K. D., Kilmer, R. P., Cauce, A. M., Watanabe, H., & Hoyt, D. R. (2000). Psychological consequences of child maltreatment in homeless adolescents: Untangling the unique effects of maltreatment and family environment. *Child Abuse and Neglect, 24*(3), 333–352.

Santrock, J. W. (2012). *A topical approach to life-span development* (6th ed.). New York, NY: McGraw Hill.

Shonkoff, J. P., Boyce, W. T., & McEwen, B. S. (2009). Neuroscience, molecular biology, and the childhood roots of health disparities building a new framework for health promotion and disease prevention. *JAMA, 301*(21), 2252–2259.

Shonkoff, J. P., Garner, A. S., The Committee on Psychosocial Aspects of Child and Family Health, Committee on Early Childhood, Adoption, and Dependent Care, & Section on Developmental and Behavioral Pediatrics. (2012). The lifelong effects of early childhood adversity and toxic stress. *Pediatrics, 129*(1), e232–e246.

Travecchio, L., Thomeer, M. A. E., & Meeus, W. (1999). Attachment, social network and homelessness in young people. *Social Behavior and Personality: An International Journal, 27*(3), 247–262.

Thorncroft, G. (2011). Physical health disparities and mental illness. The scandal of premature mortality. *The British Journal of Psychiatry*, (199), 441–442.

Thompson, S., Bender, K., Windsor, L., Cook, M., & Williams, T. (2010). Homeless youth: Characteristics, contributing factors, and service options. *Journal of Human Behavior in the Social Environment, 20*, 193–217.

van der Kolk, B., Roth, S., Pelcovitz, D., Sunday, S., & Spinazzola, J. (2005). Disorders of extreme stress: The empirical foundation of a complex adaptation to trauma. *Journal of Traumatic Stress, 18*(5), 389–399.

Wilber, K., & Wilber, K. (2000). Integral psychology: Consciousness, spirit, psychology, therapy. Boston: Shambhala.

Yoder, J. R., Bender, K., Thompson, S. J., Ferguson, K. M., & Haffejee, B. (2014). Explaining homeless youths' criminal justice interactions: Childhood trauma or surviving life on the streets? *Community Mental Health Journal, 50*(2), 135–144.

Zielinski, D. (2009). Child maltreatment and adult socioeconomic well-being. *Child Abuse and Neglect, 33*, 666–678.

Zlotnick, C., & Zerger, S. (2008). Survey findings on characteristics and health status of clients treated by the federally funded (U.S.) Health Care for the Homeless programs. *Health and Social Care in the Community, 17*(1), 18–26.

Chapter 3
Homelessness and Health Disparities: A Health Equity Lens

Elizabeth Bowen, Ryan Savino, and Andrew Irish

Introduction

The distribution and impact of health conditions across a population are always unequal. Due to a number of individual, family, and community factors, some individuals may experience multiple complex health conditions across their life spans, while others enjoy good health for all or most of their lives. The concept of *health equity* refers to the idea that all people should have equal opportunity to obtain good health (Braveman 2006). Although social workers, public health professionals, community activists, and others may seek to advance health equity, numerous health inequities currently exist in the USA and many other countries.

The term *health disparities* is used to reference differences in health conditions as experienced by different groups in society. Disparities can exist based on virtually any identifying characteristic, such as race, ethnicity, immigration status, socioeconomic status, age, gender identity, or sexual orientation. A disparity can mean that one group experiences a disease or health condition more often than another group (disparities in prevalence), that one group experiences worse outcomes due to a disease or health condition (disparities in outcomes or severity), or that one group has reduced access to care, services, or medication or receives lower-quality care (disparities in care) (Braveman 2006).

Although the causes of health disparities are complex and vary according to population, condition, and disparity type, a rich and growing body of research links disparities with *social determinants of health*. This broad term refers to the social and economic conditions that affect health, both directly and indirectly (Braveman

---

Electronic supplementary material: The online version of this chapter (https://doi.org/10.1007/978-3-030-03727-7_3) contains supplementary material, which is available to authorized users.

E. Bowen (✉) · R. Savino · A. Irish
University at Buffalo, Buffalo, NY, USA
e-mail: eabowen@buffalo.edu

H. Larkin et al. (eds.), *Homelessness Prevention and Intervention in Social Work*, https://doi.org/10.1007/978-3-030-03727-7_3

et al. 2011). It is widely recognized that safe and affordable housing is a critical social determinant of health (Thomson and Thomas 2015; Thornton et al. 2016). Stable housing provides a sense of security and is the base point from which a person can engage in a range of health-enhancing behaviors, including accessing health care, developing supportive personal relationships, safely storing and preparing food, and carrying out medication routines (Henwood et al. 2013a).

Given the recognition of housing as a social determinant of health, it is perhaps not surprising that individuals who are homeless face disparities regarding a wide range of physical and mental health conditions. In this chapter, we use a broad and inclusive definition of homelessness, incorporating children, families, and adults in a variety of living conditions, such as sleeping on the streets, living in shelters, and couch-surfing (i.e., temporarily staying with friends, relatives, acquaintances, or strangers). In many cases, the health disparities that homeless individuals experience may be related to both their status of being homeless and to other aspects of their identities, including race, gender, and sexual orientation. The following case studies of Keith and Christina, which are fictional cases based on the authors' social work practice and research experiences, provide two examples of how homeless people may experience health disparities.

Case Studies

Keith

Keith identifies as a 57-year-old, heterosexual, African American man. He has been living for decades with bipolar disorder. He previously worked as a medical technician but was laid off 10 years ago. No longer able to afford the rent on his apartment, he was evicted and found himself with few options. For the past 10 years, Keith has alternated between staying at an overnight men's shelter when the weather is bad and sleeping in an underpass beneath a highway in the warmer months. During this time, Keith began heavily using alcohol and cocaine, both to self-medicate the symptoms of his bipolar disorder and as a way of coping with the challenges of being homeless. On several occasions, he was arrested for cocaine possession and incarcerated for short periods of time as a result. Keith recently tested positive for tuberculosis while staying at the shelter and was referred to an onsite clinic for treatment. Although he successfully managed his bipolar disorder through medication and regular counseling while working, Keith has struggled to consistently take his medication and follow-up on therapy referrals during his period of homelessness.

Christina

Christina identifies as a 19-year-old, bisexual, white woman. She was removed from her birth parents' custody at age 11 by Child Protective Services, due to physical abuse and neglect, and subsequently placed in multiple foster homes. After running away from her last placement several times, her foster father beat her severely, and Christina decided to run away for good. She has spent the past year couch-surfing in the homes of friends, acquaintances, and sometimes strangers for a few days at a time. Christina did not finish high school and does not have a job; her only income is what she is able to obtain from panhandling or doing occasional odd jobs. She sometimes goes to a local soup kitchen for meals or buys snack foods from the corner store with her very limited income, but reports that she is hungry much of the time, and sometimes goes for an entire day without eating anything. A male acquaintance with whom Christina occasionally stayed coerced her into having sex with him, telling her that if she didn't, he would kick her out and lock the door, leaving her on her own on the street in the middle of the night. Christina also reports having sex in exchange for food or money. She recently tested positive at a local clinic for chlamydia, a sexually transmitted infection.

Purpose of Chapter

This chapter has three purposes. First, we describe the range of health disparities experienced by people who are homeless, including disparities regarding a variety of conditions, such as serious mental illness, addiction, infectious diseases, and food insecurity. We also review the concept of multi-morbidity. Second, we discuss the pathways or conditions that explain why homeless people experience health disparities, drawing on relevant research and theory. Lastly, we highlight promising interventions to reduce disparities and promote health equity for homeless populations.

Health Disparities Faced by Homeless Populations

Although not a comprehensive list, the types of health conditions that disproportionately affect homeless populations include serious mental illness, substance use disorders, infectious diseases (e.g., HIV/AIDS, hepatitis, and tuberculosis), food insecurity, and injuries resulting from violence and other victimization. Here, we briefly describe each of these conditions and the ways they impact people experiencing homelessness. We conclude with a discussion of multi-morbidity to demonstrate how different types of conditions may intersect, compounding their effects on a person's health.

Serious Mental Illness

Arguably, the health conditions most frequently associated with homelessness are mental illnesses and substance use disorders. Surges in the homeless population have long been attributed to pushes for psychiatric deinstitutionalization of people with mental illness (Montgomery et al. 2013). President John F. Kennedy's special message to Congress in 1963 was emblematic of this. In the message, Kennedy championed community-based mental health care as a quicker, more affordable, and more effective treatment format than institution-based care (Kennedy 1963). Kennedy (1963) set the ambitious goal of treating half of American psychiatric inpatients in the community within 10–20 years. However, the true pace of deinstitutionalization proved much more rapid. By 1975, state and county mental hospital enrollment across the USA declined by 62% (Mechanic and Rochefort 1990). Critics point out that few aspects of deinstitutionalization were cohesively coordinated (Feldman 2003; Mechanic and Rochefort 1990). Geller (2000) and Cutler et al. (2003) reflect that funding allocations for training community mental health staff were excised from 1963's Community Mental Health Center Construction Act (PL 88–164) and were not reinserted until 1965. Alternatively, Drake and Latimer (2012) suggest that community mental health centers attempted to offer too broad of a service menu even as their collective capacity swelled. Others argue that outpatient centers were initially ill-suited to take on hospitals' more ancillary roles, such as that of a long-term residence for many individuals with mental illness (Dixon and Schwarz 2013; Mechanic and Rochefort 1990). Regardless of the cause, there was a discernible lag in acknowledging deinstitutionalization's societal implications, such as increases in homelessness and incarceration among people with mental illness (Hudson 2016; Novella 2008).

In the twenty-first century, rates of serious mental illnesses remain much higher among people experiencing homelessness than their housed counterparts (Fazel et al. 2008). The Substance Abuse and Mental Health Services Administration (SAMHSA) of the US Department of Health and Human Services defines a seriously mentally ill individual as someone 18 years of age or older who possesses a current or recent (within the preceding year) diagnosable mental, behavioral, or emotional disorder that hinders at least one major life activity (SAMHSA 2013). As such, no diagnosis (according to SAMHSA) automatically qualifies an individual as seriously mentally ill, without significantly impairing their ability to function. Around 4% of housed American adults and 24% of homeless shelter dwellers were considered to have a serious mental illness in 2015 (National Institute of Mental Health 2015; US Department of Housing and Urban Development 2015b).

Several disorders, including schizophrenia, bipolar disorder, and substance use disorders, have been classified as risk factors for homelessness (Folsom et al. 2005). Others cautiously posit that homelessness can contribute to mental illness and substance use disorders or aggravate their severity (Castellow et al. 2015). Relative to patients with major depression, Folsom et al. (2005) determined that those who had schizophrenia or bipolar disorder were 2.4 and 1.6 times as likely, respectively, to become homeless. Furthermore, North et al. (1998) found that antisocial personality disorder and schizophrenia were related to aggregate lifelong time spent homeless. The US Department of Housing and Urban Development (HUD) defines a chronically homeless individual as someone who lives with a disability and has spent either 12 months continuously homeless or has experienced four or more episodes of homelessness totaling 12 months or greater (Henry et al. 2015; US Department of Housing and Urban Development 2015a). Earlier research reported that debilitating mental illnesses and substance use disorders are believed to be more prevalent among the chronically and episodically homeless than the transitionally homeless, with some variations noted by geographic setting (Kuhn and Culhane 1998; Link et al. 1994). Subsequent inquiries reached similar conclusions, depending on the diagnostic criteria and homeless typologies utilized (Brown et al. 2017; Caton et al. 2005, Patterson et al. 2012).

In addition to persons experiencing homelessness having higher rates of serious mental illness, they may experience disparities in access to care for physical and mental health needs. As the case study of Keith illustrates, without stable housing, it can be difficult for people to consistently take medication or follow through with care appointments to treat their mental health conditions. Connolly et al. (2008) obtained findings that underscore poor mental health treatment retention among homeless patients diagnosed with personality disorders, and Folsom et al. (2002) observed low levels of primary care service receipt by homeless individuals with schizophrenia. Although less likely to present to primary care, people with psychotic disorders who experience homelessness are high users of emergency psychiatric services (McNiel and Binder 2005; Cougnard et al. 2006).

Substance Use Disorders

Substance use disorders are also among the most predominant health issues affecting homeless populations (Fazel et al. 2014). Substance use disorders encompass addiction to a single substance (e.g., alcohol, cocaine, methamphetamines, marijuana, or heroin and other opioids) or multiple substances simultaneously. For example, in one study by Tsai et al. (2014), 60% of homeless veterans entering a supportive housing program met criteria for a substance use disorder. Of that group, 54% struggled with polysubstance use, meaning they were problematically using more than one substance (Tsai et al. 2014). A separate investigation revealed that 84% of men and 58% of women residing in homeless shelters or on the street met lifetime substance use disorder criteria for at least one substance (North et al. 2004). Likewise, lifetime substance use disorder rates are elevated among chronically homeless men (73%) and women (68%) (Edens et al. 2011). These figures are quite high, considering that only around 8% of all Americans above age 12 have a substance use disorder (Center for Behavioral Health Statistics and Quality 2015).

Substance use may be a contributing factor to homelessness. Thompson et al. (2013) identified substance abuse as a key predictor of first-time homelessness, and Goldfinger et al. (1999) isolated substance abuse as the most potent individual predictor of homelessness duration. Further, Linton et al. (2013) conducted a temporal analysis of homelessness and injection drug use, concluding that homelessness functioned as a predictor of relapse. Substance use disorders can frequently turn fatal for people experiencing homelessness. Baggett et al. (2013) discovered that, for homeless persons under 45 years old in Boston, Massachusetts, opioid overdose superseded HIV as the leading cause of death. In the same sample, homeless individuals were 20 times more likely to die of an overdose than the average Bostonian.

Dual Diagnoses

Many homeless individuals live with dual, or co-occurring, mental health and substance use disorders. In some cases, people may start to use substances primarily, or in part, as a way of self-medicating symptoms from their mental health disorders. The case study of Keith is an example of a person with a dual diagnosis. These individuals are particularly vulnerable. Dual diagnoses are associated with extensive emergency department use (Kushel et al. 2002), social isolation (Hawkins and Abrams 2007), high rates of psychotherapeutic treatment dropout (Ball et al. 2005), adverse clinical outcomes (Gonzalez and Rosenheck 2002), elevated hospital use, and premature death (Schmidt et al. 2011). Although only 3% of Americans were dually diagnosed in 2014 (Center for Behavioral Health Statistics and Quality 2015), rates of dual diagnosis in homeless populations may be more than 50% (Fazel et al. 2014). Research by Slesnick and Prestopnik (2005) suggests that these rates are even higher among homeless youth.

Infectious Diseases

HIV

HIV is three to nine times more prevalent among people experiencing homelessness than their housed peers (Kidder et al. 2007). That said, rates vary widely across investigations. One international meta-analysis reported HIV rates among homeless populations ranging from 0.3% to 21.1%, depending on the data collection site (Beijer et al. 2012). HIV- and AIDS-attributable deaths are also higher within populations of people experiencing homelessness. For example, in one study, 67% of AIDS-diagnosed homeless San Franciscans were alive at the 5-year follow-up, compared with 81% of AIDS-diagnosed housed persons (Schwarcz et al. 2009). HIV-positive individuals with unmet housing needs are significantly less likely to receive best practice interventions and therefore achieve poorer outcomes across a variety of health domains (Milloy et al. 2012; Schwarcz et al. 2009).

HIV/AIDS treatment can be challenging under many circumstances. About 77% of HIV patients in the USA begin treatment within 3–4 months of their diagnosis, but just over half continue (Cohen et al. 2011). Viral suppression rates (a measure of the amount of the virus in a person's bloodstream) are poorer for individuals who are homeless, with medication compliance difficulties cited as a key contributing factor (Thakarar et al. 2016). Inconsistent medication adherence can raise the risk that HIV-positive individuals will develop dangerous, drug-resistant infections (Bamberger et al. 2000). Poor treatment adherence is partially attributable to the fact that homeless individuals must make subsistence-related trade-offs in their care. For example, for HIV-positive people, being food insecure is linked with higher viral loads, poorer treatment adherence, and increased mortality (Weiser et al. 2009).

Hepatitis B and C

Hepatitis B and C are infectious diseases that affect the liver. Only 0.3% of Americans live with a chronic hepatitis B infection; however, chronic infections are much more rampant within some subgroups of people experiencing homelessness. For instance, Cheung et al. (2002) found that almost 2% of homeless veterans had a chronic hepatitis B infection and over a fifth had ever been infected with hepatitis B. Unlike hepatitis C or HIV, hepatitis B has a vaccination, yet vulnerable groups, such as homeless youth, have low vaccination rates (43%) (Roberts et al. 2016; Lifson and Halcón 2001). Given the hepatitis B vaccine's effectiveness, increasing the scope of vaccination is critical to minimizing the disease's morbidity and mortality (Nyamathi et al. 2001).

People experiencing homelessness are also disproportionately burdened by the hepatitis C virus. Around 1% of the general US population has hepatitis C (Denniston et al. 2014), compared to approximately 31% of homeless individuals (Strehlow et al. 2012). Hepatitis C is mainly transmitted through needle sharing by injection drug users (Strehlow et al. 2012). Indeed, hepatitis C infection is much more prevalent among homeless injection drug users than nonusers (approximately 70% and 16% are infected, respectively) (Strehlow et al. 2012). People who have been homeless for longer periods of time are more likely to have a hepatitis diagnosis (Stein and Nyamathi 2004). Diagnosis and treatment of hepatitis C remain elusive among many homeless individuals (Jones et al. 2015). Although 26.7% of participants in one study tested positive for hepatitis C, only about half had prior knowledge of their status (Gelberg et al. 2012).

Tuberculosis

Tuberculosis (TB) is an airborne respiratory infection that is readily communicable between individuals sharing close quarters (Deiss et al. 2009). Although TB infection rates are low in industrialized nations, they remain a concern among homeless populations (Beijer et al. 2012). Between 36 and 47 homeless people per 100,000 developed TB from 2006 to 2010 (Bamrah et al. 2013). Additional risk factors for TB include HIV diagnosis and immunosuppression, substance abuse, and malnutrition (Deiss et al. 2009; Mohtashemi and Kawamura 2010; Lönnroth et al. 2008; Semba et al. 2010; Nyamathi et al. 2007). Treatment fidelity and noncompliance are high within these populations, resulting in worse prognoses (Nyamathi et al. 2007).

Infectious Diseases and Risky Behaviors

For homeless populations, higher rates of infectious diseases—especially HIV and hepatitis C—are related to engagement in risky drug- and sex-related behaviors. For example, homeless injection drug users are more likely to needle backload (use needles to measure and divide drugs) and attend shooting galleries (locations where multiple individuals inject drugs) than stably housed users (Coady et al. 2007). Even high-risk group members, such as injection drug users, tend to underestimate their risk for infectious diseases (Norton et al. 2014). Early intervention is essential, as Garfein et al. (1996) recorded seropositivity (the presence of infection in a person's blood as measured by a virus' antibodies) rates as high as 50% for hepatitis B and 65% for hepatitis C after just 1 year of injection drug use.

Another type of risk behavior to consider is survival sex. Seeing few other options, homeless individuals and other indigent populations may engage in survival sex to meet their basic needs, such as exchanging sexual acts for money, food, shelter, or drugs (Greene et al. 1999; Walls and Bell 2011). Another study found that for each five-point increase in their score on a food insecurity assessment, marginally housed HIV-positive San Franciscans were twice as likely to engage in unprotected sex (Vogenthaler et al. 2013). Homelessness duration and severity are significantly associated with risky sexual behaviors. Respondents to a Washington, DC, area survey who were homeless beyond 90 days disclosed twice as many survival sex acts as those homeless for shorter periods, and participants who were homeless multiple times divulged similarly high levels of survival sex (Purser et al. 2017).

Survival sex is not synonymous with sexual violence, but it is seen as a risk factor for sexual victimization (Tyler et al. 2004). Some individuals, such as Christina in the case study described at the beginning of the chapter, may engage in survival sex as well as experience sexual violence. Survival sex and sexual violence can put people at increased risk of contracting or transmitting infectious diseases, including HIV and other sexually transmitted infections like herpes, chlamydia, and gonorrhea.

Violence

While not always conceptualized as such, violence is a public health issue that affects individual and community health and well-being in myriad ways. Violence—which can include physical, sexual, emotional, and structural dimensions—permeates life for many people experiencing homelessness. Often, these experiences are ongoing—stretching far back into individuals' childhoods (Goodman et al. 1997). For example, by the time they reach early adulthood, many homeless youth have already amassed extensive histories of trauma (Bender et al. 2015). Abuse perpetrated by caregivers prompts many adolescents to leave home, burdening them with the lingering effects of trauma, few economic resources, and limited housing options (Wenzel et al. 2000a). Youth who experience such abuse are vulnerable to re-traumatization, including further violence while living on the street (Bender et al. 2015). The case study of Christina illustrates one example of a young person experiencing violence both prior to and during their homelessness.

It is important to consider the intersection of gender and violence. Compared to homeless men, Wenzel et al. (2004) estimated that on average, homeless women lived through 3 times as much physical and 16 times as much sexual abuse. Intimate partner violence also disproportionately affects women and is a principal reason underlying women and their children's entry into homelessness (Henny et al. 2007; Baker et al. 2010; Ponce et al. 2014). Survivors' fears of perpetrator retribution and their experiences with unhelpful or unreceptive service providers can act as barriers to help-seeking (Huey et al. 2014; Bosick et al. 2012). Homeless men also experience significant violence, especially while living on the street (Kim et al. 2010). Masculine gender norms espousing autonomy and strength may limit male victims' reporting rates (Huey and Quirouette 2010). Finally, gender minorities, including transgender individuals and those whose gender identities do not conform to a gender binary, experience disproportionate rates of both homelessness and violence (Flentje et al. 2016).

Psychiatric symptoms can function as both risk factors for and ramifications of abuse and trauma. Persons with histories of serious mental illness or substance abuse are at an exceptionally high risk of victimization (Goodman et al. 1997; Wenzel et al. 2000b; Wenzel et al. 2004; Bender et al. 2015; Stanley et al. 2016) and psychiatric symptom aggravation (Goodman et al. 1997; Vijayaraghavan et al. 2012). The repercussions of violence on the physical health of homeless individuals are also widely documented (Padgett et al. 2006; Padgett et al. 2012; Baggett et al. 2010; Kushel et al. 2003). The physical effects of violent victimization are vast and may necessitate immediate medical attention (such as when someone is critically injured) or long-term disease management (such as when someone contracts HIV via rape or other nonconsensual sexual contact) (Dutton et al. 2006; Lin et al. 2015).

Systemic issues can drastically suppress reporting rates for homeless people who experience violence. The work of Zakrison et al. (2004) illustrated that homeless Canadians were more amenable to contacting paramedics than they were to contacting police officers. Fears of police brutality coupled with concerns regarding criminal background checks are two major deterrents to reporting violence (Huey and Quirouette 2010; Zakrison et al. 2004). Prohibitions against snitching represent another barrier to accurate and timely disclosure (Huey 2008). Presently, there is little research demonstrating whether similar reporting barriers exist within the USA. This line of investigation lends itself to further study with the goal of identifying service gaps and devising programs to improve homeless individuals' service utilization.

Food Insecurity

Another health issue that disproportionately affects homeless populations is food insecurity. Food insecurity is exemplified by uncertain access to the types and amount of food needed to facilitate an active and healthy lifestyle and that can be obtained in a socially acceptable way (Kushel et al. 2006). Close to 15% of American households struggled with food insecurity in 2013 at least once (Coleman-Jensen et al. 2014). Access to reliably sourced and nutritious food is especially challenging for many homeless or marginally housed individuals. Lee and Greif (2008) found that when compared with those who are homeless for shorter periods of time, chronically homeless individuals had less frequent access to meals (71.4% vs. 45.5%) and were more likely to fast (47% vs. 36.4%), consume inadequate food (72.5% vs. 51.7%), engage in subsistence eating (21.1% vs. 2.9%), and have difficulty affording food (45% vs. 34%). In another study, 25% of chronically homeless participants dealt with food insecurity in the previous month (Baggett et al. 2011).

People living in inadequate, unaffordable, or marginal housing are also disproportionately affected by food insecurity. If housing costs exceed 30% of a household's income, food insecurity is shown to rise (Kirkpatrick and Tarasuk 2011). And, where rental prices spike, researchers have noted concurrent upticks in food insecurity (Fletcher et al. 2009). Moreover, when households struggled to cover their housing expenses, Kirkpatrick and Tarasuk (2011) observed that they were prone to purchasing less nutritionally balanced food. Such trade-offs can be particularly risky for low-income people diagnosed with diet-sensitive diseases like diabetes (Seligman et al. 2010a). In addition, Bowen et al. (2016) found that 75% of single-room occupancy dwellers in Chicago were food insecure. Single-room occupancy units are apartments that are very small in size and typically do not include kitchen facilities, restricting residents' options for food preparation and storage (Bowen et al. 2016). The case study of Christina provides one example of how young people who are couch-surfing may experience food insecurity.

Food insecurity co-occurs with a multitude of health problems, including hypertension, major depression, diabetes, and overall low self-reported health (Seligman et al. 2010b; Siefert et al. 2001). Homeless, food insecure people are also less likely to obtain vital medical care or to consume medications as prescribed, leading to frequent emergency room use (Kushel et al. 2006). Jointly, access to food and housing may affect health-related cognitions and behaviors. Stably housed diabetic patients in one study, for example, displayed higher levels of health-specific self-efficacy (the perception that they could actualize health-promoting behaviors) (Vijayaraghavan et al. 2011).

Many communities attempt to address food insecurity among homeless and low-income populations using soup kitchens, food banks, and food pantries. But high rates of food insecurity persist even where these assets are abundant (Bazerghi et al. 2016). In some cases, capacity constraints cause pantries to turn away eligible patrons. Other barriers include restrictive hours of operation, frequently exhausted food reserves, feelings of stigmatization, long lines, geographical inaccessibility, and a dearth of nutritional foods (Miewald and McCann 2014; Tarasuk et al. 2009; Irwin et al. 2007).

Multi-morbidity

Multi-morbidity refers to individuals who live with two or more chronic health conditions, representing an intensely vulnerable subsection of the population (Barnett et al. 2012). Multi-morbidity affects homeless populations in a variety of ways. At times, having one chronic condition can complicate the treatment of another, such as when a person has both diabetes and hepatitis C (Blank et al. 2013; Maremmani et al. 2015). Individuals experiencing multi-morbidity also experience lower health-care access and use rates, magnifying their already precarious health problems (Argintaru et al. 2013). Health-care-related financial strain that is so severe it can precipitate losing one's residence is an everyday reality for many people with multi-morbid illnesses (Barnett et al. 2012; Blank et al. 2013).

Contemporary health-care systems often fall short of addressing the needs of disadvantaged and complexly ill patients. Part of this appears to stem from a long-ingrained emphasis on treating illness singularly, despite the frequent occurrence of multi-morbidity, particularly in low-income populations (Arbelle et al. 2014). Often overlooked is the immense challenge of navigating the health-care system while simultaneously struggling to acquire secure housing (Vila-Rodriguez et al. 2013). When these trying experiences converge, they can greatly impact individuals' health and well-being, often resulting in increased mortality (Vila-Rodriguez et al. 2013).

Pathways to Health Inequalities for Homeless Populations

Recognizing the numerous health disparities faced by homeless populations raises the question, "Why is homelessness associated with health disparities?" This is not a simple question to answer. Although there is not one distinct pathway linking homelessness and health disparities, several individual- and community-level factors may contribute to this association. These factors include health conditions functioning as underlying causes of homelessness, the living conditions with which homeless individuals contend, poverty and socioeconomic status, barriers to health-care access, and the notion of cumulative disadvantage.

Health Conditions as a Cause of Homelessness

In many cases, health issues can contribute to people becoming homeless. For example, since an HIV diagnosis can impact a person's relationships, employment, and finances in ways that increase susceptibility to homelessness, being HIV positive is a risk factor for homelessness (Aidala et al. 2016). In many instances, the causal relationship between homelessness and health issues is not clear-cut. One common example is that of addictions. Addiction may be a factor in a person losing their housing due to financial reasons, impaired relationships, lease violations, or incarceration related to the addiction. However, the experience of being homeless, and the stress and trauma associated with being homeless, can contribute to escalating substance use and addiction (see the case study on Keith for one illustration of this). In this sense, addiction and homelessness are mutually reinforcing.

Living Conditions

The conditions in which homeless people live may be directly related to the health disparities they experience. One clear example of this is that sleeping outdoors puts people at greater risk for weather-related health conditions, such as hypothermia or heatstroke. Because homeless people often have limited access to bathing and hygiene supplies and facilities, they are more vulnerable to infections and other skin problems (To et al. 2016).

The living conditions associated with homelessness are also directly related to problems meeting basic health needs, including food and sleep. Most homeless people lack a safe place to store and prepare food (Parpouchi et al. 2016), and getting adequate sleep is challenging in many of the conditions in which homeless people live (Chang et al. 2015). Insufficient nutrition and food access and poor sleep can then render people vulnerable to a range of health problems. In addition, storing medications (especially those that require refrigeration) and consistently adhering to complex medication regimens can prove difficult for people without a fixed residence (Kidder et al. 2007).

Other diseases that disproportionally affect homeless populations are linked with congregate living, as is the case in homeless shelters. It is much easier for communicable diseases like tuberculosis to spread when people live and sleep in close quarters. Couch-surfing can entail its own risks, such as physical and sexual assault (see the case study on Christina). Furthermore, the stress associated with residential instability or living in poor quality housing is associated with health consequences, including symptoms of anxiety and depression (Burgard et al. 2012; Suglia et al. 2011). In sum, although living conditions can vary significantly among individuals experiencing homelessness, most of the conditions are associated with increased health risks in some way.

Poverty and Socioeconomic Status

It can be difficult to distinguish the health effects associated with homelessness itself from health disparities that are linked to having a limited income and low socioeconomic status more generally. The relationship between health and income is well-studied and generally follows a linear pattern, with health improving as income increases (Braveman et al. 2011). People who are homeless typically have very limited economic resources, which can affect their health in various ways. With little or no income, it may be difficult for a person to afford health-care services or medication, purchase healthy foods, or secure transportation to attend health-related appointments. The stress associated with persistent poverty can have profound effects on physical and mental health (Santiago et al. 2011). Individual poverty also often intersects with neighborhood-level poverty. People who are homeless or low-income often live in neighborhoods of concentrated poverty, where their health may be impacted by factors such as disproportionately high levels of pollution, high crime rates, lack of health and social services, increased availability of alcohol and drugs, and limited green space and other infrastructure to encourage physical activity (Diez Roux and Mair 2010).

Health-Care-Related Barriers

Another underlying cause of health disparities is that homelessness is associated with barriers to accessing health care. In a 2010 national survey of homeless adults, nearly half of respondents experienced two or more unmet health-care needs in the preceding year—a rate 6–10 times higher than the population at large (Baggett et al. 2010). Most respondents did not have health insurance, which was independently associated with insufficient health care in multiple domains. Employed homeless individuals were at yet further risk, tending to prioritize work over health care and being less likely to be insured. Even among insured homeless persons, Brubaker et al. (2013) reported that barriers to health-care utilization were common, due to inability to afford co-payments and fees. Further, while homelessness increases risk of exposure to many health problems, it is also associated with reduced access to preventative care and use of preventative measures (Maness and Khan 2014; Bharel et al. 2011), especially regarding sexual and reproductive health services among women (American College of Obstetricians and Gynecologists 2013).

Cumulative Disadvantage

The concept of *cumulative disadvantage* encapsulates the multiple pathways through which homelessness and health are linked. Cumulative disadvantage is the idea that beginning very early in life, certain risk factors and experiences, such as living in poverty, experiencing systemic racism, or surviving a traumatic event, tend to intersect and amplify one another in ways that put individuals on a trajectory toward experiencing adverse health outcomes over the life course (Seabrook and Avison 2012). This theory is relevant to homelessness, since homeless people have often experienced a variety of individual-, family-, and community-level adversities, both prior to and since becoming homeless. In a study of formerly homeless adults with co-occurring mental illness and substance abuse problems, researchers found that participants reported an average of 8.8 adverse life events, including parental abandonment in childhood, suicidality, and incarceration (Padgett et al. 2012). In addition, racial minorities (particularly African Americans) and sexual and gender minorities, including lesbian, gay, bisexual, queer, transgender, and gender-queer individuals, are overrepresented in homeless populations; the personal and institutional discrimination experienced by these groups may combine with the adversities associated with homelessness (Gattis and Larson 2016). These adverse events, structural oppression, and related stress and trauma accumulate and intersect in ways that profoundly affect the health of vulnerable populations. Thus, rather than a single influential event or risk factor, it is likely that the accumulation of multiple forms of disadvantage underlies the health disparities faced by homeless individuals.

Interventions to Reduce Disparities and Promote Health Equity for Homeless Populations

In 2017, Physician and Hawaiian State Senator Josh Green made headlines when he introduced a bill to allow physicians to classify homelessness as a medical condition and write prescriptions for housing (Barney 2017). Sen. Green's proposed legislation reflects the idea that interventions to reduce disparities and improve the health of homeless people are fundamentally tied to housing. Given the links noted in this chapter between homelessness and health conditions, helping homeless people find and maintain safe, stable, and affordable housing is essential to effectively preventing or treating virtually any health impairment. Here, we highlight research on expanding opportunities to improve individuals' health within the permanent supportive housing model of housing services. We also discuss health care for the homeless-funded services, street medicine and mobile clinic programs, and health-care policy changes as key innovative approaches to improving the health of people experiencing homelessness.

Permanent Supportive Housing: Opportunities for Health Promotion

Permanent supportive housing (discussed in detail elsewhere in this book) is an evidence-based policy response to homelessness in the USA, particularly for homeless single adults. Permanent supportive housing combines long-term rental assistance with individualized social services to help people gain stability and meet their personal goals. Numerous studies have demonstrated that permanent supportive housing is effective in helping people maintain stable housing and is also associated with reduced hospitalizations and emergency department usage (Rog et al. 2014).

For people impacted by homelessness and serious mental illness, acquiring stable housing is associated with health and quality-of-life improvements (Henwood et al. 2014). Housing programs have also been credited with improving health outcomes for homeless individuals diagnosed with HIV/AIDS (Aidala et al. 2016; Bowen et al. 2017).

A type of permanent supportive housing known as Housing First has been particularly successful. Housing First programs emphasize helping people to quickly transition from homelessness to supportive housing and apply a harm reduction approach to substance use and mental health (Padgett et al. 2016). In other words, rather than requiring individuals to abstain from substances and achieve psychiatric stability prior to entering housing, Housing First enables people to address their physical and mental health after becoming stably housed, with an emphasis on client-driven goals and services that may or may not include abstinence from substances.

The vast body of research on Housing First suggests that this model may help to bolster residents' health in a variety of ways. Housing First programs are associated with better adherence to medications (Kidder et al. 2007; Rog et al. 2014), improvements in psychiatric symptoms and substance use outcomes (Fitzpatrick-Lewis et al. 2011; Greenwood et al. 2005), and reduced health-care costs (Wright et al. 2016). However, researchers have argued that there are opportunities for Housing First and other permanent supportive housing programs to build even greater capacity to address disparities and help their residents achieve full health equity (Henwood et al. 2013a). For example, housing programs could implement group-based and peer-led chronic disease self-management programs to help empower residents with the support, skills, and information needed to successfully manage chronic illnesses, such as diabetes, and live healthier lifestyles (Henwood et al. 2013b). Programs that provide on-site health services, such as by locating a health clinic within an apartment building or by having clinicians provide basic clinical or behavioral health services in clients' homes, may also help to reduce gaps to health-care access and ultimately improve health equity for permanent supportive housing residents (Aubry et al. 2016; Wright et al. 2016).

Health Care for the Homeless

Established as part of the 1987 McKinney-Vento Homeless Assistance Act, Health Care for the Homeless (HCH) is a federal funding program focused on community-based homeless health services. HCH covers an extensive scope of health-related projects across the USA, including outreach, primary care, and behavioral health treatment for people experiencing homelessness (US Interagency Council on Homelessness 2016). Operating on a $366 million budget in 2015, HCH grantee programs served over 840,000 homeless patients, about 70% of the total number of homeless patients seen at health clinics nationwide. This program provides a vital health safety net for those experiencing homelessness, especially when considering that 88% of those patients were at or below the federal poverty level and 38% were uninsured (National Health Care for the Homeless Council 2013, 2017). Noting the extensive range of services provided by HCH-funded programs to an extremely vulnerable population with a variety of unmet medical needs, Lebrun-Harris et al. (2013) concluded that continued financial support for such programs is an important aspect of working to combat the health disparities suffered by homeless persons.

Health-care services, including those provided through HCH funding, could be further enhanced by integrating care with other types of services, such as legal representation. Seeking disability benefits, fighting housing discrimination, or addressing disputed coverage or monetary disbursement regarding insurance claims are all common situations that may require legal representation. Recognizing this, Tsai et al. (2017) urge medical-legal partnerships in health-care programs that serve homeless populations. Like the movement toward the integration of primary and behavioral health care, the medical-legal partnership model calls for civil attorneys to be physically located at or available to patients at health-care service sites. In their study, 90% of HCH sites surveyed reported that their patients had a need for civil legal representation at least annually and, despite a clear majority of these sites desiring to implement medical-legal partnerships, only 10% actually had. This single location approach creates greater ease of access via a one-stop-shop and may help to address key social determinants of health that contribute to disparities for homeless persons, such as poverty and lack of income.

Meeting People Where They Are: Street Medicine and Mobile Clinic Programs

Another intervention used to address homeless individuals' health-care needs is the street medicine or mobile clinic model of service provision. These practices involve service providers going directly to the recipients and providing care at their location, rather than the traditional model in which services are rendered at the care provider's fixed location. Physician Jim Withers began doing street medicine work in Pennsylvania in 1992, later collaborating with fellow international street medicine providers and eventually founding the Street Medicine Institute in 2008 (Withers 2011). Reflecting on beginning his street medicine work, Dr. James O'Connell, president of the Boston HCH program, recalls that the end of his scholastic training was the beginning of his practical training in understanding the consequences of homelessness and poverty (O'Connell 2015). Extending the street medicine model, medical schools at universities such as the University at Buffalo have created student-run street medicine programs, which offer unique training opportunities for students as well as critical services to people experiencing homelessness (University at Buffalo Jacobs School of Medicine and Biomedical Sciences 2017).

Mobile clinics, in which services are provided out of a bus or van, are another common method for providing direct dental, medical, mental health, syringe exchange, and other services to clients in or near the places where they live. Chicago's Night Ministry is one well-known example. The Night Ministry's services include a health outreach bus, which visits different underserved city neighborhoods and offers a convenient place for homeless and low-income people to access medical exams, HIV testing, food, and other services (Night Ministry 2016). Beginning in San Francisco and spreading to cities across the USA, Project Homeless Connect is another program that offers homeless persons linkage to an array of services, through expo-style events at which health-care and other service providers offer short-term services and referrals in a centralized location (Project Homeless Connect 2017).

Street medicine programs, mobile clinics, and Project Homeless Connect are key illustrations of the social work dictum of "meeting people where they are." Short-term services provided at such programs may help build relationships that allow providers to successfully refer clients to housing and more intensive health-care and supportive services. However, it is critical to combine these acute and medium-term care models with continued advocacy to address the root causes of health disparities.

Health-Care Policy Innovations and Horizons

Addressing policy-level upstream determinants of health, including barriers to health-care access, is key to reducing health disparities for those experiencing homelessness. The establishment of the Affordable Care Act in 2010 offered several key provisions affecting homeless health care, including opportunities for state expansion of Medicaid eligibility, waiver programs, and funding for demonstration projects whereby agencies can provide innovative, nonstandard treatment methods, such as expansion of housing-based health programs, provided that the alternate care does not increase costs (Aykanian and Larkin 2015; Polonsky et al. 2014). For example, through the Center for Medicare and Medicaid Innovation (established by the Affordable Care Act), the National Health Care for the Homeless Council received grants to evaluate the use of community health workers in reducing emergency room care for homeless individuals and to provide care coordination for homeless Medicaid or Medicare recipients upon discharge following hospitalization (Aykanian and Larkin 2015). Some states have also applied waivers to use Medicaid funds to pay for housing-related services for formerly homeless individuals, including supports to assist individuals in transitioning from institutions to community housing and tenancy support services (Paradise and Ross 2017).

Even with these policy changes in the Affordable Care Act, as the National Health Care for the Homeless Council points out, achieving health equity may not be possible without a broader transformation of the health-care system. Alongside Physicians for a National Health Program and other major organizations across the

USA, they call for reform of the current multi-payer private health insurance system to a single-payer "Medicare for all" public insurance system, through which all individuals could access care. An international report comparing the US health-care system with other countries found that the US system is the most expensive in the world and at the same time performs worse on many key measures of efficiency and outcomes than other countries that have adopted a single-payer system (Davis et al. 2014). Single-payer universal health-care coverage would significantly reduce health-care service barriers for homeless populations and could also help to prevent homelessness through better treatment of health conditions that can contribute to people becoming homeless.

Conclusion

Striving to achieve health equity for all populations, including homeless people, is neither a simple task nor a fool's errand. Given the complex and manifold causes and consequences of health disparities, collaboration and long-term partnerships across multiple sectors and disciplines, including social work, medicine, and public health, will be necessary to make progress toward health equity. With continued research, policy advocacy, and innovative service programming, it is possible to move toward a future in which homelessness is prevented or minimized and good health is maximized for all people.

References

Aidala, A. A., Wilson, M. G., Shubert, V., Gogolishvili, D., Globerman, J., Rueda, S., et al. (2016). Housing status, medical care, and health outcomes among people living with HIV/AIDS: A systematic review. *American Journal of Public Health, 106*(1), e21–e23.

American College of Obstetricians and Gynecologists Committee on Healthcare for Underserved Women. (2013). Healthcare for homeless women. https://www.acog.org/Resources-And-Publications/Committee-Opinions/Committee-on-Health-Care-for-Underserved-Women/Health-Care-for-Homeless-Women. Accessed 27 July 2018.

Arbelle, J. E., Chodick, G., Goldstein, A., & Porath, A. (2014). Multiple chronic disorders – health care system's modern challenge in the Maccabi Health Care System. *Israel Journal of Health Policy Research, 3*(1), 29.

Argintaru, N., Chambers, C., Gogosis, E., Farrell, S., Palepu, A., Klodawsky, F., & Hwang, S. W. (2013). A cross-sectional observational study of unmet health needs among homeless and vulnerably housed adults in three Canadian cities. *BMC Public Health, 13*(1), 577–577.

Aubry, T., Duhoux, A., Klodawsky, F., Ecker, J., & Hay, E. (2016). A longitudinal study of predictors of housing stability, housing quality, and mental health functioning among single homeless individuals staying in emergency shelters. *American Journal of Community Psychology, 58*(1–2), 123–135.

Aykanian, A., & Larkin, H. (2015). Health care innovations for homeless families: Emerging opportunities under Medicaid and the Affordable Care Act. *Journal of Children and Poverty, 21*(1), 59–68.

Baggett, T. P., O'Connell, J. J., Singer, D. E., & Rigotti, N. A. (2010). The unmet health care needs of homeless adults: A national study. *American Journal of Public Health, 100*(7), 1326–1333.
Baggett, T. P., Singer, D. E., Rao, S. R., O'Connell, J. J., Bharel, M., & Rigotti, N. A. (2011). Food insufficiency and health services utilization in a national sample of homeless adults. *Journal of General Internal Medicine, 26*(6), 627–634.
Baggett, T. P., Hwang, S. W., O'Connell, J. J., Porneala, B. C., Stringfellow, E. J., Orav, E. J., et al. (2013). Mortality among homeless adults in Boston: Shifts in causes of death over a 15-year period. *JAMA Internal Medicine, 173*(3), 189–195.
Baker, C. K., Billhardt, K. A., Warren, J., Rollins, C., & Glass, N. E. (2010). Domestic violence, housing instability, and homelessness: A review of housing policies and program practices for meeting the needs of survivors. *Aggression and Violent Behavior, 15*(6), 430–439.
Ball, S. A., Cobb-Richardson, P., Connolly, A. J., Bujosa, C. T., & O'Neall, T. W. (2005). Substance abuse and personality disorders in homeless drop-in center clients: Symptom severity and psychotherapy retention in a randomized clinical trial. *Comprehensive Psychiatry, 46*(5), 371–379.
Bamberger, J. D., Unick, J., Klein, P., Fraser, M., Chesney, M., & Katz, M. H. (2000). Helping the urban poor stay with antiretroviral HIV drug therapy. *American Journal of Public Health, 90*(5), 699–701.
Bamrah, S., Yelk Woodruff, R. S., Powell, K., Ghosh, S., Kammerer, J. S., & Haddad, M. B. (2013). Tuberculosis among the homeless, United States, 1994–2010. *The International Journal of Tuberculosis and Lung Disease, 17*(11), 1414–1419.
Barnett, K., Mercer, S. W., Norbury, M., Watt, G., Wyke, S., & Guthrie, B. (2012). Epidemiology of multimorbidity and implications for health care, research, and medical education: A cross-sectional study. *Lancet, 380*(9836), 37–43.
Barney, L. (2017). Doctors could prescribe housing to the homeless under radical Hawaii bill. The Guardian. https://www.theguardian.com/us-news/2017/feb/28/hawaii-homeless-housing-bill-healthcare-costs. Accessed 27 July 2018.
Bazerghi, C., McKay, F. H., & Dunn, M. (2016). The role of food banks in addressing food insecurity: A systematic review. *Journal of Community Health, 41*(4), 732–740.
Beijer, U., Wolf, A., & Fazel, S. (2012). Prevalence of tuberculosis, hepatitis C virus, and HIV in homeless people: A systematic review and meta-analysis. *The Lancet Infectious Diseases, 12*(11), 859.
Bender, K., Brown, S. M., Thompson, S. J., Ferguson, K. M., & Langenderfer, L. (2015). Multiple victimizations before and after leaving home associated with PTSD, depression, and substance use disorder among homeless youth. *Child Maltreatment, 20*(2), 115–124.
Bharel, M., Creaven, B., Morris, G., Robertshaw, D., Uduhiri, K., Valvassori, P., et al. (2011). Health care delivery strategies: Addressing key preventive health measures in homeless health care settings. National Health Care for the Homeless Coalition. https://www.nhchc.org/wp-content/uploads/2012/02/KeyPrevHealthMeas_FINAL.pdf. Accessed 27 July 2018.
Blank, M. B., Himelhoch, S., Walkup, J., & Eisenberg, M. M. (2013). Treatment considerations for HIV-infected individuals with severe mental illness. *Current HIV/AIDS Reports, 10*(4), 371–379.
Bosick, S. J., Rennison, C. M., Gover, A. R., & Dodge, M. (2012). Reporting violence to the police: Predictors through the life course. *Journal of Criminal Justice, 40*(6), 441–451.
Bowen, E. A., Bowen, S. K., & Barman-Adhikari, A. (2016). Prevalence and covariates of food insecurity among residents of single-room occupancy housing in Chicago, IL, USA. *Public Health Nutrition, 19*(6), 1122–1130.
Bowen, E. A., Canfield, J., Moore, S., Hines, M., Hartke, B., & Rademacher, C. (2017). Predictors of CD4 health and viral suppression outcomes for formerly homeless people living with HIV/AIDS in scattered site supportive housing. *AIDS Care, 29*(11), 1458–1462.
Braveman, P. (2006). Health disparities and health equity: Concepts and measurement. *Annual Review of Public Health, 27*(1), 167–194.
Braveman, P., Egerter, S., & Williams, D. R. (2011). The social determinants of health: Coming of age. *Annual Review of Public Health, 32*(1), 381–398.

Brown, M., Chodzen, G., Mihelicova, M., & Collins, K. (2017). Applying a time-patterned typology of homelessness among individuals with mental illness. *American Journal of Community Psychology, 59*(3–4), 306–315.

Brubaker, M. D., Amatea, E. A., Torres-Rivera, E., Miller, M. D., & Nabors, L. (2013). Barriers and supports to substance abuse service use among homeless adults. *Journal of Addictions and Offender Counseling, 34*(2), 81–98.

Burgard, S. A., Seefeldt, K. S., & Zelner, S. (2012). Housing instability and health: Findings from the Michigan recession and recovery study. *Social Science and Medicine, 75*(12), 2215–2224.

Castellow, J., Kloos, B., & Townley, G. (2015). Previous homelessness as a risk factor for recovery from serious mental illnesses. *Community Mental Health Journal, 51*(6), 674–684.

Caton, C. M., Dominguez, B., Schanzer, B., Hasin, D. S., Shrout, P. E., Felix, A., et al. (2005). Risk factors for long-term homelessness: Findings from a longitudinal study of first-time homeless single adults. *American Journal of Public Health, 95*, 1753–1759.

Center for Behavioral Health Statistics and Quality. (2015). Behavioral health trends in the United States: Results from the 2014 National Survey on Drug Use and Health [HHS Publication No. SMA 15–4927, NSDUH Series H-50]. https://www.samhsa.gov/data/sites/default/files/NSDUH-FRR1-2014/NSDUH-FRR1-2014.pdf. Accessed 27 July 2018.

Chang, H., Fisher, F., Reitzel, L., Kendzor, D., Nguyen, M., & Businelle, M. (2015). Subjective sleep inadequacy and self-rated health among homeless adults. *American Journal of Health Behavior, 39*(1), 14–21.

Cheung, R. C., Hanson, A. K., Maganti, K., Keeffe, E. B., & Matsui, S. M. (2002). Viral hepatitis and other infectious diseases in a homeless population. *Journal of Clinical Gastroenterology, 34*(4), 476–480.

Coady, M. H., Latka, M. H., Thiede, H., Golub, E. T., Ouellet, L., Hudson, S. M., et al. (2007). Housing status and associated differences in HIV risk behaviors among young injection drug users (IDUs). *AIDS and Behavior, 11*(6), 854–863.

Cohen, S. M., van Handel, M. M., Branson, B. M., Blair, J. M., Irene Hall, H., Hu, X., et al. (2011). Vital signs: HIV prevention through care and treatment — United States. *Morbidity and Mortality Weekly Report, 60*(47), 1618–1623.

Coleman-Jensen, A., Gregory, C., & Singh, A. (2014). Household food security in the United States in 2013 (USDA-ERS Economic Research Report Number 173). SSRN. https://doi.org/10.2139/ssrn.2504067. Accessed 27 July 2018.

Connolly, A. J., Cobb-Richardson, P., & Ball, S. A. (2008). Personality disorders in homeless drop-in center clients. *Journal of Personality Disorders, 22*(6), 573–588.

Cougnard, A., Grolleau, S., Lamarque, F., Beitz, C., Brugère, S., & Verdoux, H. (2006). Psychotic disorders among homeless subjects attending a psychiatric emergency service. *Social Psychiatry and Psychiatric Epidemiology, 41*(11), 904–910.

Cutler, D. H., Bevilacqua, J., & McFarland, B. H. (2003). Four decades of community mental health: A symphony in four movements. *Community Mental Health Journal, 39*, 381–398.

Davis, K., Stremikis, K., Squires, D., & Schoen, C. (2014). Mirror, mirror on the wall, 2014 update: How the U.S. health care system compares internationally. Commonwealth Fund. http://www.commonwealthfund.org/~/media/files/publications/fund-report/2014/jun/1755_davis_mirror_mirror_2014.pdf. Accessed 27 July 2018.

Deiss, R. G., Rodwell, T. C., & Garfein, R. S. (2009). Tuberculosis and illicit drug use: Review and update. *Clinical Infectious Diseases, 48*(1), 72–82.

Denniston, M. M., Jiles, R. B., Drobeniuc, J., Klevens, R. M., Ward, J. W., McQuillan, G. M., & Holmberg, S. D. (2014). Chronic hepatitis C virus infection in the United States, National Health and Nutrition Examination Survey 2003 to 2010. *Annals of Internal Medicine, 160*(5), 293–293.

Diez Roux, A. V., & Mair, C. (2010). Neighborhoods and health. *Annals of the New York Academy of Sciences, 1186*(1), 125–145.

Dixon, L. B., & Schwarz, E. C. (2013). Fifty years of progress in community mental health in US: The growth of evidence-based practices. *Epidemiology and Psychiatric Sciences, 23*(01), 5–9.

Drake, R. E., & Latimer, E. (2012). Lessons learned in developing community mental health care in North America. *World Psychiatry, 11*, 47–51.

Dutton, M. A., Green, B. L., Kaltman, S. I., Roesch, D. M., Zeffiro, T. A., & Krause, E. D. (2006). Intimate partner violence, PTSD, and adverse health outcomes. *Journal of Interpersonal Violence, 21*(7), 955–968.

Edens, E. L., Mares, A. S., & Rosenheck, R. A. (2011). Chronically homeless women report high rates of substance use problems equivalent to chronically homeless men. *Women's Health Issues, 21*(5), 383–389.

Fazel, S., Khosla, V., Doll, H., & Geddes, J. (2008). The prevalence of mental disorders among the homeless in western countries: Systematic review and meta-regression analysis. *PLoS Medicine, 5*(12), e225.

Fazel, S., Geddes, J. R., & Kushel, M. (2014). The health of homeless people in high-income countries: Descriptive epidemiology, health consequences, and clinical and policy recommendations. *Lancet, 384*(9953), 1529–1540.

Feldman, S. (2003). Reflections on the 40th anniversary of the U.S. Community Mental Health Centers Act. *Australian and New Zealand Journal of Psychiatry, 37*(6), 662–667.

Fitzpatrick-Lewis, D., Ganann, R., Krishnaratne, S., Ciliska, D., Kouyoumdjian, F., & Hwang, S. W. (2011). Effectiveness of interventions to improve the health and housing status of homeless people: A rapid systematic review. *BMC Public Health, 11*(1), 638–638.

Flentje, A., Leon, A., Carrico, A., Zheng, D., & Dilley, J. (2016). Mental and physical health among homeless sexual and gender minorities in a major urban U.S. city. *Journal of Urban Health, 93*(6), 997–1009.

Fletcher, J. M., Andreyeva, T., & Busch, S. H. (2009). Assessing the effect of changes in housing costs on food insecurity. *Journal of Children and Poverty, 15*(2), 79–93.

Folsom, D. P., McCahill, M., Bartels, S. J., Lindamer, L. A., Ganiats, T. G., & Jeste, D. V. (2002). Medical comorbidity and receipt of medical care by older homeless people with schizophrenia or depression. *Psychiatric Services, 53*(11), 1456–1460.

Folsom, D. P., Hawthorne, W., Lindamer, L., Gilmer, T., Bailey, A., Golshan, S., et al. (2005). Prevalence and risk factors for homelessness and utilization of mental health services among 10,340 patients with serious mental illness in a large public mental health system. *American Journal of Psychiatry, 162*(2), 370–376.

Garfein, R. S., Vlahov, D., Galai, N., Doherty, M. C., & Nelson, K. E. (1996). Viral infections in short-term injection drug users: The prevalence of the hepatitis C, hepatitis B, human immunodeficiency, and human T-lymphotropic viruses. *American Journal of Public Health, 86*(5), 655–661.

Gattis, M. N., & Larson, A. (2016). Perceived racial, sexual identity, and homeless status-related discrimination among Black adolescents and young adults experiencing homelessness: Relations with depressive symptoms and suicidality. *American Journal of Orthopsychiatry, 86*(1), 79–90.

Gelberg, L., Robertson, M. J., Arangua, L., Leake, B. D., Sumner, G., Moe, A., et al. (2012). Prevalence, distribution, and correlates of Hepatitis C virus infection among homeless adults in Los Angeles. *Public Health Reports, 127*(4), 407–421.

Geller, J. L. (2000). The last half century of psychiatric services as reflected in psychiatric services. *Psychiatric Services, 51*, 41–67.

Goldfinger, S. M., Schutt, R. K., Tolomiczenko, G. S., Seidman, L., Penk, W. E., Turner, W., & Caplan, B. (1999). Housing placement and subsequent days homeless among formerly homeless adults with mental illness. *Psychiatric Services, 50*(5), 674–679.

Gonzalez, G., & Rosenheck, R. A. (2002). Outcomes and service use among homeless persons with serious mental illness and substance abuse. *Psychiatric Services, 53*(4), 437–446.

Goodman, L. A., Dutton, M. A., & Harris, M. (1997). The relationship between violence dimensions and symptom severity among homeless, mentally ill women. *Journal of Traumatic Stress, 10*(1), 51–70.

Greene, J. M., Ennett, S. T., & Ringwalt, C. L. (1999). Prevalence and correlates of survival sex among runaway and homeless youth. *American Journal of Public Health, 89*, 1406–1409.

Greenwood, R. M., Schaefer-McDaniel, N. J., Winkel, G., & Tsemberis, S. J. (2005). Decreasing psychiatric symptoms by increasing choice in services for adults with histories of homelessness. *American Journal of Community Psychology, 36*(3), 223–238.

Hawkins, R. L., & Abrams, C. (2007). Disappearing acts: The social networks of formerly homeless individuals with co-occurring disorders. *Social Science and Medicine, 65*(10), 2031–2042.

Henny, K. D., Kidder, D. P., Stall, R., & Wolitski, R. J. (2007). Physical and sexual abuse among homeless and unstably housed adults living with HIV: Prevalence and associated risks. *AIDS and Behavior, 11*(6), 842–853.

Henry, M., Shivji, A., de Sousa, T., Cohen, R., Khadduri, J., & Culhane, D. P. (2015). The 2015 Annual Homelessness Assessment Report (AHAR) to Congress, Part 1: Point-in-Time Estimates of Homelessness. U.S. Department of Housing and Urban Development. https://www.hudexchange.info/resources/documents/2015-AHAR-Part-1.pdf. Accessed 27 July 2018.

Henwood, B. F., Cabassa, L. J., Craig, C. M., & Padgett, D. K. (2013a). Permanent supportive housing: Addressing homelessness and health disparities? *American Journal of Public Health, 103*(S2), S188–S192.

Henwood, B. F., Stanhope, V., Brawer, R., Weinstein, L. C., Lawson, J., Stwords, E., & Crossan, C. (2013b). Addressing chronic disease within supportive housing programs. *Progress in Community Health Partnerships: Research, Education, and Action, 7*(1), 67–75.

Henwood, B. F., Matejkowski, J., Stefancic, A., & Lukens, J. M. (2014). Quality of life after housing first for adults with serious mental illness who have experienced chronic homelessness. *Psychiatry Research, 220*(1), 549–555.

Hudson, C. G. (2016). A model of deinstitutionalization of psychiatric care across 161 nations: 2001-2014. *International Journal of Mental Health, 45*(2), 135–153.

Huey, L. (2008). 'When it comes to violence in my place, I am the police!': Exploring the policing functions of service providers in Edinburgh's Cowgate and Grassmarket. *Policing and Society, 18*(3), 207–224.

Huey, L., & Quirouette, M. (2010). 'Any girl can call the cops, no problem': The influence of gender on support for the decision to report criminal victimization within homeless communities. *British Journal of Criminology, 50*(2), 278–295.

Huey, L., Broll, R., Hryniewicz, D., & Fthenos, G. (2014). "They just asked me why I became homeless": "Failure to ask" as a barrier to homeless women's ability to access services post-victimization. *Violence and Victims, 29*(6), 952–966.

Irwin, J. D., Ng, V. K., Rush, T. J., Nguyen, C., & He, M. (2007). Can food banks sustain nutrient requirements? A case study in Southwestern Ontario. *Canadian Journal of Public Health / Revue Canadienne de Sante'e Publique, 98*(1), 17–20.

Jones, A. A., Vila-Rodriguez, F., Leonova, O., Langheimer, V., Lang, D. J., Barr, A. M., et al. (2015). Mortality from treatable illnesses in marginally housed adults: A prospective cohort study. *BMJ Open, 5*(8), e008876.

Kennedy, J. F. (1963). Mental illness and mental retardation: Message from the President of the United States relative to mental illness and mental retardation. *American Psychologist, 18*(6), 280–289.

Kidder, D. P., Wolitski, R. J., Campsmith, M. L., & Nakamura, G. V. (2007). Health status, health care use, medication use, and medication adherence among homeless and housed people living with HIV/AIDS. *American Journal of Public Health, 97*(12), 2238–2245.

Kim, M. M., Ford, J. D., Howard, D. L., & Bradford, D. W. (2010). Assessing trauma, substance abuse, and mental health in a sample of homeless men. *Health and Social Work, 35*(1), 39–48.

Kirkpatrick, S. I., & Tarasuk, V. (2011). Housing circumstances are associated with household food access among low-income urban families. *Journal of Urban Health, 88*(2), 284–296.

Kuhn, R., & Culhane, D. P. (1998). Applying cluster analysis to test a typology of homelessness by pattern of shelter utilization: Results from the analysis of administrative data. *American Journal of Community Psychology, 26*(2), 207–232.

Kushel, M. B., Perry, S., Bangsberg, D., Clark, R., & Moss, A. R. (2002). Emergency department use among the homeless and marginally housed: Results from a community-based study. *American Journal of Public Health, 92*(5), 778–784.

Kushel, M. B., Evans, J. L., Perry, S., Robertson, M. J., & Moss, A. R. (2003). No door to lock: Victimization among homeless and marginally housed persons. *Archives of Internal Medicine, 163*(20), 2492–2499.

Kushel, M. B., Gupta, R., Gee, L., & Haas, J. S. (2006). Housing instability and food insecurity as barriers to health care among low-income Americans. *Journal of General Internal Medicine, 21*(1), 71–77.

Lebrun-Harris, L. A., Baggett, T. P., Jenkins, D. M., Sripipatana, A., Sharma, R., Hayashi, A. S., Daly, C., & Ngo-Metzger, Q. (2013). Health status and health care experiences among homeless patients in federally supported health centers: Findings from the 2009 patient survey. *Health Services Research, 48*(3), 992–1017.

Lee, B. A., & Greif, M. J. (2008). Homelessness and Hunger. *Journal of Health and Social Behavior, 49*(1), 3–19.

Lifson, A. R., & Halcón, L. L. (2001). Substance abuse and high-risk needle-related behaviors among homeless youth in Minneapolis: Implications for prevention. *Journal of Urban Health, 78*(4), 690–698.

Lin, W.-C., Bharel, M., Zhang, J., O'Connell, E., & Clark, R. E. (2015). Frequent emergency department visits and hospitalizations among homeless people with Medicaid: Implications for Medicaid expansion. *American Journal of Public Health, 105*(S5), S716–S722.

Link, B. G., Susser, E., Stueve, A., Phelan, J., Moore, R., & Struening, E. (1994). Lifetime and five-year prevalence of homelessness in the United States. *American Journal of Public Health, 84*, 1907–1912.

Linton, S. L., Celentano, D. D., Kirk, G. D., & Mehta, S. H. (2013). The longitudinal association between homelessness, injection drug use, and injection-related risk behavior among persons with a history of injection drug use in Baltimore, MD. *Drug and Alcohol Dependence, 132*(3), 457–465.

Lönnroth, K., Williams, B. G., Stadlin, S., Jaramillo, E., & Dye, C. (2008). Alcohol use as risk factor for tuberculosis disease – A systematic review. *BMC Public Health, 8*, 289.

Maness, D. L., & Khan, M. (2014). Care of the homeless: An overview. *American Family Physician, 89*(8), 634–640.

Maremmani, A. G. I., Bacciardi, S., Gehring, N. D., Cambioli, L., Schütz, C., Akiskal, H. S., & Krausz, M. (2015). The impact of mood symptomatology on pattern of substance use among homeless. *Journal of Affective Disorders, 176*, 164–170.

McNiel, D. E., & Binder, R. L. (2005). Psychiatric emergency service use and homelessness, mental disorder, and violence. *Psychiatric Services, 56*(6), 699–704.

Mechanic, D., & Rochefort, D. A. (1990). Deinstitutionalization: An appraisal of reform. *Annual Review of Sociology, 16*(1), 301–327.

Miewald, C., & McCann, E. (2014). Foodscapes and the geographies of poverty: Sustenance, strategy, and politics in an urban neighborhood. *Antipode, 46*(2), 537–556.

Milloy, M. J., Marshall, B. D., Montaner, J., & Wood, E. (2012). Housing status and the health of people living with HIV/AIDS. *Current HIV/AIDS Reports, 9*(4), 364–374.

Mohtashemi, M., & Kawamura, L. M. (2010). Empirical evidence for synchrony in the evolution of TB cases and HIV+ contacts among the San Francisco homeless: e8851. *PLoS One, 5*(1), e8851.

Montgomery, A. E., Metraux, S., & Culhane, D. (2013). Rethinking homelessness prevention among persons with serious mental illness. *Social Issues and Policy Review, 7*(1), 58–82.

National Health Care for the Homeless Council. (2013). Fact sheet 2013. http://www.nhchc.org/wp-content/uploads/2011/09/hch-fact-sheet-2013.pdf. Accessed 27 July 2018.

National Health Care for the Homeless Council. (2017). Frequently asked questions. https://www.nhchc.org/resources/general-information/faq/. Accessed 27 July 2018.

National Institute of Mental Health. (2015). Serious mental illness (SMI) among adults. https://www.nimh.nih.gov/health/statistics/prevalence/serious-mental-illness-smi-among-us-adults.shtml. Accessed 27 July 2018.

Night Ministry. (2016). Annual report FY 2016. https://www.thenightministry.org/TNM_Annual%20Report_2016.pdf. Accessed 27 July 2018.

North, C. S., Pollio, D. E., Smith, E. M., & Spitznagel, E. L. (1998). Correlates of early onset and chronicity of homelessness in a large urban homeless population. *Journal of Nervous and Mental Disease, 186*(7), 393–400.

North, C. S., Eyrich, K. M., Pollio, D. E., & Spitznagel, E. L. (2004). Are rates of psychiatric disorders in the homeless population changing? *American Journal of Public Health, 94*(1), 103–108.

Norton, B. L., Voils, C. I., Timberlake, S. H., Hecker, E. J., Goswami, N. D., Huffman, K. M., et al. (2014). Community-based HCV screening: Knowledge and attitudes in a high risk urban population. *BMC Infectious Diseases, 14*(1), 74–74.

Novella, E. J. (2008). Theoretical accounts on deinstitutionalization and the reform of mental health services: A critical review. *Medicine, Health Care and Philosophy, 11*(3), 303–314.

Nyamathi, A., Flaskerud, J. H., Leake, B., Dixon, E. L., & Lu, A. (2001). Evaluating the impact of peer, nurse case-managed, and standard HIV risk-reduction programs on psychosocial and health-promoting behavioral outcomes among homeless women. *Research in Nursing and Health, 24*(5), 410–422.

Nyamathi, A., Stein, J. A., Schumann, A., & Tyler, D. (2007). Latent variable assessment of outcomes in a nurse-managed intervention to increase latent tuberculosis treatment completion in homeless adults. *Health Psychology, 26*(1), 68–76.

O'Connell, J. J. (2015). *Stories from the shadows: Reflections of a street doctor*. Boston: BHCHP Press.

Padgett, D. K., Leibson Hawkins, R., Abrams, C., & Davis, A. (2006). In their own words: Trauma and substance abuse in the lives of formerly homeless women with serious mental illness. *American Journal of Orthopsychiatry, 76*(4), 461–467.

Padgett, D. K., Smith, B. T., Henwood, B. F., & Tiderington, E. (2012). Life course adversity in the lives of formerly homeless persons with serious mental illness: Context and meaning. *American Journal of Orthopsychiatry, 82*(3), 421–430.

Padgett, D. K., Henwood, B. F., & Tsemberis, S. J. (2016). *Housing first: Ending homelessness, transforming systems, and changing lives*. New York: Oxford University Press.

Paradise, J., & Ross, D. C. (2017). Linking Medicaid and supportive housing: Opportunities and on-the-ground examples [issue brief]. https://www.kff.org/report-section/linking-medicaid-and-supportive-housing-issue-brief/. Accessed 27 July 2018.

Parpouchi, M., Moniruzzaman, A., Russolillo, A., & Somers, J. M. (2016). Food insecurity among homeless adults with mental illness. *PLoS One, 11*(7), e0159334.

Patterson, M. L., Somers, J. M., & Moniruzzaman, A. (2012). Prolonged and persistent homelessness: Multivariable analyses in a cohort experiencing current homelessness and mental illness in Vancouver, British Columbia. *Mental Health and Substance Use, 5*(2), 85–101.

Polonsky, M., Aykanian, A., Records, J., & Larkin, H. (2014). Strengthening homeless services: Funding streams and emerging opportunities in Medicaid and the Affordable Care Act. http://www.albany.edu/excellencehomelessservices/assets/StrengtheningHomelessServices-ACA-2014-FINAL.pdf. Accessed 27 July 2018.

Ponce, A. N., Lawless, M. S., & Rowe, M. (2014). Homelessness, behavioral health disorders and intimate partner violence: Barriers to services for women. *Community Mental Health Journal, 50*(7), 831–840.

Project Homeless Connect. (2017). Results. https://www.projecthomelessconnect.org/about/results/. Accessed 27 July 2018.

Purser, G. L., Mowbray, O. P., & O'Shields, J. (2017). The relationship between length and number of homeless episodes and engagement in survival sex. *Journal of Social Service Research, 43*(2), 262–269.

Roberts, H., Kruszon-Moran, D., Ly, K. N., Hughes, E., Iqbal, K., Jiles, R. B., & Holmberg, S. D. (2016). Prevalence of chronic hepatitis B virus (HBV) infection in U.S. households: National Health and Nutrition Examination Survey (NHANES), 1988–2012. *Hepatology, 63*(2), 388–397.

Rog, D. J., Marshall, T., Dougherty, R. H., George, P., Daniels, A. S., Ghose, S. S., & Delphin-Rittmon, M. E. (2014). Permanent supportive housing: Assessing the evidence. *Psychiatric Services, 65*(3), 287–294.

Santiago, C. D., Wadsworth, M. E., & Stump, J. (2011). Socioeconomic status, neighborhood disadvantage, and poverty-related stress: Prospective effects on psychological syndromes among diverse low-income families. *Journal of Economic Psychology, 32*(2), 218–230.

Schmidt, L. M., Hesse, M., & Lykke, J. (2011). The impact of substance use disorders on the course of schizophrenia – a 15-year follow-up study: Dual diagnosis over 15 years. *Schizophrenia Research, 130*(1–3), 228–233.

Schwarcz, S. K., Hsu, L. C., Vittinghoff, E., Vu, A., Bamberger, J. D., & Katz, M. H. (2009). Impact of housing on the survival of persons with AIDS. *BMC Public Health, 9*(1), 220–220.

Seabrook, J. A., & Avison, W. R. (2012). Socioeconomic status and cumulative disadvantage processes across the life course: Implications for health outcomes. *Canadian Review of Sociology, 49*(1), 50–68.

Seligman, H. K., Davis, T. C., Schillinger, D., & Wolf, M. S. (2010a). Food insecurity is associated with hypoglycemia and poor diabetes self-management in a low-income sample with diabetes. *Journal of Health Care for the Poor and Underserved, 21*(4), 1227–1233.

Seligman, H. K., Laraia, B. A., & Kushel, M. B. (2010b). Food insecurity is associated with chronic disease among low-income NHANES participants. *Journal of Nutrition, 140*(2), 304–310.

Semba, R. D., Darnton-Hill, I., & de Pee, S. (2010). Addressing tuberculosis in the context of malnutrition and HIV coinfection. *Food and Nutrition Bulletin, 31*(4 Suppl), S345–S364.

Siefert, K., Heflin, C. M., Corcoran, M. E., & Williams, D. R. (2001). Food insufficiency and the physical and mental health of low-income women. *Women and Health, 32*(1–2), 159–177.

Slesnick, N., & Prestopnik, J. (2005). Dual and multiple diagnosis among substance using runaway youth. *American Journal of Drug and Alcohol Abuse, 31*(1), 179–201.

Stanley, J. L., Jansson, A. V., Akinyemi, A. A., & Mitchell, C. S. (2016). Characteristics of violent deaths among homeless people in Maryland, 2003–2011. *American Journal of Preventive Medicine, 51*(5), S260–S266.

Stein, J. A., & Nyamathi, A. (2004). Correlates of hepatitis C virus infection in homeless men: A latent variable approach. *Drug and Alcohol Dependence, 75*(1), 89–95.

Strehlow, A. J., Robertson, M. J., Zerger, S., Rongey, C., Arangua, L., Farrell, E., et al. (2012). Hepatitis C among clients of Health Care for the Homeless primary care clinics. *Journal of Health Care for the Poor and Underserved, 23*(2), 811–833.

Substance Abuse and Mental Health Services Administration. (2013). Results from the 2012 National Survey on Drug Use and Health: Mental health findings (NSDUH Series H-47, HHS Publication No. [SMA] 13–4805). https://www.samhsa.gov/data/sites/default/files/NSDUHresults2012/NSDUHresults2012.pdf. Accessed 27 July 2018.

Suglia, S. F., Duarte, C. S., & Sandel, M. T. (2011). Housing quality, housing instability, and maternal mental health. *Journal of Urban Health, 88*(6), 1105–1116.

Tarasuk, V., Dachner, N., Poland, B., & Gaetz, S. (2009). Food deprivation is integral to the 'hand to mouth' existence of homeless youths in Toronto. *Public Health Nutrition, 12*(9), 1437–1442.

Thakarar, K., Morgan, J. R., Gaeta, J. M., Hohl, C., & Drainoni, M. L. (2016). Homelessness, HIV, and incomplete viral suppression. *Journal of Health Care for the Poor and Underserved, 27*(1), 145–156.

Thompson, R. G., Wall, M. M., Greenstein, E., Grant, B. F., & Hasin, D. S. (2013). Substance-use disorders and poverty as prospective predictors of first-time homelessness in the United States. *American Journal of Public Health, 103*(2), S282–S288.

Thomson, H., & Thomas, S. (2015). Developing empirically supported theories of change for housing investment and health. *Social Science and Medicine, 124*, 205–214.

Thornton, R. L. J., Glover, C. M., Cené, C. W., Glik, D. C., Henderson, J. A., & Williams, D. R. (2016). Evaluating strategies for reducing health disparities by addressing the social determinants of health. *Health Affairs, 35*(8), 1416–1423.

To, M. J., Brothers, T. D., & Van Zoost, C. (2016). Foot conditions among homeless persons: A systematic review. *PLoS One, 11*(12), e0167463.

Tsai, J., Kasprow, W. J., & Rosenheck, R. A. (2014). Alcohol and drug use disorders among homeless veterans: Prevalence and association with supported housing outcomes. *Addictive Behaviors, 39*(2), 455–460.

Tsai, J., Jenkins, D., & Lawton, E. (2017). Civil legal services and medical-legal partnerships needed by the homeless population: A national survey. *American Journal of Public Health, 107*(3), 398–e394.

Tyler, K., Whitbeck, L., Hoyt, D., & Cauce, A. (2004). Risk factors for sexual victimization among male and female homeless and runaway youth. *Journal of Interpersonal Violence, 19*, 503–520.

U.S. Department of Housing and Urban Development. (2015a). Homeless emergency assistance and rapid transition to housing: Defining "chronically homeless". http://www.hudexchange.info/resources/documents/Defining-Chronically-Homeless-Final-Rule.pdf. Accessed 27 July 2018.

U.S. Department of Housing and Urban Development. (2015b). HUD 2015 continuum of care homeless assistance programs: Homeless populations and subpopulations. https://www.hudexchange.info/resource/reportmanagement/published/CoC_PopSub_NatlTerrDC_2015.pdf. Accessed 27 July 2018.

U.S. Interagency Council on Homelessness. (2016). The President's 2016 budget: Fact sheet on homelessness assistance. https://www.usich.gov/resources/uploads/asset_library/2016_Budget_Fact_Sheet_on_Homelessness_Assistance.pdf. Accessed 27 July 2018.

University at Buffalo Jacobs School of Medicine and Biomedical Sciences. (2017). Medical students take to streets to aid Buffalo's homeless population. University at Buffalo. https://medicine.buffalo.edu/news_and_events/news.host.html/content/shared/smbs/news/2017/01/ub-heals-street-medicine-6588.detail.html. Accessed 27 July 2018.

Vijayaraghavan, M., Jacobs, E. A., Seligman, H., & Fernandez, A. (2011). The association between housing instability, food insecurity, and diabetes self-efficacy in low-income adults. *Journal of Health Care for the Poor and Underserved, 22*(4), 1279–1291.

Vijayaraghavan, M., Tochterman, A., Hsu, E., Johnson, K., Marcus, S., & Caton, C. L. M. (2012). Health, access to health care, and health care use among homeless women with a history of intimate partner violence. *Journal of Community Health, 37*(5), 1032–1039.

Vila-Rodriguez, F., Panenka, W. J., Lang, D. J., Thornton, A. E., Vertinsky, T., Wong, H., et al. (2013). The hotel study: Multimorbidity in a community sample living in marginal housing. *American Journal of Psychiatry, 170*(12), 1413–1422.

Vogenthaler, N. S., Kushel, M. B., Hadley, C., Frongillo, E. A., Jr., Riley, E. D., Bangsberg, D. R., et al. (2013). Food insecurity and risky sexual behaviors among homeless and marginally housed HIV-infected individuals in San Francisco. *AIDS and Behavior, 17*(5), 1688–1693.

Walls, N. E., & Bell, S. (2011). Correlates of engaging in survival sex among homeless youth and young adults. *Journal of Sex Research, 48*, 423–436.

Weiser, S. D., Fernandes, K. A., Brandson, E. K., Lima, V. D., Anema, A., Bangsberg, D. R., et al. (2009). The association between food insecurity and mortality among HIV- infected individuals on HAART. *Journal of Acquired Immune Deficiency Syndromes, 52*(3), 342–349.

Wenzel, S. L., Koegel, P., & Gelberg, L. (2000a). Antecedents of physical and sexual victimization among homeless women: A comparison to homeless men. *American Journal of Community Psychology, 28*(3), 367–390.

Wenzel, S. L., Leake, B. D., & Gelberg, L. (2000b). Health of homeless women with recent experience of rape. *Journal of General Internal Medicine, 15*(4), 265–268.

Wenzel, S. L., Tucker, J. S., Elliott, M. N., Hambarsoomians, K., Perlman, J., Becker, K., et al. (2004). Prevalence and co-occurrence of violence, substance use and disorder, and HIV risk behavior: A comparison of sheltered and low-income housed women in Los Angeles County. *Preventive Medicine, 39*(3), 617–624.

Withers, J. (2011). Street medicine: An example of reality-based health care. *Journal of Health Care for the Poor and Underserved, 22*(1), 1–4.

Wright, B. J., Vartanian, K. B., Li, H. F., Royal, N., & Matson, J. K. (2016). Formerly homeless people had lower overall health care expenditures after moving into supportive housing. *Health Affairs, 35*(1), 20–27.

Zakrison, T. L., Hamel, P. A., & Hwang, S. W. (2004). Homeless people's trust and interactions with police and paramedics. *Journal of Urban Health, 81*(4), 596–605.

Chapter 4
Meeting the Diverse Service Needs of People Experiencing Homelessness

Stephanie Duncan, Ann Howard, and Calvin L. Streeter

Individuals experiencing homelessness in the USA represent a broad cross section of ages, genders, family constitutions, physical and mental health statuses, housing situations, and other demographic factors. Further, individuals and families can become homeless as a result of a broad range of systemic and individual factors. The most widely understood causes of homelessness include poverty, an absence of affordable housing, family and environmental difficulties, and fractured social supports. For young adults, homelessness may be attributed to involvement with the foster care system, a history of juvenile court or detention, abuse in the home, or family strain stemming from a youth's LGBTQ identity. However, these factors do not adequately explain the complicated structural, personal, and political factors that interact to result in homelessness (Burt et al. 2001). In other words, for some, homelessness may result from a singular cause or major event. For others, homelessness may result from a constellation of problems or a chain reaction of events.

Definitions of homelessness vary across county, state, and federal entities, as well as within agencies, suggesting that even existing demographic data may not fully represent the characteristics of people experiencing homelessness. There is no standard definition of what a homeless individual or family in the USA looks like, despite existing stereotypes. Homelessness can manifest in myriad ways, and therefore having multiple, often narrow, definitions can result in inconsistent estimates of the size of the homelessness population and certain groups or experiences being

Electronic supplementary material: The online version of this chapter (https://doi.org/10.1007/978-3-030-03727-7_4) contains supplementary material, which is available to authorized users.

S. Duncan · C. L. Streeter (✉)
University of Texas at Austin, Austin, TX, USA
e-mail: stephanie.duncan@utexas.edu; cstreeter@utexas.edu

A. Howard
Ending Community Homelessness Coalition (ECHO), Austin, TX, USA
e-mail: annhoward@austinecho.org

H. Larkin et al. (eds.), *Homelessness Prevention and Intervention in Social Work*, https://doi.org/10.1007/978-3-030-03727-7_4

excluded altogether. Because definitions of homelessness are also used to determine eligibility for specific services and funding streams, narrow definitions can also prevent homeless individuals and families from accessing housing and supports. Additionally, the strategies for addressing this social issue and for providing services to people experiencing homelessness are as complicated to define as homelessness itself. The goal of this chapter is to discuss what plans have been made in Austin, Texas, to address homelessness and to illustrate the constellation of services and supports this community's homeless service system has developed to prevent and end homelessness.

Ending Homelessness in Austin, Texas

Austin is fiercely committed to ending homelessness and over the past several years has been working toward developing a system to coordinate and adapt service delivery to meet the stated needs of clients rather than what is assumed by service providers (ECHO 2018). With the daily influx of new arrivals to Austin, there has been a trending uptick of people experiencing homelessness in the area. This increase, in part, is attributed to the lack of affordable housing and lengthy wait lists to receive supportive housing services. Austin's solution to end homelessness focuses on outreach, shelter, housing and support services, community commitment to address this public health issue, and an effective system-level response. Figure 4.1 illustrates the key elements of Austin's five-point plan to end homelessness.

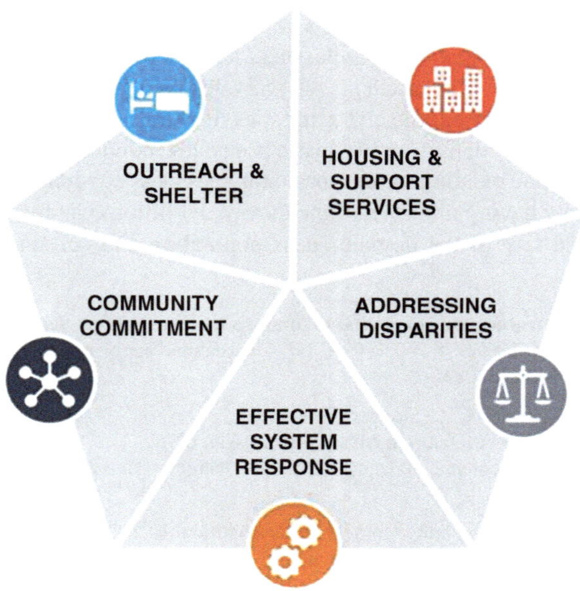

Fig. 4.1 Austin's five-point system to end homelessness (ECHO 2017)

Over 7000 people experience homelessness in Austin each year. Many factors have created this crisis, and without supporting these individuals in accessing permanent housing, this situation will remain difficult (ECHO 2018). Austin provides a framework to ending homelessness, which acknowledges long-term housing as a social determinant of health and recognizes the importance of supportive and wrap-around services to promote housing stability and overall well-being. Through the implementation of a coordinated entry process, a requirement for communities receiving funds through the US Department of Housing and Urban Development's Continuum of Care program, the community offers a common assessment to each household experiencing homelessness and makes referrals based on client needs and program eligibility requirements, all in a systemic way that prioritizes people based on needs and vulnerabilities (The Urban Institute and ICF Consulting 2002).

Communities across the country have developed their own approach to addressing the problem of homelessness. Figure 4.2 depicts Austin's core pathways to

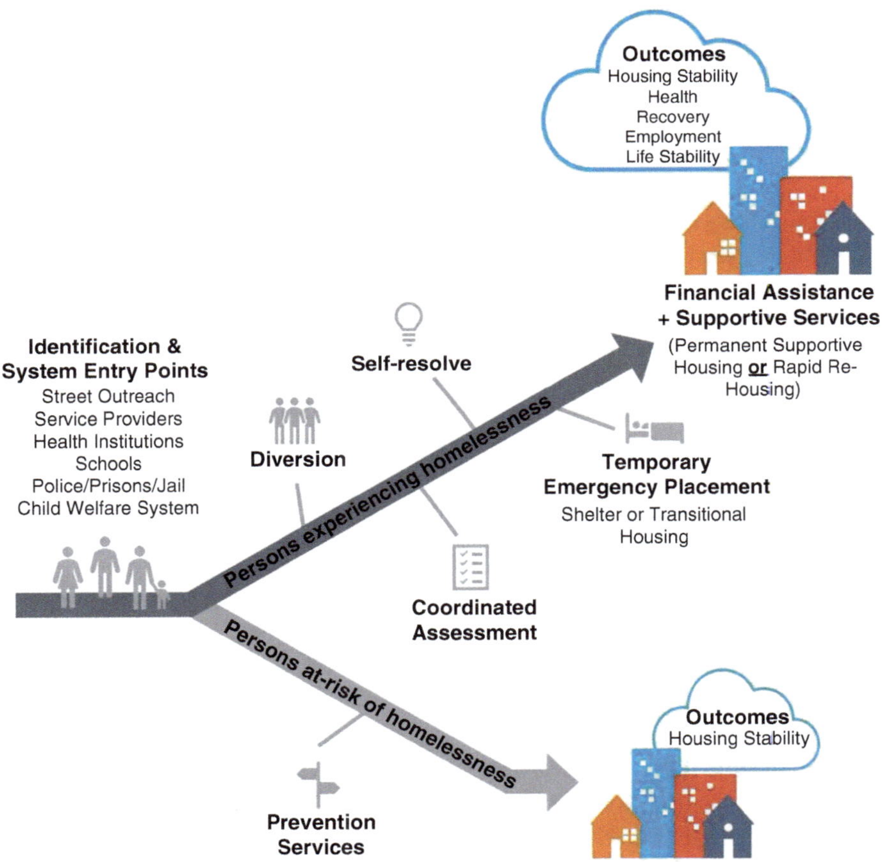

Fig. 4.2 Austin/Travis County system to prevent and end homelessness (ECHO 2017)

address homelessness and prioritize who is the most vulnerable, addressing their need for differing interventions and linking those individuals to programs, thus reducing their chances of returning to homelessness once housed.

Identification and System Entry Points

Outreach

The US Department of Housing and Urban Development (HUD) defines chronically homeless individuals as those who have a disabling condition and have been homeless for more than a year or had at least four episodes of homelessness during the past 3 years (National Alliance to End Homelessness 2015). Many individuals experiencing chronic homelessness have been homeless for years and, over time, can become service resistant, making them difficult to engage in services. Homeless outreach teams have been implemented across the USA to act as a liaison between programs and potential clients, going out to meet people where they are instead of waiting for them to come into an office. The connection between outreach services and homeless service programs or healthcare helps people experiencing homelessness access services they might not know about.

One of Austin's newer programs, the Homeless Outreach Street Team (HOST), consists of a social worker, Austin police officer, a behavioral health specialist, and a community health paramedic. The HOST team focuses on people living on the streets in downtown Austin and just west of the University of Texas campus. Some of these individuals have never been connected to services, and others are frequent users of the downtown shelters. Because of HOST's cross-disciplinary approach, they are able to assist people in crisis and meet a range of needs, such as refilling prescriptions, setting appointments, getting photo identification, and continued engagement on the street rather than requiring individuals to attend office appointments. The HOST team also links with the city's Street Medicine services to help overcome trust issues some homeless individuals have with medical providers. The Street Medicine team and HOST are part of a large continuum of outreach workers, including constables, paramedics, and social workers, who aim to meet clients where they live and provide some of the much-needed services to improve their quality of life while they wait for housing opportunities. These essential services are often the first point of contact for people not served by traditional housing services.

Case Study: HOST Meets "Patsy"

Patsy has been homeless since she was 10 years old. Through the city's coordinated assessment process, she was able to get her name on a waiting list for housing about a year ago. Patsy is known by many service providers throughout the city. When HOST developed, she was identified by the team, and they

(continued)

kept in contact with her. Patsy is an artist at heart; however, she struggles with substance use dependency and mental illness. HOST connected Patsy with a community artist who donated supplies to her and allowed her to use art studio space to practice her true passion. When Patsy's name came up for housing, HOST was able to find her, and, although she was afraid to move into a home, the team was able to support her transition into Community First Village, a housing development specifically for homeless individuals in Austin. HOST continued to follow Patsy for housing stabilization.

Many individuals who receive outreach services do not use the shelter services available in the community because of issues such as overcrowding, lack of transportation, safety concerns, or rules that prohibit pets or prevent couples from staying together. For some, there is a sense of resistance to help, perhaps because of pride, suspicion of motives, or a sense of shame about their current situation. While outreach workers often encounter this kind of resistance, there is little discussion in the literature about why such resistance occurs. Reasons may be similar to why other homeless service providers have difficulty connecting with this hard-to-reach group—lack of trust, perceptions of services being incompatible with actual needs, and other structural causes may prevent connection (Kryda and Compton 2009).

According to Tsemberis et al. (2004), the most effective time to offer housing is during the first outreach encounter. While "housing first" has gained acceptance in recent years, many agencies and service providers continue to focus on a "housing ready" approach, requiring things like sobriety and treatment and medication adherence before being considered ready to move into independent housing. The housing first model was developed by Pathways to Housing in New York City to meet the needs of chronically homeless individuals. It is based on the notion that housing is a human right and values the client's choice.

A housing first program is based on the premise that clients define their own needs and goals, and psychiatric treatment or sobriety is not a prerequisite for housing. This program posits housing first, which creates motivation to begin recovery (National Alliance to End Homelessness 2016). By contrast, housing ready programs encourage sobriety or require individuals with psychiatric concerns to become stabilized, as a prerequisite for successful transitioning into permanent supportive housing. These programs presume the client's psychiatric or substance use problems must be adequately addressed before they are able to reach independent living. Providers and clients alike are frustrated with this option, as barriers caused by service agencies and restrictions on who should be housed reduce the effort to move the most chronically homeless off the street (Kryda and Compton 2009; Tsemberis et al. 2004). Without proper housing and services being offered to address their concerns, people experiencing homelessness may perceive the services as inadequate or even meaningless.

yda and Compton (2009) conducted a qualitative study with people who are less and evaluated experiences with outreach services providers. There were two major themes discussed by people experiencing homelessness about their perception of outreach workers: (1) outreach workers are motivated primarily by their paycheck, and (2) outreach workers deliver empty promises. The belief that outreach workers gain commission, or that the agency capitalizes on a person's homelessness, led these particular participants to refuse services. Moreover, the same individuals reported having been promised services they were never delivered, which undermined their trust in the workers and their agencies.

Homeless service professionals in Austin collaborate around a system of care that is client centered and uses a shared database to track assessment, referrals, and housing outcomes. First, everyone experiencing homelessness is encouraged to complete a coordinated assessment. A coordinated assessment is an evaluation process used to determine which type of housing intervention best matches the needs of individuals experiencing homelessness, whether connecting them to community resources or referring them to housing programs. This process standardizes access for all clients and coordinates program referrals across all providers in the system (ECHO 2018). HOST fits in this system of care by building relationships and trust with individuals who otherwise may not receive services because of stigma, distrust, or the inability to get to appointments.

Ending Youth Homelessness

Homeless youth have unique struggles compared to homeless adults, including higher rates of risky sexual behaviors and barriers to healthcare and services (Slesnick et al. 2016). Often shelters are the first service contact for those experiencing homelessness. But homeless youth are less likely to use a crisis shelter. Research found that only 20–30% of homeless youth report ever having stayed at a crisis shelter (Slesnick et al. 2016; Springfield's Housing Collaborative 2007). Drop-in programs were developed to overcome the restrictions of the shelter, increase engagement of youth, and are low demand (Slesnick et al. 2016). The first connection with drop-in centers and service programs is often through outreach. According to Slesnick et al. (2016), drop-in services increase service use overall and are preferred by youth.

However, not all youth are connected with service providers, so Austin created a set of guiding principles to prevent and end youth homelessness. The goal is to intentionally imbed these principles into interventions, which will support youth and make a youth response system once connected with services (Varnell and Shoenfeld 2017; ECHO 2016). Special populations, such as LGBTQA+, minors, transition age youth, victims of sex trafficking, and immigrants who are unstably housed and may need specific pathways to enter services, are especially vulnerable. Mainly, the community is promoting more cultural competency trainings for service providers, as well as linking in other systems, such as Child Protective Services and the juvenile justice system. For example, Austin has created programs focused specifically on transition aged youth who have aged out of the foster care system and are in need of housing.

Having secured a $5.2M grant through HUD's Youth Homelessness Demonstration Program, Austin is connecting homeless youth with housing, jobs, and support services so they can heal from past trauma and strengthen their resolve for self-sufficiency. Service providers are connecting to school districts, foster care, and juvenile justice systems to build the connections needed to both prevent and end youth homelessness by the end of 2020. Through this initiative, Austin will model how to design programs for young adults experiencing homelessness that include these four elements:

1. Stable housing includes a safe and reliable place to call home.
2. Permanent connections include ongoing attachment to families, communities, schools, and other positive social networks.
3. Education/employment includes high performance in and completion of educational and training activities, especially for younger youth, and starting and maintaining adequate and stable employment particularly for older youth.
4. Social-emotional well-being includes the development of key competencies, attitudes, and behaviors that equip a young person to succeed across multiple domains of daily life, including school, work, relationships, and community.

Temporary and Emergency Shelter

In recent years, the USA has shifted focus from emergency shelter to interventions that emphasize permanent housing and support services to help people stabilize and maintain their housing. However, often the entry point into supportive housing programs is through the emergency shelter (Brown et al. 2017). In cities like Austin, where there is an influx in the population, shelter space is limited. Emergency shelter, however, remains a necessary component of the system because of the lack of permanent housing options and lengthy wait lists for subsidized housing. Procedures for who enters the shelter vary based on the community and typically are first come first serve, or, as in Austin, a lottery system is in place for some shelter beds. This type of system does not guarantee the most vulnerable receive a bed and in many cases those who have employment or other appointments that interfere with being present when doors open will lose out on the opportunity of sleeping in the emergency shelter.

Emergency shelters offer temporary placement for those who do not have alternative options available (U.S. Department of Housing and Urban Development 2017). The Austin Resource Center for the Homeless (ARCH) functions as a day resource center and a night shelter, and, like many other city shelters across the USA, it lacks enough resources to ensure that everyone using the shelter has access to housing programs. Instead, the Austin shelter traditionally offers housing programs only to those who are assigned a bed and participate in case management. The process of bed assignment creates yet another barrier to accessing long-term shelter (Brown et al. 2017). As such, people who are homeless who attempt to connect with case management services through the shelter to support them in securing long-term housing may have a delay in these services until they receive a bed assignment. Much work is being done across the country and in Austin to re-scope shelter services to better align with housing programs. Austin is discussing reducing the number of people who stay at the shelter at any one time but increasing the number of clients enrolled in housing programs to improve the rate of flow through the shelter and into housing. Austin recognizes that emergency shelter is not the end but a key component in a system that makes homelessness rare, brief, and a onetime event.

Diversion

Much of the literature only looks at shelter entries and not plausible prevention strategies (Goodman et al. 2014). One strategy that has been implemented in order to support individuals who are not able to gain an emergency shelter bed is diversion. Creating a successful diversion plan helps those who need immediate shelter to access alternate housing arrangements and, if necessary, connects them to financial assistance to return to permanent housing (National Alliance to End Homelessness 2015). In systems like Austin's that use a coordinated entry process, a designated intake process is used to assess level of need and acts as the service entry point to determine the appropriate programs to support an individual or family with housing and services. During intake, specific questions are asked, and often individuals are found appropriate for diversion, and immediate housing arrangements are sought to avoid a shelter stay. Staff who work in the diversion program are familiar with the assessment process and are trained in landlord mediation and conflict resolution (NAEH, 2018). In Austin, funding for diversion services comes primarily from local resources.

What Diversion Looks Like: Adapted from the National Alliance to End Homelessness

A 59-year-old man goes to a local shelter because he has been evicted after losing his job and being unable to pay rent. He is temporarily living in his car and runs the risk of being ticketed for loitering overnight in the local Walmart parking lot. During his intake interview, he shares with the intake worker that he would like to return to his old apartment, but he fears the relationship is damaged with his landlord and is ashamed to face him. The intake worker first discusses short-term options with this individual and learns his family is local,

(continued)

but he is too ashamed to ask to stay with them. The intake worker helps him strategize about how to ask family members to let him stay with them and encourages him to call from the office, so he feels supported. Once his family confirmed he could stay short-term, the intake worker discussed long-term housing plans. The intake worker collects contact information for the landlord and sets up a meeting to discuss the situation. In this meeting, the worker learns the man had a positive rental history and was previously well-regarded by the landlord. The intake worker tells the landlord her agency will pay the costs for him to return to his old apartment and that she will continue to work with this individual short-term to provide housing stabilization services. After a few days of staying with family, the man was able to move back into his old apartment.

Case Management

Homelessness is a serious public health issue in the USA and is often accompanied by other problems. As such, almost 40% of homeless people are dependent on alcohol and 25% on drugs (de Vet et al. 2017). Moreover, people who are homeless suffer from extreme poverty and lack of social support, as well as mental health and physical health problems (de Vet et al. 2017). The housing first approach is a shift away from people who are homeless going through the requirement to prove housing readiness. Through the process of helping clients gain housing stability, case managers have the important role of providing practical support, assessing needs, and linking with care and advocacy resources, especially for those with psychiatric and health problems.

de Vet et al. (2017) discusses four models of case management: standard case management (SCM), intensive case management (ICM), assertive community treatment (ACT), and critical time intervention (CTI). SCM, ICM, and ACT are distinguished from one another based on caseload, whether outreach is offered and whether a person reports to a single case manager versus a multidisciplinary team. CTI is a time-limited, strengths-based approach that works with people to prevent homelessness after transitioning from the street, shelter, or an institutional setting into community-based living. According to the literature, CTI is proven to be most effective with people experiencing homelessness when the primary goal is to bridge the gap between services and increase connections with social and professional supports. When working with people experiencing homelessness, CTI is used during the vulnerable transition from shelter or street to independent housing (de Vet et al. 2017). de Vet's (2017) review of case management literature reveals CTI decreased length of stay in the shelter and increased days housed. The transition from homelessness to housing can be difficult, and CTI provides the emotional and practical support necessary for those losing services through the shelter as well as the termination of their social support through other shelter members.

Locating individuals, effectively engaging them in services, and working with them toward independent housing and stability are not always done in an office setting. As such, Austin has established several paths for people who are homeless to connect with services, such as Pop-Up Resource Clinics, in order to bring services in areas of need where clinics are not accessible. Additionally, the Downtown Austin Community Court has case managers who use creative methods to connect with clients and work with defendants to complete court requirements and increase clients' stability to reduce the risk of re-offense. And, local libraries have recognized the need to assist with connecting people who are homeless with services, whereas providers come to the library to connect with those who are in need and aren't willing or able to go to an office appointment.

The experience of a person who was formerly homeless affects the transition into housing in different ways; some may feel elation or denial, and others may not be ready to settle. According to the US Department of Housing and Urban Development, a housing plan provides a framework for the housing referral process and serves as a means by which to measure progress toward goals (U.S. Department of Housing and Urban Development 2018). Created collaboratively, the housing plan takes into consideration the unique strengths, weaknesses, and desires of the person who is homeless. This involves an assessment of their individual living skills and identification of the supports they may need in order to thrive. Considerations may include, but are not limited to, applicant preferences, medical and mental health status, daily living skills, motivation, substance abuse, social skills, and social history.

A housing plan is considered a living document subject to change after its creation. Plans are reviewed regularly as more relevant information is brought to light. The plan is to be client driven and not influenced by the provider's beliefs. This necessitates self-awareness and control on the part of the service provider assisting the individual. It also requires honesty, as foreseen challenges should not be washed over during this process, and patience, as it takes time for people to share personal information. The individual is entitled to know what they are entering into and that they have a support system to turn to in times of need. Negotiation, if needed, should be handled mindfully.

Part of the housing plan developed with clients is a discussion concerning neighborly behavior, sensitivity to and respect for the needs and rights of others, the expected rules of tenancy in the new housing, avoidance of conflict, and ways to get to know people (U.S. Department of Housing and Urban Development 2018). Reluctance to engage with neighbors and the community may be a common response for newly housed individuals, especially those in recovery from drug and alcohol abuse. Time should be granted to allow the individual to warm to the changes that have taken place. Being a good neighbor can take on many forms; it includes a commitment to a respectful standard of conduct, open communication, and safety for oneself and others.

Elements of an individual's housing history to take into consideration when developing a housing plan include causes of homelessness, experiences in long-term institutionalization, and experiences in other housing situations or programs (e.g., un-serviced housing; serviced or supportive housing; living with roommates;

living with family, friends, or significant others) (United States Interagency Council on Homelessness 2014). Clients' experiences in these different settings should be discussed at length in order to determine the best housing option for them. Obstacles to overcome may include mental illness, substance use, and changes in daily activities and relationships. An additional barrier is that of shelterization, a learned dependency on the routine structure of how transitional facilities are run that may create reluctance to leave (United States Interagency Council on Homelessness 2014).

Housing interviews may consist of questions related to mental health, substance use, criminal history, and employment. According to a curriculum produced by HUD concerning the transition into housing, housing providers generally want to know four things about their potential residents: (1) will they pay their rent, (2) can we meet their service needs, (3) will they fit into our housing community and make a good neighbor, and (4) is this person going to be honest with me, or are they hiding something (United States Interagency Council on Homelessness 2016). Interviewing is a stressful process, so it is essential that applicants feel prepared and comfortable.

According to HUD's Homeless Services System, there are levels of barriers that should be considered. Level One consists of no barriers related to things like evictions, criminal history, or active chemical dependency or abuse issues. These are individuals who may be experiencing a temporary financial or personal crisis. Level Two consists of low to moderate housing barriers, where families or individuals have two or more of the following: no rental history, poor rental history, insufficient savings, poor credit history, sporadic employment history, no high school diploma/GED, recent or current abuse and/or battering, a head of household under 18 years old, a large family, or a criminal background. Level Three consists of high barriers where families or individuals have two or more of the following: no income, recent history of substance abuse, serious health conditions, and some of the barriers from Level Two. Finally, Level Four denotes extreme barriers, where individuals have severe mental illness and/or substance abuse problems, are living on the street, and have been unable or unwilling to participate in supportive services (United States Interagency Council on Homelessness 2015).

Recruiting landlords and cultivating relationships with them is an important step for housing organizations that takes time and commitment. Community Solutions, an organization that helps communities optimize their existing resources to make measurable social change, has outlined tips for working with landlords. These include the establishment of a landlord advisory group, attending meetings of one's local landlord organization, targeting "medium-sized" landlords, divide and conquer, screen clients appropriately, think like a salesperson, be honest, be strategic about placements, remain neutral, and practice patience (Community Solutions 2016).

The establishment of a landlord advisory board will let landlords speak about their fears and concerns with accepting formerly homeless individuals and offering suggestions for how to make it more appealing. Medium-sized landlords are those that have just the right amount of capacity to consider being a part of housing programs. For example, smaller units may not have high turnover rates and vacancies, and larger units may have stricter screening policies (Community Solutions 2016). Enlightening possible landlords to the benefits they would receive from joining the housing program is an effective way to persuade participation. Possible benefits include elimination of advertising costs, the presence of a neutral party to mitigate potential conflicts, and renters who come with a safety net—in some cases there is a guaranteed security deposit, and clients may have access to time-limited subsidies (Community Solutions 2016).

Financial Assistance and Supportive Services

Two types of established evidenced-based housing programs—rapid rehousing and permanent supportive housing—are central to Austin's efforts to end homelessness and are increasingly being used throughout the nation. These housing and service interventions have been proven to end homelessness for individuals and families (ECHO 2018; U.S. Department of Housing and Urban Development 2011, 2013). Rapid rehousing is meant to provide intensive case management and short-term rental assistance to link those who are homeless to sustainable, permanent housing as quickly as possible. In this program, case managers are in the position to directly address specific issues, such as unemployment or medical conditions, that may have led to homelessness. This program also connects individuals with longer-term needs, such as education programs, counseling, and other effective interventions for families with children (Oliva 2014).

Permanent supportive housing (PSH) is a combination of long-term financial assistance with intensive case management and support services. PSH is focused on those who have the longest history of homelessness and who are in need of services and supports to address complex needs, including mental or physical health concerns. Austin's high occupancy rates and tight rental market have proven challenging when trying to locate affordable housing, as well as landlords who are willing to overlook possible poor credit and criminal backgrounds. These housing programs provide leverage with landlords through incentives and mitigation tools to create housing opportunities, which otherwise would not be available (Substance Abuse and Mental Health Services Administration 2010).

Healthcare Meets Homelessness

Many people experiencing homelessness rely on Austin's "safety net hospital" for healthcare when they inevitably become ill. In a 2016 review compiled by Austin ECHO, nearly 64% of people who are homeless reported having used the local emergency department for care within the last 6 months (ECHO 2017). In most case scenarios, these patients are then discharged to the streets or sent to the local shelter without support or guaranteed follow-up in the earliest days of their convalescence.

On the national level, respite care—or recuperative care as it is sometimes called—has become an increasingly popular means by which medical providers may ensure a smoother transition out of the hospital for homeless men and women.

Compared to their housed counterparts, the homeless are already more likely to utilize the emergency room, and once hospitalized they remain for a longer duration on average. Evidence from a number of studies has shown that those who are discharged back to the streets have higher rates of readmission for the same chronic condition (Feldman et al. 2017). Respite care offers those recovering from acute illnesses or needing post-acute care (e.g., patients receiving intravenous antibiotics or physical therapy for debility) a sustained but temporary degree of step-down medical care that continues beyond the acute hospitalization. While there exists a broad spectrum of respite care based on inclusion and exclusion criteria, medical capabilities, and physical location (e.g., freestanding facilities, existing homeless shelters, church basements, post-acute care hospital beds), the common core principles include ensuring a healthy transition out of the hospital and optimization of available social services for the patient.

Respite care is less expensive than an extended hospital stay and can therefore result in cost savings. A study done by the Chicago Housing for Health Partnership showed an annual cost savings of $6307 for a group receiving respite care accompanied by case management and supportive housing following hospitalization versus the control group. Buchanan et al. (2006) concluded that the cost of 1 day of respite care was approximately half of a given hospital day. Unlike traditional homeless shelters, which require people to vacate each morning and live on the street, medical respite programs provide around-the-clock room and board for people in need of posthospital rehabilitation. Respite services not only reduce the utilization of inpatient services, but individuals are often linked to housing from this resource and avoid returning to the street because of the supportive services available. Respite care is not available in every community; however, it is recognized as a need by many service providers where respite care is provided individually by local agencies. For example, social work students who interviewed several agencies in Austin found several organizations that provided respite informally for their clients once they were discharged from the local hospitals if it did not seem safe to return to the streets. Housing services integrated in the healthcare system benefit the community and provide a holistic approach for clients who are likely the most vulnerable.

Another concept relevant to promoting health in homeless services is harm reduction. Harm reduction has a wide range of practices, such as needle exchange, safer sex supplies, and overdose prevention. It may also include services for medical concerns that are able to be addressed at a mobile site by a licensed practitioner. The harm reduction strategy, coupled with motivational interviewing, has been shown effective with people struggling with substance use concerns (Homeless HUB 2018). The literature suggests that harm reduction can help improve public order, reduce HIV risk behaviors, and has been a conduit for many individuals seeking substance use treatment. In many communities, harm reduction remains controversial, and there are many misconceptions about the concept. Harm reduction is about choice and is often a step toward cessation of substance use while teaching safe practices and support change over time (Homeless HUB 2018).

Harm reduction has also served as end-of-life care for those who are homeless and use alcohol or illicit drugs. We know homelessness is strongly correlated with adverse health outcomes and often leads to early mortality, which can be exacerbated by substance use. People who are homeless and use substances have complex end-of-life care needs, which are aggravated by the challenges of day-to-day survival (McNeil et al. 2012). Medical staff often encounter many challenges linking people who are homeless to end-of-life care because of social and structural barriers. Harm reduction programs have helped these individuals establish contact and develop trusting relationships without judgment about their continued use of drugs or alcohol (McNeil 2012). For this incredibly marginalized group of individuals, harm reduction programs have linked up with end-of-life care services to address the gaps that exist. With harm reduction strategies not being supported in many parts of the country, action is needed to fill these significant gaps in services for homeless individuals experiencing medical problems and in need of end-of-life care.

Conclusion

Communities across the nation are dedicated to successfully ending homelessness, and from the literature we know this requires systemic change that is client centered and data driven. This requires services and providers who have a shared vision of connecting people who are homeless with housing and stabilization services to maintain this housing. This commitment not only has to be with individual service providers but across networks of agencies, linking data and information, so individuals who are homeless are supported and do not have to repeat the process of telling their story every time they connect with a new service. The community of providers, including social workers, needs to continue to advocate for this kind systemic change.

References

Brown, M., Vaclavik, D., Watson, D. P., & Wilka, E. (2017). Predictors of homeless services re-entry within a sample of adults receiving Homelessness Prevention and Rapid Re-Housing Program (HPRP) assistance. *Psychological Services, 14*(2), 129–140.

Buchanan, D., Doblin, B., Sai, T., & Garcia, P. (2006). The effects of respite care for homeless patients: A cohort study. *American Journal of Public Health, 96*(7), 1278–1281.

Burt, M. R., Aron, L. Y., & Lee, E. (2001). *Helping America's homeless: Emergency shelter or affordable housing?* Washington, D.C.: Urban Institute Press.

Community Solutions. (2016). Tips for working with landlords (outreach and engagement strategies). https://www.community.solutions/landlord-toolkit. Accessed 2 Oct 2018.

de Vet, R. D., Beijersbergen, M. D., Jonker, I. E., Lako, D. A. M., van Hermert, A. M., Herman, D. B., & Wolf, J. R. (2017). Critical time intervention for homeless people making the transition to community living: A randomized controlled trial. *American Journal of Community Psychology, 60*(1-2), 175–186.

ECHO. (2016). Youth homelessness needs assessment. http://www.austinecho.org/wp-content/uploads/2016/11/161214-FINAL-youth-homelessness-needs-assessment-1.pdf. Accessed 1 Oct 2018.

ECHO. (2017). Current needs and gaps report. http://www.austinecho.org/wp-content/uploads/2017/01/170901-Austin-Homelessness-Needs-Gaps-Analysis-2017.pdf. Accessed 18 Sept 2018.

ECHO. (2018). Austin's action plan to end homelessness. www.austintexas.gov/edims/document.cfm?id=292841. Accessed 1 Sept 2018.

Feldman, B. J., Calogero, C. G., Elsayed, K. S., Abbasi, O. Z., Enyart, J., Friel, T. J., & Greenberg, M. R. (2017). Prevalence of homelessness in the emergency department setting. *Western Journal of Emergency Medicine, 18*(3), 366–372.

Goodman, S., Messeri, P., & O'Flaherty, B. (2014). How effective homelessness prevention impacts the length of shelter spells. *Journal of Housing Economics, 23*, 55–62.

Kryda, A. D., & Compton, M. T. (2009). Mistrust of outreach workers and lack of confidence in available services among individuals who are chronically street homeless. *Community Mental Health Journal, 45*(2), 144–150.

McNeil, R., Guirguis-Younger, M., Dilley, L. B., Dilley, L. B., Aubry, T. D., Turnbull, J., & Hwang, S. W. (2012). Harm reduction services as a point-of-entry to and source of end-of-life care and support for homeless and marginally housed persons who use alcohol and/or illicit drugs: A qualitative analysis. *BMC Public Health, 12*, 312.

National Alliance to End Homelessness. (2015). Assessment tools for allocating homelessness assistance: State of the evidence. *U.S. Department of Housing and Urban Development*. https://www.huduser.gov/publications/pdf/assessment_tools_Convening_Report2015.pdf. Accessed 2 Oct 2018.

National Alliance to End Homelessness. (2016). Housing first. https://endhomelessness.org/resource/housing-first/. Accessed 2 Oct 2018.

NAEH (2018). The Role of Emergency Shelter in Diversion. National Alliance to End Homelessness, September 27, 2018. https://endhomelessness.org/resource/role-emergency-shelter-diversion/. Accessed 14 January 2018.

Oliva, A. M. (2014). SNAPS in focus: Rapid re-housing as a model and best practice. *U.S. Department of Housing and Urban Development*. https://www.hudexchange.info/news/snaps-in-focus-rapid-re-housing-as-a-model-and-best-practice/. Accessed 2 Oct 2018.

Slesnick, N., Feng, X., Guo, X., Brakenhoff, B., Carmona, J., Murnan, A., Cash, S., & McRee, A. L. (2016). A test of outreach and drop-in linkage versus shelter linkage for connecting homeless youth to services. *Prevention Science, 17*(4), 450–460.

Springfield's Housing Collaborative. (2007). *High risk and homeless youth survey*. Springfield, MO: Community Partnership of the Ozarks, Christian, Greene, and Webster Counties Continuum of Care.

Substance Abuse and Mental Health Services Administration. (2010). Permanent supportive housing evidence-based practices (EBP KIT). https://store.samhsa.gov/product/Permanent-Supportive-Housing-Evidence-Based-Practices-EBP-KIT-/SMA10-4510. Accessed 2 Oct 2018.

The Homeless Hub. (2018). Harm reduction. http://homelesshub.ca/about-homelessness/substance-use-addiction/harm-reduction. Accessed 2 Oct 2018.

The Urban Institute, & ICF Consulting. (2002). Evaluation of continuums of care for homeless people: Final report. *U.S. Department of Housing and Urban Development*. https://www.huduser.gov/publications/pdf/continuums_of_care.pdf. Accessed 1 Sept 2018.

Tsemberis, S., Gulcur, L., & Nakae, M. (2004). Housing first, consumer choice, and harm reduction for homeless individuals with a dual diagnosis. *American Journal of Public Health, 94*(4), 651–656.

U.S. Department of Housing and Urban Development. (2011). Homelessness prevention and rapid re-housing program year 2 summary. https://www.hudexchange.info/resources/documents/HPRP_Year2Summary.pdf. Accessed 2 Oct 2018.

U.S. Department of Housing and Urban Development. (2013). Making the transition to permanent housing. https://www.hudexchange.info/resources/documents/shptransitionpermanenthousing.pdf. Accessed 2 Oct 2018.

U.S. Department of Housing and Urban Development. (2017). Coordinated entry core elements. https://www.hudexchange.info/resources/documents/Coordinated-Entry-Core-Elements.pdf. Accessed 2 Oct 2018.

U.S. Department of Housing and Urban Development. (2018). Homeless services system: Program referral guidelines. https://www.hudexchange.info/resources/housingsearchtool/?housingsearchtoolaction=public:main.client-intake-and-case-management-resources. Accessed 2 Oct 2018.

United States Interagency Council on Homelessness. (2014). Implementing housing first in permanent supportive housing. https://www.usich.gov/resources/uploads/asset_library/Implementing_Housing_First_in_PermanentSupportive_Housing.pdf. Accessed 2 Oct 2018.

United States Interagency Council on Homelessness. (2015). Rapid re-housing. https://www.usich.gov/solutions/housing/rapid-re-housing. Accessed 2 Oct 2018.

United States Interagency Council on Homelessness. (2016). Housing first checklist: Assessing projects and systems for a housing first orientation. https://www.usich.gov/resources/uploads/asset_library/Housing_First_Checklist_FINAL.pdf. Accessed 2 Oct 2018.

Varnell, W., & Shoenfeld, E. A. (2017). Ending youth homelessness in Austin/Travis County. *The College for Behavioral Health Leadership.* https://www.leaders4health.org/images/uploads/files/Lifeworks_Youth_Homelessness.pdf. Accessed 1 Oct 2018.

Part II
Individual, Community, and System Responses to Homelessness

Chapter 5
Affordable Housing and Housing Policy Responses to Homelessness

Linda Plitt Donaldson and Diane Yentel

Introduction

The lack of affordable housing is a core contributing factor explaining why more than a half million people, 20% of whom are children, experience homelessness on any given night in the USA (HUD 2018). The US Department of Housing and Urban Development (n.d.) considers housing affordable when households pay no more than 30% of their monthly gross income in housing costs (i.e., rent, mortgage, and utilities). Sociologist Matthew Desmond (2016) describes the affordable housing crisis as "among the most urgent and pressing issues facing America today" (p. 5). Study after study has shown that access to affordable housing makes a fundamental difference in whether a family or individual is simply poor or homeless. In her review of the research on family homelessness, Shinn (2009) observes, "For the vast majority of [poor] families, affordable housing… is sufficient to assure housing stability" (p. 1). In a national, 12-city study of 2300 families who experienced homelessness, families who received long-term housing subsidies had "by far the best outcomes for reducing family homelessness 3 years after random assignment" (Gubits et al. 2016, p. 4). Similarly, numerous studies have demonstrated the effectiveness of the Housing First model (see Chap. 8 for a discussion of Housing First) in ending homelessness for individuals experiencing long-term homelessness and struggling with chronic mental illness and/or addiction (Henwood et al. 2015)

Electronic supplementary material: The online version of this chapter (https://doi.org/10.1007/978-3-030-03727-7_5) contains supplementary material, which is available to authorized users.

L. P. Donaldson (✉)
Catholic University of America, Washington, DC, USA
e-mail: donaldson@cua.edu

D. Yentel
National Low Income Housing Coalition, Washington, DC, USA
e-mail: dyentel@nlihc.org

H. Larkin et al. (eds.), *Homelessness Prevention and Intervention in Social Work*, https://doi.org/10.1007/978-3-030-03727-7_5

showing that housing can end homelessness for the most vulnerable people. In addition to ending homelessness, affordable housing offers other advantages to the health and well-being of society.

Affordable Housing Increases Economic Mobility

Affordable housing is a long-term asset that helps families and children climb the economic ladder. A wide body of research shows that all areas of life, from employment and economic mobility to health and education, are improved when individuals and families have access to a decent and stable home (NLIHC n.d.). According to the How Housing Matters survey, 70% of Americans agree that "investing in affordable, quality housing is investing in kids and their future (Hart Research Associates 2016, p. 35)."

Increasing the supply of affordable housing and rental assistance—especially in areas connected to good schools, well-paying jobs, healthcare, and transportation—helps families climb the economic ladder and leads to greater economic and community development. In addition, children who live in a stable, affordable home have better health and educational outcomes, gain greater access to economic opportunities, enjoy better mental and physical well-being, and benefit from stronger communities. Research shows that increasing access to affordable housing is the most cost-effective strategy for reducing childhood poverty in the USA (Ginnarelli et al. 2015).

Groundbreaking research by Harvard economist Raj Chetty offers persuasive evidence of the impact of affordable housing on upward mobility for children. Using tax data, Chetty and his colleagues assessed the long-term outcomes for children who moved at a young age to lower poverty neighborhoods. Chetty's study found that children who were younger than 13 when their family moved to lower poverty neighborhoods saw their earnings as adults increase by approximately 31%, an increased likelihood of living in better neighborhoods as adults, and a lower likelihood of becoming a single parent (Chetty et al. 2014).

Other research shows that children living in stable, affordable homes are more likely to thrive in school and have greater opportunities to learn inside and outside the classroom. Children in low-income households that live in affordable housing score better on cognitive development tests than those in households with unaffordable rents (Newman and Holupka 2015). Researchers suggest that this is partly because parents with affordable housing can invest more in activities and materials that support their children's development (Newman and Holupka 2014). Having access to affordable housing allows the lowest-income families to devote more of their limited resources to other basic needs. Families paying large shares of their income for rent have less money to spend on food, healthcare, and other necessities than those with affordable rents (Joint Center for Housing Studies 2015).

Affordable Housing Spurs Economic Growth

Beyond the broad benefits to economic mobility, investments in affordable housing for the lowest-income households bolster productivity and economic growth. By connecting workers to communities with well-paying jobs, good schools, and transit, investments in affordable housing can spur local job creation and increase incomes. Research shows that the shortage of affordable housing in major metropolitan areas costs the American economy about $2 trillion annually in wages and productivity (Hsieh and Moretti 2017). The lack of affordable housing acts as a barrier to entry, preventing lower-income households from moving to communities with more economic opportunities. Without the burden of higher housing costs, these families would be better able to move to areas with growing local economies where their wages and employment prospects may improve.

High housing costs constrain opportunities for families to increase earnings, causing slower gross domestic product (GDP) growth. In fact, researchers estimate that the growth in GDP between 1964 and 2009 would have been 13.5% higher if families had better access to affordable housing. This would have led to a $1.7 trillion increase in income or $8775 in additional wages per worker (Hsieh and Moretti 2017). Moreover, each dollar invested in affordable housing infrastructure boosts local economies by leveraging public and private resources to generate income—including resident earnings and additional local tax revenue—and support job creation and retention. In fact, building 100 affordable rental homes generates $11.7 million in local income, $2.2 million in taxes and other revenue for local governments, and 161 local jobs in the first year (NAHB 2015).

Affordable Housing Improves Health Outcomes

Research also shows that access to affordable housing improves health outcomes. For example, in their nationally representative sample of non-disabled adults between 18 and 64, Simon et al. (2017) found that people who received housing assistance were less likely to be uninsured and had lower levels of unmet health needs than people who had not received housing assistance. In their summary of research examining the link between affordable housing and health, Moqbook et al. (2015) reported that affordable housing enabled families to spend more on healthy food and healthcare, reduces stress and related mental health problems for household members, and improves health outcomes for those suffering from chronic illness. They also report on research showing improved health and mental health outcomes when survivors of domestic violence have access to affordable housing. The importance of housing in improving the stability and quality of life for individuals and families does not diminish the importance of other supports to help households exit poverty, such as employment, education, living wages, healthcare, child care, and mental health or substance abuse treatment (Bassuk and Geller 2006).

However, access to affordable housing has been shown to prevent homelessness, improve health outcomes, and provide a base from which household members can have the space and security to improve their life situations.

Affordable Housing Reduces Income and Racial Inequality

Research from the Brookings Institution has found a direct relationship between income inequality and the rental housing affordability crisis. In addition to finding that income inequality in the USA is higher than before the Great Recession of 2007, the Brookings Institution found that housing is less affordable for low-income households in cities with higher levels of inequality. Their findings also suggest that housing markets in cities with high inequality are more responsive to the demand for rental housing for higher-income households and less responsive to the demand for housing that is affordable for lower-income households (Holmes and Berube 2016.)

People of color are disproportionately impacted by the housing affordability crisis. Households of color and foreign-born households account for half of renter households. Over the next decade, it is projected that people of color will contribute virtually all the net increase in renters, with Hispanics alone accounting for more than half of the total (Joint Center for Housing Studies 2013). By investing in affordable homes for the lowest-income people, our nation can lift families with the greatest needs, help close the gap between rich and poor, and level the playing field for families of color.

Despite the broad-based evidence for the benefits of affordable housing, the supply and accessibility of affordable housing is growing scarcer. The rest of this chapter describes the growing housing affordability crisis by first defining affordable housing and reviewing some of the historical and contemporary trends showing the decreasing supply of affordable housing. Next, the chapter reviews some of the policies and programs that make housing more affordable for low- and middle-income people, including specific strategies used by jurisdictions to build more affordable and inclusive housing strategies. Finally, the chapter concludes by describing next steps in terms of addressing affordable housing in the USA and other policy initiatives that could be combined with housing to make a meaningful dent in reducing poverty and ending homelessness.

Growing Scarcity of Affordable Housing

The US Department of Housing and Urban Development (n.d.) defines affordable housing as housing costs (i.e., rent, mortgage, and utilities) that do not exceed 30% of a family's monthly gross household income. Households that pay more than 30% of their monthly gross income for housing costs are considered cost-burdened.

Households that pay more than 50% of their monthly gross income for housing costs are considered severely cost-burdened. In their annual report, *The State of the Nation's Housing*, the Joint Center for Housing Studies (2017) at Harvard University reported that in 2015, one-third of US households (39 million households) paid more than 30% of their income in rent or mortgage payments and renters, versus homeowners, were disproportionately represented in these cost-burdened households (21 million versus 18 million). In fact, 48% of all renters were cost-burdened, and those in the two lowest income groups (i.e., incomes at $15,000 and below and incomes between $15,000 and $29,999) had cost burden at rates of 83% and 77%, respectively. Moreover 70% of those with incomes below $15,000 were severely cost-burdened (i.e., paying more than 50% of their income to rent). Figure 5.1 (National Low Income Housing Coalition 2017a, p.6) shows the rental burdens for households by income level.

In 2015, there were 8.1 million extremely low-income (ELI) renters in the USA. This number represents an increase of 38.7% of renters with worst case housing needs since 2007 and 63.4% since 2001 (Watson et al. 2017). As one might expect, households of color experience greater cost burdens than white households; 47% of black households are cost-burdened, as are 44% of Hispanic households, 37% of Asian households, and 28% of white households. Twenty-five million children are among those in cost-burdened households, and one-third of older adults experience cost burden, 54% of them are renters and 43% of them are homeowners (Joint Center for Housing Studies 2017). Contributing to the high rates of families who are cost-burdened is the diminishing supply of affordable

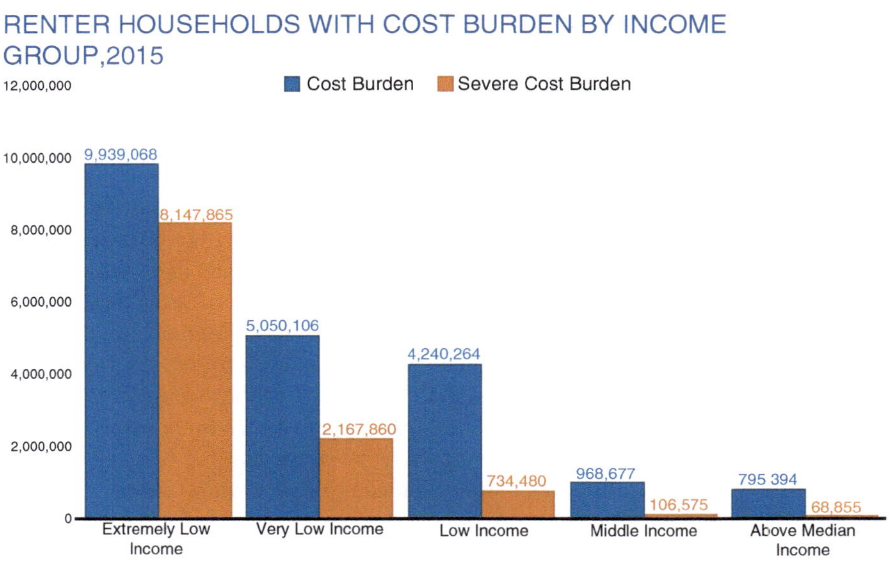

Fig. 5.1 Renter households with cost burden by income group (National Low Income Housing Coalition 2017a)

homes for the lowest-income people, while wages for the lowest-income earners have stagnated or even declined. When the rental housing market is tight and wages stagnate or decline, the cost of housing grows further out of reach for millions of American families.

The National Low Income Housing Coalition (2017a) reports that there are 11.4 million ELI households, accounting for 25% of all US renter households and 10% of all US households overall. The NLIHC observes, "The United States has a shortage of 7.4 million affordable and available rental homes for extremely low-income (ELI) renter households, resulting in 35 affordable and available units for every 100 ELI renter households nationally" (NLIHC 2017a, p. 2). Every state and every major metropolitan area in the USA have a shortage of affordable and available homes for the lowest-income renters. The shortage of affordable and available rental units for ELI renters ranges from roughly 8700 in Wyoming to 1.1 million in California. In the state of Nevada, there are just 15 homes affordable and available for every 100 of the lowest-income renters, and in Alabama there are only 61 affordable and available rental units for every 100 extremely low-income renters (NLIHC 2017a).

Low Wages, Low Public Benefit Levels, and Affordable Housing

The affordability of housing is directly related to the wages households earn. Every year, the National Low Income Housing Coalition calculates the "housing wage" or the amount one must earn per hour to afford to rent a modest, two-bedroom apartment at HUD's fair market rent, paying 30% of income toward rent (2017b).[1] Fair market rent refers to the 40th percentile of gross rents for standard rental units. FMRs are determined by HUD on an annual basis and reflect the cost of shelter and utilities. FMRs are used to determine payment standards for the Housing Choice Voucher Program and Section 8 contracts (NLIHC 2017b, p. 1).

In 2017, NLIHC calculated the national housing wage as $21.21/hour for a two-bedroom unit and $17.14 for a one-bedroom unit. Comparing the cost of housing with the minimum wages across the country, NLICH found that "in no state, metropolitan area, or county can a full-time minimum-wage worker afford a modest two-bedroom rental home. In only 12 counties can a full-time minimum-wage worker afford a modest one-bedroom rental home" (p. 1). It's not just minimum wage workers for whom the rent is out of reach. NLIHC estimates that the average hourly wage of renters in the USA is $16.38, $4.83 less than the two-bedroom housing wage. In many states, the gap between the average renter's wage and the housing wage is even higher. Figure 5.2 illustrates the 2017 housing wage in all 50 states.

Many of the low-income renters for whom housing is not affordable work in low-wage jobs, such as retail, food service, and housekeeping. Edin and Shaefer (2015) document the impact of low-wage work combined with the lack of affordable

[1] The housing wage is available for every state, metropolitan area, and zip code.

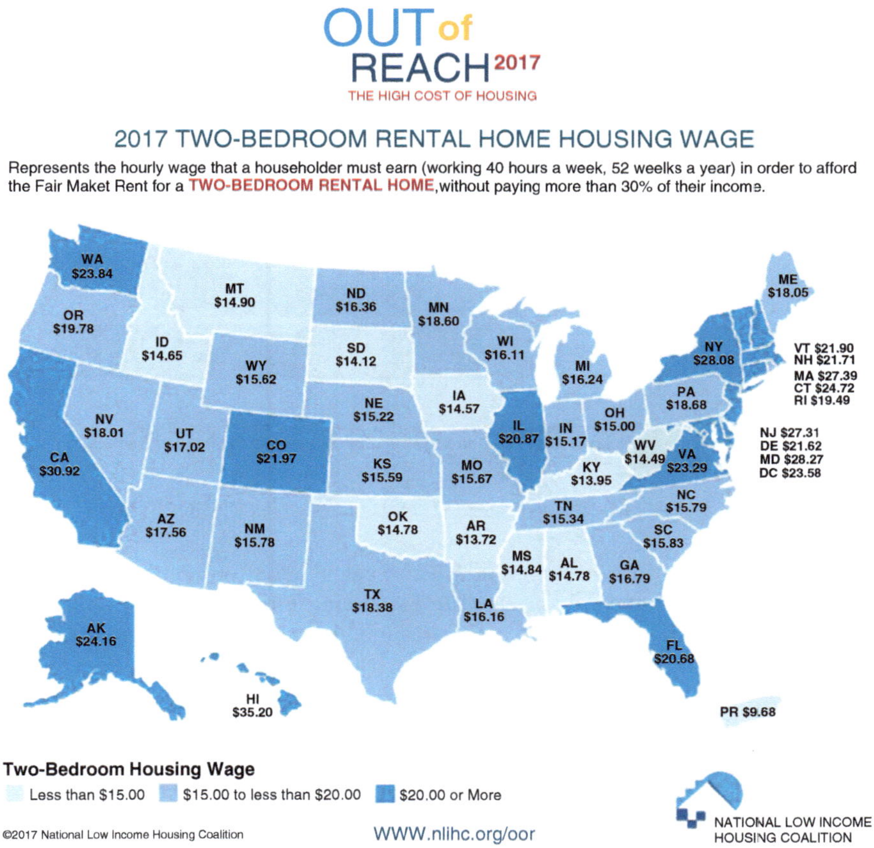

Fig. 5.2 2017 Two-bedroom rental home housing wage (NLIHC 2017b)

housing on low-income families showing that approximately 1.5 million households, including 3 million children, live on virtually 2 dollars a day. NLICH (2017b) observes that "six of the seven occupations projected to add the greatest number of jobs by 2024 provide a median wage that is not sufficient to afford a modest one-bedroom rental home" (p. 1). Figure 5.3 shows the amount of rent affordable to various types of low-income renters as compared to the HUD fair market rent rate for a one- and two-bedroom unit.

Supplemental Security Income (SSI) is the federal program for low-income individuals who are over age 65, blind, or disabled. Many people who are chronically homeless either receive or would qualify for this federal benefit. In 2017, the Social Security Administration calculated the monthly SSI benefit to be $735/month. Using the standard formula of 30% of one's income as being an affordable rent payment, an adult who is receiving SSI should pay no more than $221/month in rent. Few, if any, units exist at that level without some type of private or federal housing

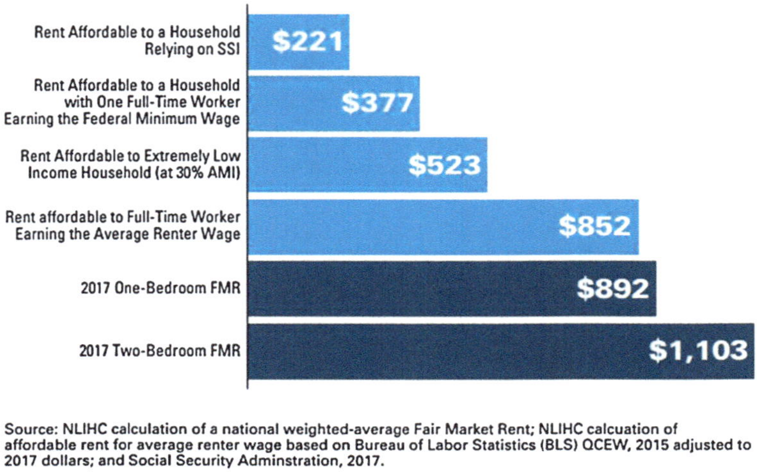

Fig. 5.3 Rents affordable for different categories of income source (NLIHC 2017b)

subsidy. Using this same formula, Fig. 5.3 also calculates affordable rents for households with one full-time worker earning the federal minimum wage ($7.25/hour), households with incomes at 30% of the area median income,[2] and households with one full-time worker earning the average renter wage.[3]

Diminishing Federal Investments in Affordable Housing

Federal investments in affordable housing—at the US Departments of Housing and Urban Development (HUD) and Agriculture (USDA)—have lifted millions of families out of poverty. Without these investments, many of these families would be homeless, living in substandard or overcrowded conditions, or struggling to meet other basic needs because too much of their limited income would go to paying rent. Despite their proven track record, federal affordable housing investments have been chronically underfunded as is illustrated in Fig. 5.4. Today, of the families who qualify for housing assistance, only a quarter will get the help they need.

Families use a variety of strategies to cobble together the funds needed to provide a roof over their head, which sometimes means living in substandard housing

[2] The area median income (AMI) is the income level within a particular jurisdiction within which half of all household incomes in that area fall above and half of all household incomes in that area fall below. HUD considers households whose income is 30% of the AMI are considered "extremely low income." Those with incomes at 50% of the AMI are considered very low income, and households with incomes at 80% of AMI are considered low income.

[3] Renter wage is the mean hourly wage earned by US renters derived from the Bureau of Labor statistics wage data (NLIHC 2017a).

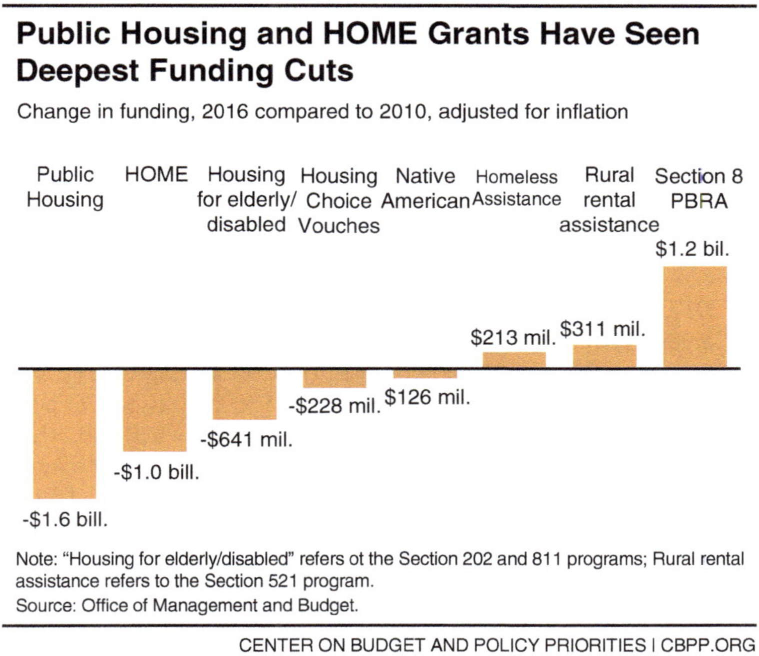

Fig. 5.4 Funding cuts to federally assisted housing programs (Center for Budget and Policy Priorities 2016)

or living doubled- or tripled-up with other families in units designed to hold fewer people. Many household bread winners work two or three jobs to make ends meet. Millions of households live in precarious conditions and are at risk of eviction. Desmond (2016) documented that between 2009 and 2011, 25% of the moves undertaken by low-income families in Milwaukee were involuntary, meaning that families were forced to move or were evicted from their homes. He also documented the toll eviction takes on families, including loss of community (e.g., neighborhood and school), possessions, job, self-worth, and government assistance. Yet, many low-income families can thrive through a variety of programs that make housing more affordable. Many of these programs are described in the next section.

Sources of Affordable Housing

This section describes the most commonly applied strategies to make housing more affordable for and available to American families. Such strategies include offering tax benefits (e.g., mortgage interest deduction), providing government-run housing (i.e., public housing), providing government subsidies for housing on the private market (e.g., housing choice vouchers), and other efforts to increase the supply of affordable housing units (e.g., low-income housing tax credits, housing trust funds, and inclusionary zoning).

Mortgage Interest Deduction

In 2015, the federal government spent $190 billion to support or defray housing costs for American families (Fischer and Sard 2017). However, a disproportionate share of these dollars helped higher-income homeowners, primarily through the mortgage interest deduction (MID). The MID allows homeowners to subtract the value of the interest they have paid on their mortgage from their taxable income. The federal government spends over $60 billion on this housing benefit each year, of which 84% goes to households with incomes over $100,000 (Joint Committee on Taxation 2017). "The seven million households with incomes of $200,000 or more receive a larger share of [federal housing spending] than the more than 509 million households with incomes of $50,000 or less" (Fischer and Sard 2017, p. 2). The average benefit for households with incomes over $200,000 is $6076, nearly four times the average benefit for households with incomes below $20,000, who receive an average benefit of $1529 (Fischer and Sard 2017). Those with the most severe cost burden for housing (i.e., low-income renters) receive less than 30% of federal housing spending (see Fig. 5.5).

In fact, three out of four families who qualify for housing assistance do not receive it because the funding levels do not support the level of need (Fischer and Sard 2017). As a result, most low-income families are severely cost-burdened or experiencing homelessness. However, some lucky families can benefit from the modest investments in federal and state initiatives that make housing more affordable. The most common of these programs are described below.

Housing Choice Vouchers: Tenant-Based

The Housing Choice Voucher Program, formerly known as Section 8, is the largest federal rent subsidy program for very low-income families. It is administered by local public housing agencies (PHA). "More than five million people in 2.2 million low-income families use vouchers" (CBPP 2017a, p. 1). As shown in Fig. 5.6, most people who benefit from vouchers are children, older adults (Section 202), and people with disabilities (Section 811).

Theoretically, families who qualify for the program receive a voucher that can be used to rent an apartment, townhouse, or single-family home from a participating landlord whose property meets the health and safety standards of the local PHA. In some cases, vouchers can be used to purchase a modest home. Families are responsible for finding their own units based on their needs (e.g., family size and composition). The PHA pays the value of the subsidy to the landlord, and families pay the difference between the rent and the subsidy. That difference should be no more than 30% of the family's income.

In addition to the Housing Choice Voucher (HCV) Program for the general population, there are voucher programs for special populations, such as veterans (HUD-

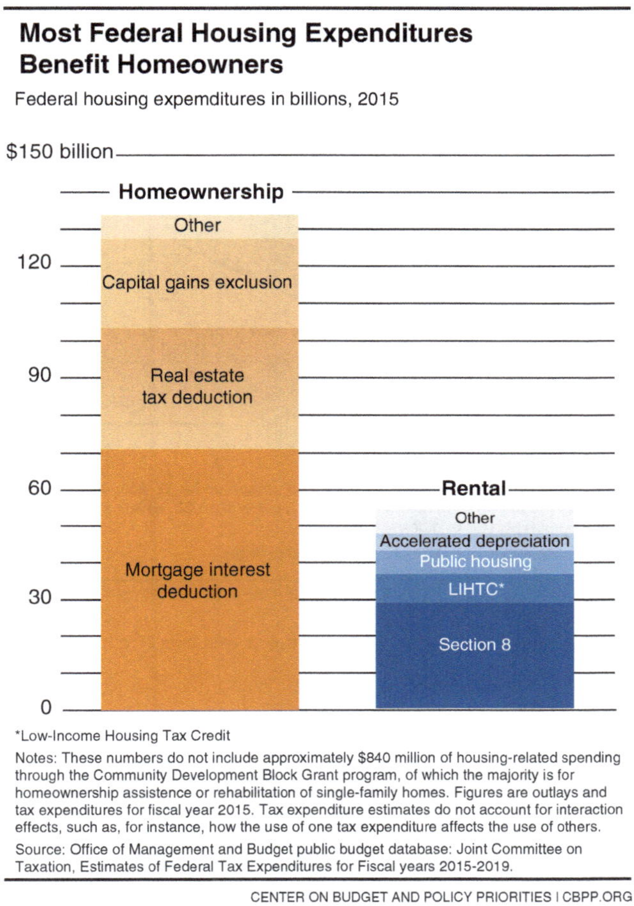

Fig. 5.5 Most federal expenditures benefit homeowners (Fischer and Sard 2017)

Veterans Affairs Supportive Housing), people with disabilities, people in rural areas, tribal communities, and family reunification vouchers (to support families involved in the child welfare system). Investments in the HUD-VASH program, combined with the Housing First model, have been largely credited with the success in ending veteran homelessness in a variety of cities (US Interagency for the Council 2017).

Many families who qualify for HCVs are not able to receive them because the program is not funded sufficiently to meet the need. In addition, for every 100 extremely low-income and very low-income renters, only 38 and 62 affordable units are available, respectively (HUD 2017). Furthermore, although PHAs may maintain a waiting list for housing, many of them don't maintain a waiting list because these lists can grow to tens of thousands of households, and since they know they cannot meet the need, they don't bother to maintain a list. In their national

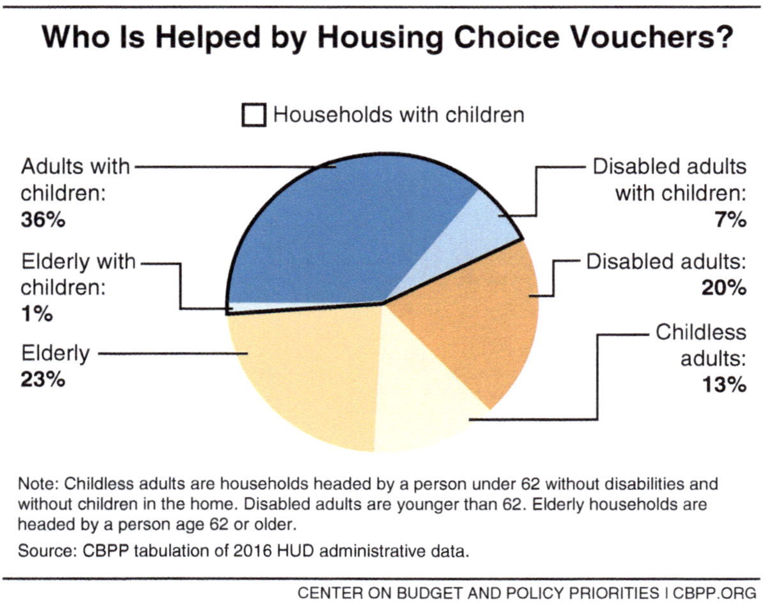

Fig. 5.6 Households who benefit from housing choice vouchers (Center for Budget and Policy Priorities 2017a)

PHA survey, the National Low Income Housing Coalition (2016) found that the HCV waiting lists of 53% of 320 participating PHAs were closed to new applicants, and 63% of those had been closed for at least 1 year. Furthermore, for 25% of waiting lists, the wait times were more than 3 years, and 74% of families on the waiting lists were in the extremely low-income category. In Washington, D.C., the centralized waiting list for subsidized housing includes more than 40,000 families and is currently closed (Harrison 2017). Given the lack of affordable housing, vouchers don't turnover that often.

To supplement the federal HCV Program, states may offer local housing subsidy programs. For example, in 2007, Washington, D.C., created a Local Rent Supplement Program (LRSP) that offers a limited number of housing subsidies to qualifying D.C. residents. In fiscal year 2016, D.C. spent $48 million to assist 3530 low-income families through the LRSP (D.C. Fiscal Policy Institute 2016a). A local subsidy program is an example of how states and local jurisdictions can help address the housing affordability gap in their communities. A challenge with rent subsidy programs is that as rents rise, the subsidy dollars don't go as far, so if funding for the program remained level, fewer households would be served by the subsidies. To that end, jurisdictions need to consider strategies that curb overall housing costs, so all housing investments can help more families in need.

Housing Choice Vouchers: Project-Based

As part of the Housing Choice Voucher Program, local PHAs and nonprofit housing developers can tie a portion of their vouchers to specific existing or developing housing units. This makes the unit available only to applicants whose household income is low enough to qualify. Unlike tenant-based vouchers, project-based vouchers are attached to the unit. In other words, when the tenant moves out, the subsidy does not follow them, and it remains with the unit. Typically, for-profit and nonprofit developers enter into multi-year contracts with HUD to allocate a portion or all the units in a building for low-income tenants. Applicants who meet the income criteria are eligible to access these units if they are available, and pending other screening requirements which may serve as barriers to housing. For example, affordable housing models that do not follow a Housing First approach, may have requirements related to sobriety and mental health treatement compliance, which are common barriers to accessing project-based housing for people struggling with chronic homelessness.

Approximately two million people in 1.2 million households benefit from the project-based voucher program (Center for Budget and Policy Priorities 2017b). As with the tenant-based vouchers, older adults, people with disabilities, and children are the primary beneficiaries of the project-based program. However, continued availability of these units is contingent on landlords renewing their contracts when they expire. From 2005 to 2014, nearly 45,763 project-based units were lost due to landlords opting out of their contracts (Ray et al. 2015). Housing markets in denser areas are more vulnerable to losing affordable housing through contract opt-outs. Typically, when landlors opt-out of a contract to provide low-income housing, they renovate their units as high-end apartments or condominium units because the market will bear it.

Public Housing

HUD oversees approximately 1.1 million public housing units across the USA. Public housing units are apartments that are managed and administered by the 2900 Public Housing Authorities across the country (CBPP 2017c), and they are heavily subsidized by government funding. Like the tenant-based and project-based voucher programs, the 2.1 million low-income residents who live in public housing are primarily older adults (31%), people with disabilities (30%), and families with children (34%). Only 14% of residents in public housing are single, childless adults (CBPP 2017c).

The supply of public housing units has diminished by more than 250,000 since the mid-1990s (CBPP 2017c). Housing assistance strategies have shifted to public-private partnerships to deconcentrate poverty. Therefore, money to build new public housing units has not been provided since the mid-1990s. The costs of public housing are funded by two primary streams: the Public Housing Operating Fund (to support the administration of PHAs) and the Public Housing Capital Fund (to support the rehabilitation and maintenance of public housing facilities). However, the

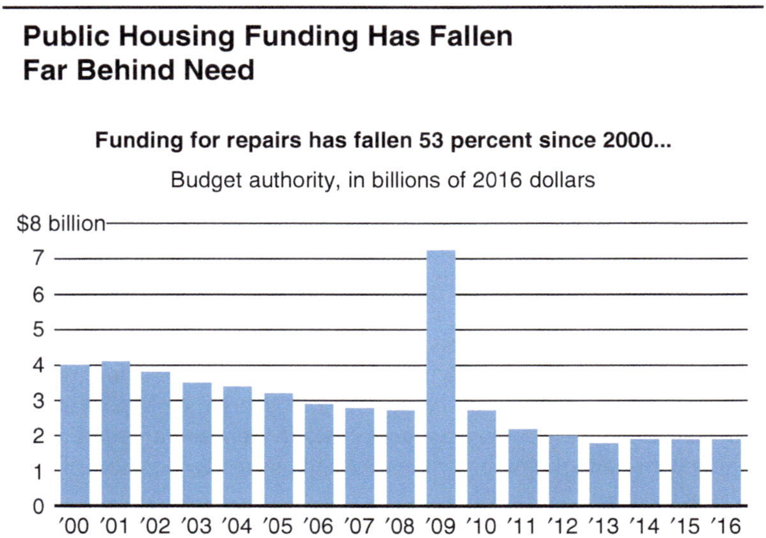

Fig. 5.7 Diminishing funding for public housing repairs (Center for Budget and Policy Priorities 2016, April 12)

funding level for these streams has not kept pace with the need, resulting in a backlog of maintenance and repairs for public housing buildings (CBPP 2016) (see Fig. 5.7). As the financial investment has deteriorated, many PHAs have opted to tear down public housing communities, with few being replaced with similarly affordable units.

Low-Income Housing Tax Credits

Tenant-based vouchers, project-based vouchers, and public housing are the primary forms of federal assistance to make rental housing more affordable for low-income households, particularly extremely low-income renters. For residents to be able to find decent, safe, and quality homes where they can use their vouchers, there must be a supply of affordable housing available to them. The low-income housing tax credit (LIHTC) is the largest source of federal assistance for developing rental housing for low-income families and financed nearly three million rental units between 1987 and 2015 (HUD 2017). Each year, the federal government allocates a limited supply of LIHTCs to states on a per capita basis, spending roughly $8 billion each year on the LIHTC program (HUD). State Housing Finance Agencies administer the LIHTC program based on their local needs and priorities. The LIHTC program[4] incentivizes individuals and corporations to invest in the production and rehabilita-

[4] Details on the nuts and bolts of this complicated program can be found in Gramlich's (2017) entry in the NLIHC Advocacy Guide and Keightley (2017) Congressional Research Service overview.

tion of low-income housing by offering them a tax credit. The cash used from these investments is used by housing developers to provide equity for housing projects, thus lowering the financing costs associated with the project. Lower financing costs help developers keep housing more affordable for low-income families. Many non-profit housing developers use this equity to build single-room occupancy (SRO) housing and other project-based housing targeted directly to low-income or special populations.

In their analysis of the HUD data on LIHTC tenants as of December 31, 2014, the New York University Furman Center (2017) found that nearly half of LIHTC households were in the extremely low-income category, and 60% of tenants had annual household incomes of less than $20,000. However, in a 2012 study of tenants in 15 states representing 30% of all LIHTC units, researchers found that tenants who benefit from LIHTC had higher incomes than those who accessed other federal assistance (e.g., housing choice vouchers and public housing). Furthermore, 70% of the extremely low-income tenants living in LIHTC properties were also receiving other forms of rental assistance, such as housing choice vouchers (NYU Furman Center 2012). So, while LIHTC is a core engine in the creation of low-income, multifamily housing, many of the families accessing those units are also using housing choice vouchers to afford them. Therefore, the LIHTC program does not necessarily create housing units that are affordable without the support of federal or local subsidy programs, but it does provide additional housing where voucher holders and those who qualify for project-based units can live.

Housing Trust Funds

In addition to the LIHTC, housing trust funds are another mechanism states and the federal government use to invest in the construction of affordable housing. Housing trust funds provide dedicated funding to support the construction and rehabilitation of affordable housing in communities. Currently, 47 states have housing trust funds and most fund them by dedicating a percentage of real estate transaction fees to build a fund for the development of affordable housing (Center for Community Change 2016). In Washington, D.C., since 2001, the Housing Production Trust Fund (HPTF) has helped build or renovate 9900 affordable housing units (DCFPI 2016b). In 2016, 2017, and 2018, Washington, D.C., leaders added additional funding from general revenues to the HPTF to bring the funding level up to $100 million. Other states and local communities are doing the same thing.

On the federal level, the national Housing Trust Fund (HTF) was established in 2008 and funded for the first time in 2016 at the level of $174 million (NLIHC 2017c); in 2017, it was funded at the level of $220 million. The HTF is funded with dedicated sources of revenue and does not compete with existing HUD programs funded by appropriations. At its current funding level, all the national HTF dollars must be used to renovate, operate, or develop affordable rental housing for extremely low-income households or those earning 30% or less of the annual median income. The HTF funds are administered by HUD and distributed to states through formula block grants based on factors that consider only renter household needs: the number of extremely low-income (ELI) and very low-income (VLI) households with severe cost burden (i.e., paying more than half of their income for rent and utilities), as well as the shortage of rental properties affordable and available to ELI and VLI households. Seventy-five percent of the value of the formula goes to the two factors that reflect the needs of ELI renters, because the statute requires the formula to give priority to them. The other two factors concern the renter needs of VLI households. Regardless of these factors, no state or the District of Columbia receives less than three million dollars.

Inclusionary Zoning

Inclusionary zoning (IZ) is a strategy used by state and local governments to increase the supply of affordable housing in mixed-income communities. Inclusionary zoning policies require private developers to dedicate a certain percentage of the units in a new housing development for low-income households. IZ policies vary across the country regarding whether they are mandatory or voluntary, what percentage of units are set aside for low-income families, income level requirements for those set-aside units, and the length of time the set-aside units are required to remain affordable. In cases where IZ policies are voluntary, developers are typically offered incentives to participate in the program, such as waived fees and expedited permit review access.

In their study of the impact of IZ in 11 jurisdictions, Schwartz et al. (2012) found that IZ policies did tend to provide low-income families access to low-poverty neighborhoods and public schools with a lower proportion of students qualifying for free or reduced meals. However, most IZ jurisdictions served families with relatively high incomes (e.g., 6 of the 11 jurisdictions served families with incomes at 80% or less of the annual median income, only three of which reserved housing for families with incomes at 30% of the area median income). Five of the programs were for households earning up to 100% or 120% of the area median income. In 2016, HUD calculated the area median income for a family of four in Washington, D.C., to be $108,600; 80% of the AMI is $86, 880 for a family of four. So, in 8 of 11 cases, families of more moderate incomes benefited from IZ policies. This does not mean that IZ policies are a bad approach to growing the supply of affordable housing. Rather, it means that advocates and administrators need to ensure that a higher proportion of IZ units are available to extremely low-income and very low-income families.

Affordable Housing Policy Solutions

As described above, a range of federal, state, and local strategies are used to make housing more affordable (e.g., housing subsidies, public housing, housing trust funds, and inclusionary zoning). Evidence for these programs making housing more affordable is clear. Evidence also exists that these programs help end homelessness, increase family stability, improve health and education outcomes, and may even provide access to higher-income neighborhoods and schools. Therefore, among the solutions to the affordable housing crisis is to fund these programs at much higher levels, particularly the housing subsidy programs for general and special populations.

As mentioned above, funding could be made available to support housing assistance for low-income households by reducing the mortgage interest deduction for high-income households and redirecting savings to housing assistance for extremely low-income and very low-income households. Modest changes to the mortgage interest deduction could allow for a greater tax break for 25 million low- and moderate-income homeowners while saving the federal government $241 billion over 10 years (NLIHC 2017a). Investing these savings into affordable rental housing solutions for the lowest-income people could mean 2.4 million new affordable rental housing units built through the national Housing Trust Fund or 3.3 million additional households receiving housing choice vouchers. State and local governments can better target LIHTC and units created through inclusionary zoning to ELI and VLI families.

Proposals to establish a renters' tax credit offer a promising opportunity to address the affordable housing challenges of many of the lowest-income households that go without assistance.[5] A renters' tax credit could complement the existing LIHTC, which works well as a subsidy for affordable housing development but is rarely sufficient on its own to push rents down to levels poor families can pay, and rental assistance programs such as Housing Choice Vouchers, which are highly effective but meet only a modest share of the need.

Any renters' tax credit should be tailored to primarily benefit families with the lowest incomes. Opportunities to provide monthly rather than annual credit payments, adapt the credit to reflect local housing costs, and ensure that the lowest-income households that are not required to file tax returns with the IRS receive the benefit should be explored further. Efforts to ensure that extremely low-income households do not pay more than 30% of their incomes on housing should be prioritized. Community land trusts[6] and housing preservation[7] approaches are additional strategies communities can use to preserve affordable housing in their neighborhoods.

Conclusion

Affordable housing is the fundamental support all human beings need to provide the stability and safety needed for household members to improve their lives and pursue their dreams. Stable, affordable housing improves academic outcomes for children,

[5] Proposals have been developed by the Center on Budget and Policy Priorities (CBPP) and the Terner Center for Housing Innovation at the University of California Berkeley. Details on the CBPP proposal can be found here: http://www.cbpp.org/research/housing/renters-tax-credit-would-promote-equity-and-advance-balanced-housing-policy. The Terner Center proposal can be found here: http://ternercenter.berkeley.edu/fair-tax-credit.

[6] The National Community Land Trust Network offers support in pursuing this approach to affordable housing, http://cltnetwork.org/.

[7] The National Housing Preservation Foundation can help communities identify next steps to preserving affordable housing in their neighborhoods: http://www.nhpfoundation.org/.

fosters employment prospects, and minimizes vulnerability to violence and trauma. Research has shown that housing ends homelessness, and the Housing First model has demonstrated that even people struggling with mental illness, addiction, or both can be stably housed with the proper supports in place.

Despite the intuitive and empirical evidence for the importance of safe, decent, affordable housing, investments in federal housing assistance for the lowest-income households are modest, especially compared to the housing benefits received by families making more than $100,000 per year. Proposed cuts to 2017 federal housing assistance programs would further reduce investments in low-income housing, including significant reductions in funding for public housing, elimination of the community development block grant program, and 4% and 17% cuts in housing choice vouchers and subsidies for people with disabilities, respectively.

State and local governments supplement federal housing assistance with their own rental subsidy programs and investments in affordable housing production, like the housing trust fund models. Social workers must continue to advocate within their own communities for investments in decent affordable housing. Their advocacy must include ensuring that scarce housing dollars get directed to the most vulnerable populations, including households with extremely low incomes, people with disabilities, older adults, and children. Social workers must also fight against housing discrimination based on race, sexual orientation, gender identity, eviction history, criminal record, credit scores, and sources of income. Finally, the degree to which households can afford housing is related to their income, access to employment opportunities, child care, and transportation. Social workers must give attention to the constellation of structural factors that maintain individuals and families in poverty, with housing being at the intersection of those issues.

References

Bassuk, E. L., & Geller, S. (2006). The role of housing and services in ending family homelessness. *Housing Policy Debate, 17*, 781–806.

Center for Budget and Policy Priorities. (2016). Chart book: Cuts in federal assistance have exacerbated families' struggles to afford housing. https://www.cbpp.org/research/housing/chart-book-cuts-in-federal-assistance-have-exacerbated-families-struggles-to-afford. Accessed 30 June 2018.

Center for Budget and Policy Priorities. (2017a). The housing choice voucher program. https://www.cbpp.org/sites/default/files/atoms/files/PolicyBasics-housing-1-25-13vouch.pdf. Accessed 30 June 2018.

Center for Budget and Policy Priorities. (2017b). Policy basics: Section 8 project-based rental assistance. https://www.cbpp.org/research/housing/policy-basics-section-8-project-based-rental-assistance. Accessed 30 June 2018.

Center for Budget and Policy Priorities. (2017c). Public housing. https://www.cbpp.org/sites/default/files/atoms/files/policybasics-housing.pdf. Accessed 30 June 2018.

Center for Community Change. (2016). State housing trust funds 2016. http://housingtrustfund-project.org/wp-content/uploads/2016/10/State-htfund-admin-and-date-2016-1.pdf. Accessed 30 June 2018.

Chetty, R., Hendren, N., Kline, P., & Saez, E. (2014). Where is the land of opportunity? The geography of intergenerational mobility in the United States. *The Quarterly Journal of Economics, 129*, 1553–1623.

D.C. Fiscal Policy Institute (2016a). The local rent supplement program. http://www.dcfpi.org/wp-content/uploads/2016/04/16-04-LRSP-Brief.pdf. Accessed 30 June 2018.

D.C. Fiscal Policy Institute (2016b). The housing production trust fund. http://www.dcfpi.org/wp-content/uploads/2016/04/16-04-HPTF-Brief.pdf. Accessed 30 June 2018.

Desmond, M. (2016). *Evicted: Poverty and profit in the American city*. New York: Penguin Random House.

Edin, K., & Shaefer, L. (2015). *$2.00 a day: Living on almost nothing in America*. Boston: Houghton Mifflin Harcourt.

Fischer, W., & Sard, B. (2017) Chart book: Federal housing spending is poorly matched to need. Center for Budget and Policy Priorities. https://www.cbpp.org/research/housing/chart-book-federal-housing-spending-is-poorly-matched-to-need. Accessed 30 June 2018.

Ginnarelli, L., Lippold, K., Minton, S., & Wheaton, L. (2015, January 30). Reducing child poverty in the United States: Costs and impacts of policies proposed by the Children's Defense Fund. Urban Institute. http://www.urban.org/research/publication/reducing-child-poverty-us. Accessed 30 June 2018.

Gramlich, E. (2017). Low income housing tax credits. National Low Income Housing Coalition. http://nlihc.org/sites/default/files/2017_Advocates-Guide.pdf. Accessed 30 June 2018.

Gubits, D., Shinn, M., Wood, M., Bell, S., Dastrup, S., Solari, C., et al. (2016). Family options study: 3-year impacts of housing and services interventions for homeless families. U.S. Department of Housing and Urban Development. https://www.huduser.gov/portal/sites/default/files/pdf/Family-Options-Study-Full-Report.pdf. Accessed 30 June 2018.

Harrison, B. M. (2017). The role of access to counsel in preventing eviction. Presentation at the Congressional Briefing on Children and Families Facing Eviction.

Hart Research Associates. (2016). How housing matters: Key findings from a nationwide survey among adults conducted April–May 2016 for MacArthur Foundation. Mac Arthur Fund. https://www.macfound.org/media/files/E-How_Housing_Matters_National_Full_Report.pdf. Accessed 30 June 2018.

Henwood, B. F., Wenzel, S. L., Mangano, P. F., Hombs, M., Padgett, D. K., Byrne, T., et al. (2015). The grand challenge of ending homelessness. American Academy of Social Work and Social Welfare. http://aaswsw.org/wp-content/uploads/2015/12/WP9-with-cover.pdf. Accessed 30 June 2018.

Holmes, N., & Berube, A. (2016). City and metropolitan inequality on the rise, driven by declining incomes. Brookings Institute. https://www.brookings.edu/research/city-and-metropolitan-inequality-on-the-rise-driven-by-declining-incomes/.

Hsieh, C., & Moretti, E. (2017, May 18). Housing constraints and spatial misallocation. The University of Chicago Booth School of Business. http://faculty.chicagobooth.edu/chang-tai.hsieh/research/growth.pdf. Accessed 30 June 2018.

Joint Center for Housing Studies. (2013). America's rental housing: Evolving markets and needs. http://www.jchs.harvard.edu/sites/jchs.harvard.edu/files/jchs_americas_rental_housing_2013_1_0.pdf. Accessed 30 June 2018.

Joint Center for Housing Studies. (2015). America's rental housing: Expanding options for diverse and growing demand. http://www.jchs.harvard.edu/sites/jchs.harvard.edu/files/americas_rental_housing_2015_web.pdf.

Joint Center for Housing Studies. (2017). The state of the nation's housing. http://www.jchs.harvard.edu/research/state_nations_housing, Accessed 30 June 2018.

Joint Committee on Taxation. (2017). Estimates of federal tax expenditures for fiscal years 2016–2020. https://www.jct.gov/publications.html?func=startdown&id=4971. Accessed 30 June 2018.

Keightley, M. (2017). An introduction to the low-income housing tax credit. Federation of American Scientists. https://fas.org/sgp/crs/misc/RS22389.pdf. Accessed 30 June 2018.

Maqbook, N., Viveiros, J., & Ault, M. (2015). *The impacts of affordable housing on health: A research summary*. Washington, D.C: Center for Housing Policy, National Housing Conference.

National Association of Home Builders. (2015, April). The economic impact of home building in a typical local area: Income, jobs and taxes generated. https://www.nahb.org/~/media/Sites/

NAHB/Economic%20studies/1-REPORT_local_20150318115955.ashx?la=en. Accessed 30 June 2018.

National Low Income Housing Coalition. (2016). The long wait for a home. http://nlihc.org/sites/default/files/HousingSpotlight_6-1.pdf. Accessed 30 June 2018.

National Low Income Housing Coalition. (2017a). The gap: A shortage of affordable homes. http://nlihc.org/sites/default/files/Gap-Report_2017_interactive.pdf. Accessed 30 June 2018.

National Low Income Housing Coalition. (2017b). Out of reach. Available: http://nlihc.org/sites/default/files/oor/OOR_2017.pdf. Accessed 30 June 2018.

National Low Income Housing Coalition. (2017c). The housing trust fund. http://nlihc.org/sites/default/files/HTF_Factsheet.pdf. Accessed 30 June 2018.

National Low Income Housing Coalition. (n.d.). A place to call home. http://nlihc.org/sites/default/files/A-FiPlace-To-Call-Home.pdf. Accessed 30 June 2018.

New York University Furman Center. (2012). What can we learn about the low-income housing tax credit program by looking at the tenants? http://furmancenter.org/files/publications/LIHTC_Final_Policy_Brief_v2.pdf. Accessed 30 June 2018.

New York University Furman Center. (2017). The effects of the low-income housing tax credit (LIHTC). http://furmancenter.org/research/publication/the-effects-of-the-low-income-housing-tax-credit-lihtc. Accessed 30 June 2018.

Newman, S., & Holupka, C. S. (2014). Affordable housing is associated with greater spending on child enrichment and stronger cognitive development. https://www.macfound.org/media/files/Affordable_Housing_Child_Enrichment_Stronger_Cognitive_Development.pdf. Accessed 30 June 2018.

Newman, S. J., & Holupka, C. S. (2015). Housing affordability and child well-being. *Housing Policy Debate, 1*, 116–151.

Ray, A., Kim, J., Nguyen, D., & Choi, J. (2015, May). Opting in, opting out a decade later. U.S. Department of Housing and Urban Development. https://www.huduser.gov/portal/sites/default/files/pdf/508_MDRT_Opting%20In_Opting%20Out.pdf. Accessed 30 June 2018.

Schwartz, H. L., Ecola, L., Leuschner, K. J., & Kofner, A. (2012). *Is inclusionary zoning inclusionary?* RAND Corporation. http://www.rand.org/content/dam/rand/pubs/technical_reports/2012/RAND_TR1231.pdf. Accessed 30 June 2018.

Shinn, M. (2009). Ending homelessness for families: The evidence for affordable housing. National Alliance to End Homelessness. https://b.3cdn.net/naeh/b39ff307355d6ade38_yfm6b9kot.pdf. Accessed 30 June 2018.

Simon, A. E., Fenelon, A., Helms, V., Lloyd, P. C., & Rossen, L. M. (2017). HUD housing assistance associated with lower uninsurance rates and unmet medical need. *Health Affairs, 36*, 1016–1023.

U.S. Department of Housing and Urban Development. (2018). Annual homeless assessment report. https://www.hudexchange.info/resource/5783/2018-ahar-part-1-pit-estimates-of-homelessness-in-the-us/ Accessed 23 January 2019.

U.S. Department of Housing and Urban Development. (2016). Annual homeless assessment report. https://www.hudexchange.info/resources/documents/2016-AHAR-Part-1.pdf. Accessed 30 June 2018.

U.S. Department of Housing and Urban Development. (2017). Low-income housing tax credits. https://www.huduser.gov/portal/datasets/lihtc.html. Accessed 30 June 2018.

U.S. Department of Housing and Urban Development. (n.d.). Resources. https://www.huduser.gov/portal/glossary/glossary_a.html. Accessed 30 June 2018.

U.S. Interagency Council on Homelessness. (2017). Ten strategies to end veteran homelessness. https://www.usich.gov/tools-for-action/10-strategies-to-end-veteran-homelessness. Accessed 30 June 2018.

Watson, N. E., Steffen, B. L., Martin, M., & Vandenbroucke, D. A. (2017, August). Worst case needs preview. U.S. Department of Housing and Urban Development. https://www.huduser.gov/portal/sites/default/files/pdf/Worst-Case-Needs-Preview.pdf. Accessed 30 June 2018.

Chapter 6
Street Talk: Homeless Discourses and the Politics of Service Provision

Arturo Baiocchi and Tyler M. Argüello

Why are people homeless?
How can the richest country in the world have so many homeless people?
What's causing the "rise" in homelessness in America today?

As researchers and professors of social work, we often face the above questions about the causes of homelessness—from our students as well as through our work with community members and policymakers. In the ensuing conversations, we inevitably hear about people's own folk theories of why homelessness exists—their own personal explanations of why certain people find themselves in a housing-insecure situation. These explanations touch on issues spanning from underprivileged upbringings to mental illness and chemical dependency, as well as to other economic and social factors, like the lack of affordable housing, the dearth of well-paying jobs, and society's disregard for human well-being. While we find that most people acknowledge that homelessness is *complicated* and that there are *different types* of homeless people, we are nonetheless taken aback by the persistence of certain narratives of homelessness we encounter.

Still, we find some resonance in many of the folk explanations and homeless caricatures espoused; undoubtedly, bad luck, personal decisions, the economy, mental health, fragmented families, and the housing market, among other factors, all contribute to homelessness at some level and speak to some aspect of the experience. However, what we find more interesting is how people persist to emphasize one factor over another (e.g., it's a lack of affordable housing *or* mental illness and not a lack of affordable housing *and* mental illness). From a critical perspective, we come to view these explanations and their commonalities as less unique and

Electronic supplementary material: The online version of this chapter (https://doi.org/10.1007/978-3-030-03727-7_6) contains supplementary material, which is available to authorized users.

A. Baiocchi (✉) · T. M. Argüello
California State University, Sacramento, Sacramento, CA, USA
e-mail: arturo.baiocchi@csus.edu; tyler.arguello@csus.edu

H. Larkin et al. (eds.), *Homelessness Prevention and Intervention in Social Work*, https://doi.org/10.1007/978-3-030-03727-7_6

insightful as people might take them to be. Rather, we see these folk explanations as part of a broader, long-standing cultural conversation, if not dilemma, that Americans have had about poverty for some time. In other words, we believe these discussions about homelessness reflect an entrenched set of beliefs and shared language in Western society about what it means to be poor and in this case without a home; in turn, they function to simplify, if not neutralize, the complexities of these lived experiences.

A central argument of this chapter is that people experiencing homelessness are more complicated and layered—like all people—than the stories we often hear and tell ourselves about them. Most of us implicitly know this, yet, we are often tempted to relegate people experiencing homelessness to individualizing narratives that frame them as hapless victims of the economy, their (mental) illness, or their own moral or ethical failings. These narratives have considerable traction in society because they may reflect some truths, or aspects of truth, about homelessness, but they also latch onto enduring ideologies about poverty that we hold dear in Western culture (as we will elaborate below). And while these narratives are in some sense practical because they simplify homelessness into talking points, they are also problematic because of how they obscure and reframe the lived realities of homelessness. We suspect that most people deploying these narratives are unaware, at least consciously, of the political ideologies and socio-history implicated in their folk theories of homelessness. The truths being highlighted about homelessness in these discussions, and the truths being silenced, undoubtedly serve broader political and economic interests, even if we ourselves are unaware of what those may be when we engage in these conversations.

To be sure, the field of social welfare has attempted to resist these types of linear explanations by embracing ecological perspectives of practice (e.g., person-in-environment; Gitterman and Germain 2008). Nonetheless, we suspect that social workers still face significant institutional pressure and cultural temptation to simplify homelessness into one-dimensional issues, much like we do when we engage in these conversations with the public and our students. One way to confront this challenge, we contend, is for social workers to be more attentive to the language we use when discussing our work with clients experiencing homelessness and more pointedly to understand how the common caricatures of homelessness dominant in society have become taken for granted and used in different political contexts.

A recent ethnography of homelessness in San Francisco provides a powerful lens for highlighting these issues and one that introduces a useful typology for identifying the three most common homeless narratives we are often confronted with in modern society. Teresa Gowan's *Hobos, Hustlers, and Backsliders* (2010) identifies three central narratives of homelessness that she describes as *sin-talk*, *sick-talk*, and *system-talk*, which form the basis of how most Americans—including social workers—frame and understand how individuals find themselves in housing-insecure situations. Beyond tracing the institutional history of each narrative structure, and their different orientations to poverty management, Gowan's ethnography also powerfully shows how these talks get taken up (unwittingly) even by people experiencing homelessness. Through their interactions with social workers, police, homeless advocates, and the broader institutions that these professionals represent, homeless people are encouraged to use these talks as a way of making sense of themselves and their situation, along with strategizing survival and solutions. While Gowan's book is an academic project of homelessness, it nonetheless can offer social workers a useful strategy to deepen their understanding of their work with people experiencing poverty and inequality as well as their work with colleagues and communities.

In this chapter, we draw out Gowan's general argument of how these discourses of homelessness and poverty more broadly have coalesced during the last two centuries in the USA. We particularly highlight the basic typology for understanding the underpinning of most discussions about homelessness in the current political climate. In the end, we highlight the value and challenges that social workers face if they incorporate an analysis of discourse into their practice; this is achieved through an expansion of Gowan's typology as set into applied work.

Discourse: What Are We Talking About?

Before reviewing Gowan's typology, it is useful to first delineate what exactly is meant by the term *discourse*—the simultaneously analytical and methodological framework Gowan deploys to understand sin-talk, sick-talk, and system-talk. Indeed, discourse is widely used across several disciplines (e.g., linguistics, sociology, cultural studies, anthropology), and not surprisingly, there are varying approaches to its specific meaning and application.

Contemporarily, discourse is perhaps most frequently associated with the French theorist Michel Foucault, who used the concept to explore the taken-for-granted ways societies construct knowledge and everyday practices related to various issues, such as mental illness, child rearing, prisons, and sexuality (Foucault 1990, 1995). For Foucault, the language we use to understand these issues gives rise to specific narrative structures (i.e., how we implicitly frame things), which in turn shape how we accept the reality of these issues and our responses to them. In short, how we define and describe a problem—or if we consider it a problem at all—ultimately shapes how we deal with it. For example, framing homelessness as *purely* an affordable housing issue may result in policy interventions to increase housing stock and expand housing subsidies—but may not spark efforts to increase access to mental health or substance use services for people experiencing or at risk of homelessness. Whether *homelessness* is described as resulting from personal-level factors (e.g., mental health problems, substance use) or system-level ones (e.g., lack of affordable housing), the discourse animates assumptions we make about homeless individuals (e.g., as dangerous or deserving), and, in turn, it works to circumscribe the policies and programmatic responses we might consider necessary.

On one level, the Foucauldian concept of discourse is like the assertion by social constructionists that the *accepted reality* of a situation is malleable to different frames of interpretation. But this approach to discourse goes further to implicate an analysis of power. Indeed, discourse is what Foucault described as *knowledge/power*, a cultural form of power that has been institutionalized in society to legitimate certain realities while obscuring others (Foucault 1980). According to Foucault, specific narratives have been codified and perpetuated over time by institutions (e.g., schools, the church, the state, psychiatric/hospitals, prisons, media); as a result, these narratives are often experienced by people as if they are natural or normal (i.e., *just the way things are*). These explanations seem so common sense that we often feel like they came from our own personal experiences and not from broader institutions in society. For example, many people have their own explanations about why other people experience homelessness. Foucault would argue that most of these explanations are driven by broader structural interests: the real power of discourse is how it permeates our thinking and feeling to the level that we often believe that these explanations derive from ourselves.[1]

Foucault was particularly interested in the emergence of medical knowledge/power over the centuries, and the way it provided a new scientific language to make meaning about behaviors that seemed out of the norm. According to Foucault, medical institutions have increasingly consolidated power and influence in our modern society to frame social deviants and their vices and, in turn, the nature of vice itself. For example, drinking excessive amounts of alcohol is considered an *addiction* or even a disease; such a framing relies on a certain discourse of the dangers of alcoholism but also makes a knowledge claim of how humans behave and why. In other words, when we use the language of medicine to understand a situation, we are implicitly conjuring up a purely corporeal view of human nature, often based within the individual, at the expense of other explanations (e.g., community-wide factors, trauma). The problem per Foucauldian thought is that the realities of these situations are often more complex than the naturalizing language we use to understand them. In this vein, human situations often consist of more than one reality and perspective: context is key. One may indeed have a chemical dependency to alcohol or suffer from a genetic predisposition, but other factors likely also contribute to excessive drinking, such as a job loss, isolation, or other life stressors. Importantly, the lived experiences of individuals—especially those who are cast as deviant characters within these discourses—too often are disregarded. An attention to discourses and their analysis, then, works to not only re-/conceptualize social issues but also critically assess and deconstruct the social world. And in the context of homelessness, Gowan argues (2010) that this type of engagement with discourse helps us "unflatten" (p. 25) the otherwise one-dimensional representations that we often see of homelessness in society—which itself is an intervention.

[1] Indeed, Foucault argues that discourse shapes our perspectives but also our relationship and interactions to the world itself, which he terms as our subjectivities or the process of *subjectivation*.

A Typology for (Homeless) Talk: Sick, Sin, and System

With this understanding of discourse, we now turn to the work proper of *Hobos, Hustlers, and Backsliders.* According to Gowan (2010), her extended ethnography[2] of homelessness arose out of her experiences in San Francisco, in the South of Market area, and volunteering in various social service agencies in the Tenderloin. Her experience in these two impoverished areas led to a scholarly project initially focused on the varied lived experiences of homeless recyclers. As she describes, however, her systematic observations of recyclers' day-to day interactions with different social networks, communities, and social service agencies eventually evolved into a full-scale ethnographic inquiry into the discursive practices and identities of homelessness throughout the Bay Area. In total, Gowan's multi-year project included prolonged interactions with 38 single men and their daily routines as well as their involvement with a myriad of disconnected safety net and social services. As Gowan (2010) came to know these men over time, she learned that many identified themselves within the subculture of homelessness as either *modern day hobos* (recyclers), *hustlers* (petty criminals), or *backsliders* (addicts), appreciating that individuals could straddle different identities overtime.

Accordingly, Gowan organizes her analysis around a discursive typology that she argues undergirds these identities as well as modern conceptions of homelessness across the USA: *sin-talk*, *sick-talk*, and *system-talk* (see Table 6.1). These three *talks* have allowed for various organizations and institutions—along with the individuals interacting with and between them—to make sense of the issue of homelessness. Each discourse provides and constructs a commonsense notion, or *truth*, of why homelessness and poverty occur in the USA. And, as her analysis demonstrates, these discourses have distinctive social and institutional lineages that can be traced back to the earliest efforts to provide poor relief in the Western world and to the evolution of the modern welfare state. Each discourse circumscribes the complexity of homelessness and prescribes an appropriate reaction to, or set of strategies against, the social problem. Generally, these strategies are either oriented

Table 6.1 Discursive typology

Construction of homelessness discourse	Moral: Sin-talk	Disease: Sick-talk	Systemic: System-talk
The central cause and truth of homelessness	A person's sin	A person's illness or disease	Social structure, inequality
Fundamental strategy	Exclusion	Treatment	Social change

[2] Originally derived within anthropology, ethnography is a sustained inquiry into a topic sometimes characterized as prolonged participant observation. These observations often include verbal interviews, continuous note-taking, multimedia texts (e.g., photographs), and real-time encounters (e.g., engaging in everyday tasks with research participants). Depending on the theoretical motivations of the researcher, ethnography can serve a variety of ends, though largely to provide in-depth, rich description of cultural practices often of poorly understood cultural groups.

toward punishing and excluding individuals from public spaces (*sin-talk*), increasing access to treatment for those afflicted with conditions that made them homeless (*sick-talk*), or pursuing large-scale social change to redress societal inequities (*system-talk*). As her analysis ebbs and flows across time and space, Gowan asserts that these discourses are neither insular nor static. In fact, as we discuss, they intersect, synergize, and potentiate depending on the historical and social context.

In the rest of this chapter, we present each talk, deconstructing their inner workings. We start each discussion by highlighting an example of the talk from our own experiences of presenting our research and engaging with this discourse within the public sphere. Next, we present an overview of the tenets of that discourse and review its historical basis. Then, we discuss the social practices that have worked to maintain each discourse. Within each section, we work to expose some of the constraints, particularly from the perspective of applied practitioners. Ultimately, this is the intention and intervention of this chapter's work: just as Gowan sought to articular the "grammar of action" of homelessness, we seek to translate such a lived grammar into tools for applied practice.

Sin-Talk

The public park should belong to normal people in the community, those who have jobs, families, and homes. Homeless in the park make the park dangerous for everyone else.

If we want to help the homeless, we have to let them help themselves and let them learn from their own decisions and mistakes. A lot of homeless choose to be homeless, which is their decision.

What Is Sin-Talk?

The above passages paraphrase the types of comments that we have often heard at community meetings and forums where we have presented our research, and they represent examples of what Gowan calls sin-talk. The discourse of sin-talk is closely associated with what Gowan describes as a moral construction of poverty—a moralistic understanding of poverty that emphasizes the poor choices made by individuals, their character weaknesses, and a general moral laxity in modern society toward hard work and other responsibilities. In other words, sin-talk comprehends homelessness as another indicator of moral decay in modern society, a society that has become too accepting of deviant lifestyles and personal failings, particularly with respect to obtaining and maintaining employment. While sin-talk acknowledges the difficulties faced by the poor, the discourse reduces these challenges to the natural consequences of a person's lack of integrity and their improper upbringing. Indeed, sin-talk constructs the individual as having ultimate agency in their own fate and as victims of their own choices. Sin-talk also purports that homeless individuals are dangers to themselves and others because of their proclivity toward deviant acts (e.g., stealing from law-abiding citizens). Homelessness, then, represents a more fundamental threat because its very presence erodes the moral fabric and social order, sowing discord and dysfunction in public spaces and rendering these places unsafe and crime-ridden. In response, sin-talk calls for a re-establishment of social order, often via strict policing of areas wherein the homeless reside. While sin-talk can lead to efforts toward (moral) rehabilitation (e.g., to encourage individuals to repent and amend their ways, particularly with respect to their unemployment), it largely prescribes exclusion and punishment, justifying that homeless individuals are primarily outsiders to the community (no matter their tenure therein) and must be excommunicated, symbolically or literally.

Sin-Talk History

Gowan's (2010) historical account of sin-talk highlights how the discourse has played a recurring, dominant role in shaping what she described as "poverty management" in the West (p. 27). Indeed, sin-talk and its concerns with managing deviance have come in and out of dominance as a guiding principle to various forms of social welfare, from the limited poor relief provided by communities in the seventeenth century to later forms of charity work in the late nineteenth century and, more recently, during the emergence of the welfare state during the twentieth century. In this sense, sin-talk is the most enduring of the three discourses on poverty, which Gowan traces its inceptions back to the Protestant Reformation of sixteenth century Europe and Martin Luther's early writings on the vices of the begging poor. In his infamous "beggar book", *Liber Vagatorum*, Martin Luther articulated a dramatic reformation of how the church should address the impoverished and wandering vagabonds of his day. Rather than being recipients of charity and almsgiving, Luther proposed that the poor should be chastised for their idleness and be encouraged to work. Underlying this reorientation was an evolving religious doctrine that celebrated the virtues of hard work and of finding *one's calling* and connection to God through everyday toil (Weber 2002). From this perspective, beggars and vagabonds represented a willful rejection of the virtue that hard work was both a duty and an end to itself. Accordingly, charity and almsgiving—traditions of Catholicism—represented licentious, if not corrupt, practices that enabled the inherent vices of idleness and dereliction, if not a rejection of God's calling.

Gowan argues that in the years following the Protestant Reformation, Martin Luther's moralistic ideas of how the poor should be treated gradually spread throughout Europe. By the mid-sixteenth century, several municipalities had adopted restrictive ordinances that explicitly outlawed public forms of begging within their jurisdictions, and some even barred individuals from entering the community if they were unemployed. In many Protestant regions, traveling vagabonds could also be arrested and conscripted to work in nearby farms if they were found wandering the countryside without work papers. In short, if being out of work was a vice *in the community*, then naturally being conscripted to work *for the com-*

munity could be one way to make amends for moral transgression. Over time, Protestant values and practices gradually spread to Catholic regions of Europe, particularly in areas facing periodic shortage of farm labor due to famine and disease. As Gowan argues, the emergence of various vagabond work laws across Europe reflected not only a shift in the religiosity associated with hard work but conveniently also functioned to mitigate the vacillating demands of the agricultural labor market.

Notably, the English Poor Laws of 1601, which became a model of early safety-net provision across Europe and colonial America for addressing periodic famine in the countryside, further institutionalized a moralistic discourse of poverty. Key to most of these local systems of poor relief, Gowan notes, were settlement requirements that barred community outsiders, and vagabonds in particular, from receiving assistance. Moreover, consistent with Protestant tenets, poor relief was restricted only to local residents deemed too ill or old to *work* (e.g., the *impotent poor*). This moralistic distinction between the deserving and undeserving poor became more refined over the subsequent centuries, according to Gowan, as various helping institutions emerged to address the shifting group distinctions of the worthy and non-working poor (e.g., orphaned children, the mad, the derelict). Indeed, the workhouses, asylums, and orphanages that came into prominence in the mid-nineteenth century, in both the USA and Europe, often provided recipients a blend of religious teachings and rigorous activities designed to reform and embed the poor with the virtues of hard work. Though these moral treatments evolved through periods of reform—and at times resembled an early therapeutic form of sick-talk, at least on the surface, Gowan claims—the moralistic distinctions between the deserving and undeserving "able-bodied" poor nonetheless remained a cornerstone of the American social welfare tradition (Katz 2013). As we elaborate in the next section, Gowan primarily identifies the expansion of the welfare state with a different discourse of system-talk; nonetheless, here she makes a convincing argument that, in the most current era of welfare retrenchment (e.g., federal entitlement reforms in the late 1990s) or what some might frame as neoliberal welfare reform (Soss et al. 2011), sin-talk has experienced a revival in reorganizing welfare as an implement of support and discipline.

Beyond the legacy of a restrictive social welfare tradition, Gowan suggests that moral constructions of poverty may have also become more salient in American culture, compared to other Western countries, due to the heightened values and ethics of colonialism and capitalism practiced in the USA. As other scholars have commented (Myers 2001), American culture has often cultivated an ideology of rugged individualism (i.e., the virtuous individual overcoming extreme challenges through hard work) as this notion pays tribute to USA's frontier westward expansion and acceptance of laissez-faire capitalism. As Belcher and Deforge (2012) have similarly argued, Americans have largely embraced (or become accustomed to) a free market way of life because it paints a vision of America as the land of (equitable) opportunity for those willing to work hard for it, despite the evidence of inequitable outcomes for many hardworking Americans. Moreover, the ideology of "meritocracy," which asserts that success and wealth are generally earned in

America (McNamee and Miller 2009), has allowed Americans to dismiss the poor and homeless as victims of their own vices and poor economic decisions while obscuring the various structural advantages of more economically successful classes. While it is beyond the scope of this chapter to fully summarize the historical permeations of this ideology,[3] notions of rugged individualism, meritocracy, and free market capitalism have contributed to the moralistic lens through which many US citizens understand poverty today, particularly as a function of lifestyle and poor choices, if not a broader "culture of poverty."

How Sin-Talk Is Perpetuated

In the contemporary context, Gowan argues that moral constructions of poverty and, in turn, homeless sin-talk continue to be perpetuated by a broad set of institutions in US society, including the media, religion, and even the social welfare system—which increasingly emphasize the importance of reinforcing a strong work ethic among the poor.[4] But of all, the US criminal justice system is the dominant institution by which sin-talk is promulgated, particularly as a lens to understand homelessness as a function of personal decisions. At large, the criminal justice system emphasizes the responsibility of the individual to manage their own behavior and the role of the state to occasionally administer punishment for the sake of law and order. And, as Gowan argues, individuals experiencing homelessness are likely to have regular encounters with law enforcement, and the broader criminal justice system, due to their compromised, and often criminalized, status in many public spaces. Indeed, Gowan contends many homeless individuals are well versed in sin-talk and may even use the discourse as an identity, because of their regular encounters with police and ensuing bouts of incarceration. In the US era of mass incarceration, Gowan and other scholars contend that *punishment and exclusion* have become the dominant interventions by which the state addresses most problems associated with poverty (e.g., the ongoing War on Drugs). Recent work by Wacquant (2009) and Soss, Fording, and Schram (2011) similarly highlights a growing conflation and

---

[3] Gowan suggests that these enduring US values also stem from the colonial founding of the country as well as its eventual expansion throughout the continent. Moreover, during the late nineteenth century, these sentiments at times blended with Social Darwinist theories that not only rationalized the imperial pursuits of the USA but were also used to make sense of the unequal outcomes of unfettered capitalism.

[4] Despite the expanding role of the federal government during the twentieth century to provide social welfare services, many safety-net programs continued to be wedded to notions of deservingness and virtues of hard work. The emergence of social welfare programs was largely predicated on a *system-talk discourse*, as Gowan discusses, but in the US context, the *moral construction of poverty* has nonetheless continued to periodically shape the more restrictive aspects of the welfare state, particularly in comparison to other industrialized countries (Esping-Anderson 1990). One of the clearest examples of this was the federal welfare reforms in 1996, which ended a number of safety net entitlement programs for poor families under the banner of *welfare-to-work* reform.

collusion between the punitive and welfare functions of the state: social services increasingly serve the goals of disciplining the poor, rather than helping them transition out of poverty.

Gowan highlights that one of the clearest examples of contemporary sin-talk has been recent efforts by local municipalities to more closely monitor and restrict public spaces where homeless people reside. Under the premise that homeless individuals commit "quality-of-life" crimes (e.g., minor acts of public deviance that contribute to social disorder and more serious crimes), many municipalities have passed a variety of ordinances that target the survival strategies of homeless individuals (e.g., panhandling, soliciting, sleeping in public spaces) (Snow and Anderson 1993). While concerns about public safety can be justified, the rise of these laws has been motivated by an enduring theory of criminal behavior often described as *broken windows theory* (Kelling and Wilson 1982). This theory asserts that a community's permissiveness toward norm violations (e.g., allowing homeless people to sleep on a park bench) can signal an erosion of social control, thus inviting more serious deviant acts to occur in an area. Under the premise that homeless individuals threaten the social harmony of certain spaces, local ordinances to restrict public spaces where homeless individuals can panhandle for money, sleep, or simply be have been embraced by many jurisdictions across the USA over the last 20 years (National Law Center on Homelessness and Poverty 2016; Aykanian and Lee 2016). For Gowan, however, the underpinning logic of these policies is a contemporary rendition of sin-talk. Indeed, her urban ethnography highlights how *quality-of-life* ordinances are often promulgated by local business interests (e.g., business improvement districts) and their desire to sanitize the aesthetics of downtown areas. For Gowan, these ordinances harken back to a more punitive construction of homelessness, one in which the poor are reimagined as perpetual outsiders and threats to community life and thus must be expelled from public spaces. Sadly, Gowan (2010) recounts that by the 1990s nearly 75% of US cities had passed some version of these laws criminalizing panhandling and other survival strategies (p. 52).

System-Talk

The issue of homelessness is too difficult to solve at the local level. The federal government has to fund subsidized housing for people who can't maintain income for a home. We've had this problem before in our country and solved it by building housing for the poor. The amount of money to do this can't come from local governments. We need a national solution to this problem.

Instead of further criminalizing the city's displaced residents, maybe we should look at the causes: skyrocketing rents, stagnant and falling wages, and a lack of reasonable services and housings options.

What Is System-Talk?

As highlighted above, in our work in the community, we sometimes encounter a broader discourse on homelessness that foregrounds the social and structural factors underpinning poverty. Indeed, while sin-talk frames poverty primarily as a moral issue, system-talk takes a wider lens on the structural constraints and barriers that disadvantaged groups experience in everyday life. These disadvantages implicate the precarious employment opportunities, the high cost of housing in the community, and the dearth of social welfare supports. As the name implies, system-talk centers on the more *systemic* ways that housing insecurity and marginalization operate in an unequal society. Indeed, behaviors are largely viewed as irrelevant by system-talk, if not interpreted as acts of defiance, within a capitalistic society that naturally mistreats those within lower economic strata. Similarly, system-talk argues that efforts to address homelessness must target the broad policies and structural arrangements that allow homelessness to grow in the USA

It is important to note that system-talk coincides with a progressive, if not socialist, understanding of political economy. The discourse not only asserts that economic factors are important but also critiques the effects of laissez-faire capitalism and its misdistribution of resources and power across society. This discourse purports that the stark inequities between the rich and poor are not anomalies of free market capitalism—rather an effect of capitalism itself.[5] From this standpoint, homelessness is just another manifestation, albeit an extreme one, of the broader exploitative nature of capitalism. While sin-talk is sympathetic to social movements attempting to revolutionize the system, more pragmatically, system-talk attempts to mobilize the government to pursue policies that directly redress the ill effects of capitalism on society's very poor. In this way, system-talk emphasizes the preeminent role of the state to protect citizens from the vicissitudes of the market via pursuing redistributive policies, establishing regulations to ensure affordable housing, and enforcing a livable wage. The site of intervention, then, is not the individual but government itself.

System-Talk History

While the discursive register of system-talk would cohere decades after the New Deal era, Gowan links its inception back to the social activism of the late nineteenth century and the broader Progressive Movement in the USA. As a number of scholars have similarly argued, the Gilded Age of industrial capitalism not only exemplified the dramatic accumulation of wealth in the USA, it also highlighted the growing disparity between the rich and poor, worsening living conditions, and a rise of urban

[5] Similar to a Marxist analysis, system-talk purports that laissez-faire capitalism inevitably perpetuates systemic inequities because class interests will always be misaligned and in conflict with one another, given that the broader economic system demands that groups, in a word, exploit one another for survival.

homelessness (Katz 2013). In the aftermath of the Civil War, combined with the consequent boom-and-bust economic cycles, the USA saw a dramatic increase of unemployment and abject poverty throughout many urban centers (Skocpol 1992).

The stark contrast between the grim realities of urban poverty and the opulence made possible by industrial capitalism gave rise to a discourse of ambivalence in Western culture about the apparent limitations, if not contradictions, of the free market system itself (Katz 2013; Zelizer 1985; Skocpol 1992). If capitalism meant more wealth and opportunities, it was also clear that it had contributed to high levels of inequality and precarious working conditions for the masses. Such apparent contradictions clearly resonated with a Marxist, class-based analysis of the unfolding ills of industrial capitalism, popular among the working classes. But even within upper-class culture, a distrust of unfettered markets emerged during the late nineteenth century (Zelizer 1985), which at times colluded with a variety of early progressive efforts to expand the regulative powers of the state, such as the campaigns at the end of nineteenth century to establish children's rights and abolish child labor (Platt 1977). While these campaigns were not outwardly radical, or particularly popular among urban elites, they nonetheless helped formulate a distinctive system discourse for the need of large-scale governmental interventions to curtail the negative impacts of capitalism. Indeed, as Gowan (2010) describes, these movements were significant because they represented a vocal "minority of elite social reformers" who promoted a new perspective on the structural inequalities of modern society, as, for example, the insight "that unemployment itself was indeed a systematic problem beyond the control of poor people themselves" (p. 40).

Similarly, Gowan (2010) points out that during this time the USA saw the rise of active and violent conflicts between industrialists and workers, the latter beginning to organize into more collective efforts to demand better wages and improved working conditions. As an organized labor movement began to take shape in the USA during the first decades of the twentieth century, a number of unions mobilized explicitly on issues related to the state's ill treatment of the unemployed. Particularly in urban areas facing an influx of unattached, placeless, wandering single men in the aftermath of economic calamites of the late nineteenth century, unions challenged the rise of anti-vagrancy laws and "anti-tramp" sentiments (p. 38) that punished unemployed workers for their own predicament. According to Gowan (2010), union campaigns, such as those by the Industrial Workers of the World (aka, the *Wobblies*), were effective because they provided a "radical analysis of homelessness, eloquently blaming the greed of the employing class for destitution of the hobo army" (p. 40). In short, efforts by these and other unions reflected and contributed to a *rising consciousness* among different classes of workers of their collective, shared interests with the unemployed.

These disparate forms of activism eventually coalesced into a coherent system-talk discourse that guided the Progressive Movement through several successful efforts to mobilize the state to intervene on issues related to working conditions, public education, suffrage, and social welfare more broadly. These progressive sentiments eventually promulgated the American welfare state, following the economic and social upheaval of the Great Depression, when the federal government became more committed to funding social insurance and broad-based entitlement programs (e.g., passage of the Social Security Act of 1935).[6] In the decades that followed, older Americans and women with children more generally would benefit from these programs as poverty rates dropped in most urban areas (Skocpol 1992). Interestingly, as the USA enjoyed broad economic revival during and after World War II, issues pertaining to urban poverty and displaced poor largely fell out of public discourse for the next several decades. Indeed, Gowan argues that even in the height of Johnson's War on Poverty and expansion of the welfare state during the late 1960s, homelessness was not a salient concern in the public sphere.

This would dramatically change in the 1980s, according to Gowan, as a new homelessness crisis surfaced in the last decades of the twentieth century. The economic malaise of the late 1970s, combined with the gradual deindustrialization of the US economy, saw a rise of unemployment throughout the manufacturing sectors (Blau 1992; Rossi 1991). Moreover, the eventual cuts to social entitlements and welfare that would take place throughout the 1980s (i.e., trickle down *Reaganomics*) contributed to growing inequality in the USA not seen in several decades (Heathcote et al. 2010). Punctuating this situation, many state-run mental health hospitals were closed during the preceding decades; a policy of *deinstitutionalization* that had begun in the late 1950s and resulted in hundreds of thousands of patients being discharged into the community.[7] As we discuss later, while there is debate as to what extent deinstitutionalization should be seen as a direct cause of the homelessness crisis in the 1980s, it was nonetheless clear that the cuts to mental health funding, and the underfunding of nascent community programs meant to provide supportive services—including housing—for former patients, undoubtedly contributed to the rise of individuals experiencing homelessness across the USA (Lamb 1984; Mechanic 2008). Therein, the discursive register of system-talk emerged, and

---

[6] Welfare scholars of this era stress that progressive sentiments were far from universally accepted in the USA and were in fact actively resisted by many segments of society. Welfare theorists, particularly those informed by Marxist frameworks, have often discussed the emergence of welfare regimes through the lenses of class conflict (in particular the disputes between labor and capital). Accordingly, the state, in the face of acute civil strife and disorder, will initiate and extend social supports in attempts to appease and placate constituents. For example, Piven and Cloward (1971) suggest that welfare expansion in the 1930s was the government's response to widespread fear of growing social disorder and economic calamity. Other theories of welfare expansion emphasize the role that social movements play in mobilizing the state to counteract the inequities of the market.

[7] Deinstitutionalization broadly refers a number of initiatives during the late 1950s through the early 1980s that dramatically altered the institutional landscape by which large mental health institutions operate in the USA. Generally speaking, these varied state and federal initiatives (e.g., the *Community Mental Health Act* of 1963) sought to (1) dramatically reduce the number of persons residing in state mental hospitals and transfer them into the community, (2) expand community-based mental health and supportive services, and (3) decrease the use of prolonged institutionalization by diverting inappropriate hospital admissions and shortening inpatient stays in psychiatric hospitals (Lamb 1984). As a result of these initiatives, mental health institutions in the USA declined dramatically in the last half of the twentieth century, as did the number of individuals residing within them—national estimates from 550,000 in the mid-1950s to less than 100,000 in 1980 (Mechanic 2008).

indeed the term *homelessness* itself, due to a broad coalition of housing advocates struggling to mobilize around the alarming rates of people living on the streets. Estimates suggest that more than 100,000 citizens lived outdoors by 1980, rising to over 450,000 by the next decade (Jencks 1995).

Churches and other philanthropic organizations throughout the country were quickly overwhelmed by the sheer number of adults and families needing shelter, and, reminiscent of the economic crash of the 1930s, social workers and advocates gravitated toward a more systemic explanation of both the causes and solutions to homelessness. These advocates emphasized that shelter from the elements should be a right of all Americans, if not an entitlement. Activist organizations like the Community for Creative Non-Violence, and more formal organizations like the National Housing Alliance, similarly advocated that the federal government play an interventionist role in funding homelessness services. Despite some resistance by policymakers, this anti-homelessness movement based on rights and entitlement was surprisingly successful; for example, Gowan cites that after the establishment of a tent city called *Reaganville* outside of the White House, along with other direct action, the federal government began funding emergency shelters around the country by the mid-1980s. The passage of the McKinney-Vento Act of 1987 formally established stable federal funding for the creation of an entire emergency shelter apparatus. Though Gowan critiques that these efforts led to a new shelter industry, or *shelterization* of homelessness, the 1980s would see considerable investments by the federal government into a variety of homeless programs. All this said, system-talk discourse eventually became undercut by charity and religious-based organizations that inadvertently blended more moralistic framing of homelessness within the services they provided. And, by the 1990s, a new discourse about the pathology of some homeless (and in particular their mental health and substance use) would largely supplant system-talk with a more medicalized conception of poverty (i.e., *sick-talk*), as will be discussed below.

How System-Talk Is Perpetuated

Gowan paints a rather cynical view of the successes and perpetuation of system-talk since the 1980s. While system-talk advocates were effective in initially mobilizing local and federal support for new programs and services, these developments ironically became victims of their own success as the more radical elements of the anti-homeless movement became supplanted by more pragmatic voices. As new homeless programs became more established with federal funding and embedded within the bureaucratic state apparatus, their orientation toward challenging the status quo and housing inequities—the core of system-talk—gradually became replaced by a conciliatory logic of working within the system rather than against it. In short, homeless advocacy became replaced by a professionalized homeless industrial complex, concerned with maintaining itself rather than challenging structural injustices. Indeed, Gowan's interviews with several executive directors of homeless organizations, individuals who often began their careers in system-talk, saliently show some of their own disillusionment toward their organizations' misaligned goals today, which often run counter to the objectives of the rights-based movement of the early 1980s. Moreover, her ethnography highlights how system-talk has gradually become undercut by a more punitive, moralistic construction of service provision from the more conservative and religious sectors. For example, religious-based programs sometimes encourage participants to pray to absolve their sins or require more stringent behavioral requirements as a condition for access to housing or meals. From another side, social workers working within the homeless industrial complex—and particularly within Gowan's dubbed *archipelago* of disjointed service programs—have become voices of another discourse altogether, emphasizing pathology (i.e., the sick-talk discourse we discuss below).

Despite this cynical lens, system-talk can still be found today—primarily perpetuated by the few homeless advocacy organizations that still hold true to their social justice roots. There are homeless programs and services, Gowan seems to contend, and then there are true homeless *advocates* who continue to promote a system-talk construction of poverty. To be sure, Gowan makes a point that organizations tackling homelessness exist within a spectrum and that programs can hold drastically different ideological positions about solutions. Moreover, Gowan also makes an important insight that while programs and policies may sound like system-talk on the surface, their implementation will often take on a more sin- or sick-talk orientation. Gowan shows, for example, how some *street outreach programs* in San Francisco—designed to help homeless people readily access services and emergency housing (e.g., temporary housing vouchers)—in reality function to move homeless individuals away from commercial and retail sectors of the city, where they are put onto extended waiting lists for permanent housing, which rarely materialize. Rather than providing individuals experiencing homelessness with quick access to services, Gowan argues that many street outreach programs simply guide these individuals to relocate to areas where they are less visible. Similarly, Gowan argues that Housing First programs, which assert housing as a right and are touted as a radical departure from the conventional service models established in the 1980s and 1990s, are often compromised in their actual application. One shortcoming of Housing First that Gowan highlights is how most of these programs require participants to first establish a verified diagnosis and/or disability before they can be admitted. Even though Housing First is supposedly underpinned by a philosophy that "housing is a human right" (Tsemberis 2011. p. 1), it is a right primarily mediated by one's medical diagnosis and/or disability status. As a result, only a small percentage of individuals who experience homelessness are eligible for a Housing First program. And so, despite the system-talk underpinning of Housing First programs, Gowan argues, they are relatively expensive compared to funding of general public housing as well as more restrictive as who they can house.

Both cases of Housing First and street outreach programs, then, highlight how policy applications of system-talk can be easily co-opted given the broader sociopolitical landscape. Indeed, Gowan seems to suggest that one way policymakers neutralize the radical extension of system-talk (with respect to challenging the status quo) is to deploy a more humanistic version of sin-talk that reframes the deviance of homelessness from a moral issue to a medical one—*sick-talk*. In this way, policymakers are able to pursue a more palatable policy of social exclusion by deploying programs that seem progressive, and even system-talk oriented, but in practice function to sequester the homeless to less desirable parts of city—what Gowan (2010) eloquently describes as programs that merge the goals of "clearance with treatment" (p. 244). Indeed, for Gowan the "diplomatic claim of sick-talk that the homeless deserve services" (p. 192) often resembles more a conciliatory sin-talk goal of exclusion, as we discuss below.

Sick-Talk

They need to be institutionalized as most of them are mentally ill. They are either manic depressives or schizophrenics and are a danger to themselves and to others.

Ninety percent of homeless have mental problems. They need to be put away and supervised by a professional mental health staff who will make sure that they will receive their medications and therapy.

What Is Sick-Talk?

In many of the community meetings we attend about homelessness, the issue of mental illness is perhaps the most common discussion that we encounter. Similar to the paraphrased quotes above, however, concerns about mental health and homelessness are distinctive from discussions we hear about mental health more generally. Indeed, when the topic of mental illness emerges, we notice discussions are often less about the psychological suffering of individuals or their general well-being, as they are about identifying the deviant abnormality of homelessness itself. Similar to the purported deviance at the heart of *sin-talk*—that homelessness stems from the abnormality of individuals themselves—discussions about homelessness and mental health are often centered on a more socially acceptable register for identifying deviance. We also notice that these discussions about mental health often point to the need to sequester these individuals from the community and place them in treatment *for their own good.*

In a similar way, Gowan (2010) introduces sick-talk as a more *therapeutic* discourse about the deviance of homelessness, akin to sin-talk, but one that has also perpetuated a "medicalization of poverty" more broadly (p. 193). What was once the issue of moral failings or the system's lack of stable employment has now become reframed as occasions for clinical introspection and therapeutic practices. In this frame, homelessness is simply another symptom of one's inner sickness, one's undiagnosed and typically inadequately (or untreated) treated pathology. Housing is now a psychiatric intervention, addressing a medical issue rather than just a social justice one.

This shift toward *sick-talk* has been both a problem and an opportunity according to Gowen (2010): from a moral lens, it is better to be sick than bad; unlike sin-talk, one cannot be blamed for their mental and physical disabilities. Yet, it also creates certain obligations among the sick to manage their conditions. And so, while someone with insecure housing is certainly better regarded as an *alcoholic*, *psychotic*, or *addict*, they must nonetheless be assessed, diagnosed, and agree to be (medically) treated—preferably treated *somewhere else from here*. Even more, professionals are essential for making such judgments and doling out indicated interventions. And in this era of therapy, the homeless individual must learn to forego their own "street agency" (p. 194) and become "clients" who simultaneously divulge their pain, helplessness, and inner experiences—as well as embrace the more modern clinical practice of self-examination.

Sick-Talk History

Gowan (2010) asserts that a rendition of sick-talk has always existed as an "unspoken accusation" that those without secure housing need reform and rehabilitation (p. 185). Yet, Gowan asserts that this more medicalized discourse about homelessness only rose to prominence toward the later part of the twentieth century, when psychiatry became more widely accepted. While in our opinion Gowan sidesteps a thorough review of medicalization in Western culture, or at least its complexities vis-à-vis social work practice, which we discuss below, she nonetheless provides a convincing description of how sick-talk cohered and expanded in the 1990s.

As we already discussed above, initial responses to the rise of homelessness in the late 1970s and early 1980s, particularly by homeless advocates and social workers, had already pointed to the deinstitutionalization of mental health services as a significant driver of the crisis. Though Gowan seems to de-emphasize how these voices often focused on the failed promises of the community mental health movement, which had been articulated as early as in the *Community Mental Health Act* of 1963 as a more humane and effective way for helping individuals with mental health challenges (Bloom 1984; Caplan 1961; Langsley 1985a; Langsley 1985b), undoubted concerns about deinstitutionalization helped solidify a link between homelessness and untreated mental health conditions. Indeed, the underfunding of supportive services in the community—including transitional housing programs—had been often discussed in the mental health literature as one of the central failures of deinstitutionalization (Langsley 1985a; Langsley 1985b). This policy failure was evidenced in various studies that highlighted the dearth of community-based mental health programs across the country and the disproportionate number of individuals living on the streets who struggled with mental health challenges and/or substance abuse/use (Lamb 1984). And so, the perception that many homeless struggled with untreated mental illness was already firmly established both in public consciousness and research by the 1980s.

But for Gowan these trends would only cohere as a dominant discourse, and in turn policy shift, after the 1993 publication of *A Nation in Denial: The Truth about*

Homelessness by Baum and Burnes—a manifesto of sorts, seeking to discredit the dominance of system-talk being perpetuated by anti-homeless advocates. As we discussed, system-talk advocates had initially been successful in reframing the discussion of people living on the streets as about the structural situations that individuals found themselves in *as people without a home*, hence the new term *homeless*. But according to Gowan, Baum and Burnes (1993) articulated a convincing counter argument that many homeless were primarily victims of medical conditions that prevented them from living independently. The homeless were not in need of housing per se but (medical) treatment. This emerging discourse, which was soon taken up by both policymakers and strategic advocates, not only promoted an explicit medicalization of poverty but also emphasized that housing provisions and subsidies were, at best, partial solutions to homelessness.

Indeed, as the Clinton administration took hold in the early 1990s, the Department of Housing and Urban Development (HUD) reorientated itself to prioritize rehabilitation services that purportedly helped the homeless become more *housing-ready* as opposed to just sheltering them temporarily. Specifically, HUD's new Continuum of Care (CoC) Program outlined a three-tiered set of programs, which graduated individuals from shelters to transitional housing-ready programs and, finally, to subsidized housing. Central to the CoC model throughout the 1990s was the notion that housing programs should be coupled with varied allied service professionals who could diagnose, assess, and treat clients. Housing was now directly coupled with addiction counseling, psychotherapy, vocational rehabilitation, and other supportive services.

From an institutional perspective, these new programs created a need and space for a professionalized workforce to exist within the pathway toward housing; housing programs now had to be filled with various social workers, licensed clinicians, and paraprofessionals who could all engage in the discourse of sick-talk and frame the medical necessity for housing. In this sense, sick-talk became a compromising discourse between the broad interventionist scope of system-talk, with the individualistic frame of sin-talk. In short, sick-talk became a dominant way for social workers to frame housing as a legitimate intervention for the poor and legitimized social service providers themselves while adhering to the notion that the central problem of homelessness resided within the homeless themselves. In this context, Gowan argues, federal funding for public housing—the third tier of the CoC model—has substantially decreased during this time, despite the increased expenditures on homeless supportive services more generally.

How Sick-Talk Is Perpetuated

According to Gowan, sick-talk continues to be perpetuated by the *archipelago* system of disconnected service providers that offer the homeless a variety of interventions related to addiction counseling, psychotherapy, vocational rehabilitation, and case management more generally. At the "street level," Gowan (2010) asserts that "the most powerful strand of sick-talk within the homelessness industry is the language of the twelve-step movement" (p. 126), long promoted by peer groups like Alcoholic Anonymous. Interestingly, this nonprofessional resource and contingent discourse now can be part of the gateway ritual of confession to access resources. As Gowan documents, interactions among these resources and professional services are today often structured by explicit discussions of assessments, diagnoses, treatment plans, and other professionalized technologies. Particularly with concerns regarding program resources (i.e., cost, reimbursements, and insurance eligibility), the discursive practice of clinically diagnosing "disability" and "medical necessity" can take center stage in discussions about access to housing and services. It is important to keep in mind this continuum is populated by a bevy of peers, paraprofessionals, trained clinical professionals, and administrators. Moreover, the overt medicalizing discourse is propelled by the need to reframe housing and income assistance as part of one's broader medical story, one which makes occasional references to their need for drug rehabilitation, vocational training, social skill development, therapy, inpatient stays, and outpatient services for co-occurring conditions. In other words, as individuals learn to transverse the resources available to them through the archipelago, they must also learn how to strategically engage in versions of introspective sick-talk. As Gowan (2010) describes, each person "had to learn to tell the right kind of story for each given situation–to emphasize job possibilities here, disability there…stories of deprivation and disability inevitably became a skill" (p. 214).

Across the continuum of providers, a wide gamut of staff propel individuals to engage in different forms of sick-talk(s)—from paraprofessional staff and licensed professionals to newly *graduated* clients of these services now turned volunteers. Depending on several variables, including education and training, acumen, and (clinical) approach, these frontline and clinical staff mediate access or barriers for clients depending on their sick-talk rendition. In some cases, however, Gowan shows how sin-talk can become wrapped up in sick-talk, which has the effect of stigmatizing if not restricting clients' access from services, as in the case when staff turn away individuals who are disabled but also *resistant*.

Gowan asserts that the weaknesses of this housing continuum derive from (social) workers not providing the *environment* for clients to transform their lives without being boxed into having to atone for pathologies or moral failings. This is punctuated by the ineffective training of workers along the gamut of providers, from lay workers to trained professionals. Ironically, what is being argued as the cause for entering homelessness and therefore the continuum of services—that is, mental illness based on the discourse of sick-talk—is possibly creating mental health problems anew or in addition to what clients have in the first place. Sick-talk straddles mental health (problems) as both the cause and the effect of homelessness.

Bringing It All Together: Discourse as/in Practice

We suspect that at first reading Gowan's discursive and historical analysis of homelessness may be difficult for practitioners to find direct application, given the intentional academic tone and broad scope. Indeed, Gowan is not a practitioner rather an academic sociologist who is not overtly concerned with applied practice nor translational science. Nonetheless, we contend that her analysis of homelessness unwittingly contributes to the field and professional training of social work, all the while having some limitations.

The overarching insights by Gowan that homelessness is complex, and in particular that individuals experiencing homelessness are more complex than the narratives we hear about them, are largely consistent with the ethos of modern social work practice. Indeed, the ecological and person-in-environment perspectives, dominant in US social work, posit that problems and issues faced by clients are multifaceted and rarely arise from one location (e.g., mental disorders are not simply a problem of neurology, nor is homelessness just caused by a moral attribute or economic insufficiency). And so, in this way, Gowan's (2010) ethnographic effort to "unflatten" the caricatures of homelessness (p. 25) reinforces social work's commitment to understand people's lived experiences as intersecting identities, complex biographies, and negotiated relationships across systems of family, community, society, and more. Understanding how certain discourses serve to oversimplify the realities of clients and lived experiences helps social workers avoid the pitfalls of engaging in *talks* that stereotype, objectify, and disempower clients.

From a similar perspective, the typology of sin-, sick-, and system-talk also has much potential to be both useful and insightful for conceptualizing the day-to-day language social workers often hear about homelessness, whether in public or in our practice. This rubric offers a concise language to identify the contours of these discourses—how they shape certain truths about homelessness—but also their social and historical legacies in social welfare provision in the USA. The history of social welfare is complex and layered, as are our attitudes and beliefs toward state programs to address poverty and homelessness. As such, we contend that Gowan adds to the field of social work, in both theory and in practice, a concise language for understanding the parallel factors that have shaped, and continue to shape, the provision of social welfare services in the USA. Sin-talk, system-talk, and sick-talk serve as convenient heuristics for mapping the explicit limits and constraints of these dominant discourses.

Moreover, social work is principally concerned with maneuvers of power and oppression in people's lived experiences and how they perpetuate social, economic, and health inequities. Critical to this understanding is that marginalization is maintained through the un-/intentional actions across the levels of the individual, institutional policies and practices, and sociocultural norms and assumptions (Johnson 2006; Mullaly 2002). As such, when Gowan implies that homeless people are objectified through the (pseudo) clinical gaze of sick-talk, she has a point. Oppression can be perpetuated through well-intentioned, but nonetheless uncritical, uses of language, which in turn can inadvertently contribute to exploitation, marginalization, and symbolic violence (Adams et al. 2013).

In this way, Gowan's research highlights the fundamental power of language—and, that discourse can itself be an intervention of social work. In various points in her ethnography, Gowan shows how power plays out through the communication between people experiencing homelessness (*clients*) and social service staff (*social workers*). This is an important insight, as too often discourse is regarded as a singularly top-down social process (e.g., institutional and professional practices). Yet Gowan's analysis holds the important potential to acknowledge that discourse is also a bottom-up dynamic (Jaworski and Coupland 1999; Wetherell et al. 2004). Her respondents not only reflected on the dominant discourses that purportedly explained their predicaments, but they also took up these discourses in their own way, reshaping these *talks* for their own needs and interests. In this sense, Gowan's analysis demonstrates how discourse can be both a site for oppression (i.e., top-down, the patient must submit to medical and mental health systems) and also simultaneously as a site for resistance and empowerment (i.e., bottom-up, the person holds agency and self-determination and can resist). Setting Gowan's academic project in conversation with recent research on microaggressions (Sue 2010) adds depth to her analysis of how power and oppression work through language practices. If microaggressions are day-to-day communications that perpetuate social divisions and marginalization, they can also be occasions—or discursive moments—in which social workers can help actively resist and push back against these divisions through the use of counter-discourses.

Despite these strengths, however, we note two central limitations of Gowan's work, particularly as it applies to the field of social work practice. First, while we agree with Gowan's overall description of sick-talk and her critique of its myopic application to frame and dominate discussions of homelessness, her conception of this mental health discourse is perhaps a bit un-nuanced for a social work audience. Specifically, Gowan seems to conflate any discussion of mental health and/or addiction as explicit efforts to medicalize and disempower clients. From our point of view, this minimizes the reality that *some* people experiencing homelessness may also be struggling with addiction or other challenges. And, we contend that it is possible, particularly for social workers, to accept both the reality of mental health and the reality that social and environment factors are involved in perpetuating homelessness; these are not mutually exclusive realities. Though mental health is often framed in individualistic terms, many mental health professionals, especially social workers, acknowledge the complex interplay between individuals and their environment in promoting (or not) mental health. As such, to dismiss any discussion of mental health as simply a discursive tactic and discount the social effects of context grossly oversimplifies the realities faced by people experiencing homelessness. For us, the critical issue is not whether mental health is ever discussed as a factor in homelessness but rather how that discourse is deployed. Depending on the frame, mental health discussions can be empowering and contribute to self-determination, as well as engage with the broader issue of context.

A second related critique of Gowan's analysis is her apparent dismissive attitude toward social work itself. Social workers are noticeably absent in her telling of how social welfare emerged and evolved in the USA (e.g., Jane Addams, Frances Perkins, Edith Abbott, among many others). Instead, the profession of social work and its impact on the discourses of poverty are largely footnoted in Gowan's (2010) text and relegated to the limited roles of "elite reformers" in the early part of the twentieth century (p. 40) or "ideologists of medicalization" at the end of the century (p. 191). And, even when individual social workers are discussed in her ethnographic analysis of social services, she seems to conflate *social workers* as any persons working in the capacity of shelter staff or case managers. Indeed, it is unclear to us still how many of the "social worker" research subjects whom she interviewed were professionals with a degree in social work. And so, in her analysis of these, how discourses are deployed in professional settings is somewhat limited to what she mainly heard from "frontline staff" (p. 191), "shift-manager(s) at the shelter" (p. 200), or the occasional "drug counselor" and "case manager" (p. 194). Gowan acknowledges that what she observed in shelters was at most an "inexpert" therapeutic discourse—or "pop medicalization" (p. 193)—and not the "expert-led…process of doctor-centered medicalization" (p. 193). But even in this acknowledgment, Gowan misunderstands that most expert-trained therapists are not medical doctors and that the majority are, in fact, master's degree social workers (NASW 2017). As such, Gowan's analysis is somewhat of a missed opportunity to directly engage, and put her *talks* in dialogue, with arguably one of the central professions in the USA working on issues of poverty and homelessness. Indeed, despite this shortcoming of her analysis, Gowan's insights and findings raise important, and difficult, issues for professional social workers to consider.

Expanding the Typology: Social-Talk

Perhaps one way to reconcile some of the limitations of these talks, despite their usefulness, is to consider the need for a new, more social work-focused discourse on homelessness, one that amends and builds from Gowan's tripartite typology. Indeed, embedded within Gowan's methodology and analysis is a tendency to paint a series of false dichotomies: homeless or housed, client or worker, sane or (mentally) sick, able or disabled, or (dutiful) citizen or sinner. As evidenced in her participants' narratives, living on the streets is anything but black and white but rather consists of complex realties that resemble different shades of gray. From a more critical standpoint, we assert that her rubric is missing an appreciation for the relational and functional qualities of the experiences she is so eager to critique. In particular, a core value of social work is to understand people and both their challenges and strengths within context. Social work practice is relational and concerned about the lived negotiations we, as professionals and clients, engage with every day.

As such, we conclude this chapter by proposing the need for a new talk: *social-talk*. It is beyond the scope of this chapter to completely outline and flesh out fully this new discourse; we are proposing an emerging theory for practice and a future research-practice agenda that we ourselves are already taking up—and encourage our colleagues to do so as well. Nonetheless, we conclude our discussion by highlighting the key, broad contours of what we believe *social-talk* should touch on. Following are the broad goals of social-talk:

- *Social-talk* discusses micro, mezzo, and macro issues simultaneously.

Table 6.2 Expanding the discourse

Construction of poverty and homelessness discourse	Moral: Sin-talk	Disease: Sick-talk	Systemic: System-talk	Relational: Social-talk
The central cause and truth of homelessness	Sin	Sickness, disease	Social structure, inequality	Social oppression
Fundamental strategy	Punishment and exclusion	Treatment	Social change	Collaboration, solidarity
Focus of cause	Individual	Individual	Structural	Multilevel
Level of agency	Strong	Weak	Weak	Contextual

- *Social-talk* engages discussions of mental illness, mental health, well-being, and biopsychosocial issues without disempowering clients.
- *Social-talk* deals with the fact that clients need help today and acknowledges that this help must challenge the status quo, which may be at the micro, mezzo, and/or macro levels.

In concert with the analytic framework of Gowan's presentation, we frame *social-talk* in the following way (see Table 6.2). The *central problem* or cause of homelessness is an effect (or symptom) of the fact that people live within a matrix of power and oppression; and, the (focus of) *cause* for such a problem is *multilevel*, not simply relegated to within the individual nor endemic of *the structure*. Moreover, social-talk asserts that through helping relationships, clients have the potential to make meaning of themselves and their world. Implicit in this is that it is assumed clients have *agency*, and the struggles they go through and the strategies they determine to be effective (or at least attempt) are *contextual*: their lived experience is in context. Part of the work of social workers, therefore, necessarily needs to be, as we assert, actively *collaborating* with clients to re-/negotiate the meanings of the discourses in which they circulate; social workers stand in *solidarity* with their clients and communities. Moreover, the express mission of social work would suggest a tendency toward fostering counter-discourses. A stance such as that derives from ethics, theory, and practice.

Social-talk would also turn back to the original works that constructed social work itself. Jane Addams and Hull House are a prescient example of the potential for working in and with discourse, specifically regarding insecure housing, poverty, and inequalities. Counter to the allegation that "social workers" were unable to create an environment through which clients could prosper as found by Gowan, Hull House was exactly about place-making strategies to empower participants as well as reconfigure the discourses about indigent, downtrodden, mentally unwell, and marginalized persons. Indeed, Addams' social-talk became social work.

In the end, we call for social welfare researchers and social work practitioners to stand in solidarity with Gowan. We do not encourage social workers to overgeneralize discourses about the most marginalized and vulnerable in our society. Rather, through this chapter, we have attempted to marshal a call for social workers to take very seriously the constructions and effects of discourse, historically and contemporarily. Discourse and its analysis must be included in the arsenal of interventions used in our profession. To be obvious, for many of our communities, clients, and justice-seeking collaborators, language pregnant with challenges as well as possibilities often is the foundational thing to make sense of those very conditions that marginalize them. To that point, Gowan offers much advocacy and import to social work.

References

Adams, M., Blumenfeld, W., Castaneda, C., Hackman, H. W., Peteres, M. L., & Zuniga, X. (Eds.). (2013). *Readings for diversity and social justice*. New York: Routledge.

Aykanian, A., & Lee, W. (2016). Social work's role in ending the criminalization of homelessness: Opportunities for action. *Social Work, 61*(2), 183–185.

Baum, A. S., & Burnes, D. W. (1993). *A nation in denial: The truth about homelessness*. Ann Arbor: Westview Press.

Belcher, J. R., & DeForge, B. R. (2012). Social stigma and homelessness: The limits of social change. *Journal of Human Behavior in the Social Environment, 22*(8), 929–946.

Blau, J. (1992). *The visible poor: Homelessness in the United States*. New York: Oxford University Press.

Bloom, B. L. (1984). *Community mental health: A general introduction* (2nd ed.). Monterey: Brooks/Cole.

Caplan, G. (1961). *An approach to community mental health*. New York: Grune & Stratton.

Esping-Andersen, G. (1990). The three political economies of the welfare state. *International Journal of Sociology, 20*(3), 92–123.

Foucault, M. (1980). *Power/knowledge: Selected interviews and other writings, 1972–1977*. New York: Pantheon.

Foucault, M. (1990). *The history of sexuality* (Vol. 1). New York: Random House.

Foucault, M. (1995). *Discipline and punish: The birth of the prison* (2nd ed.). New York: Random House.

Gitterman, A., & Germain, C. B. (2008). *The life model of social work practice: Advances in theory and practice*. New York: Columbia University Press.

Gowan, T. (2010). *Hobos, hustlers, and backsliders: Homeless in San Francisco*. Minneapolis: University of Minnesota Press.

Heathcote, J., Perri, F., & Violante, G. L. (2010). Unequal we stand: An empirical analysis of economic inequality in the United States, 1967–2006. *Review of Economic Dynamics, 13*(1), 15–51.

Jaworski, A., & Coupland, N. (Eds.). (1999). *The discourse reader*. London: Routledge.

Jencks, C. (1995). *The homeless*. Boston: Harvard University Press.

Johnson, A. G. (2006). *Privilege, power, and difference*. Boston: McGraw Hill.

Katz, M. B. (2013). *The undeserving poor: America's enduring confrontation with poverty: Fully updated and revised*. Oxford: Oxford University Press.

Kelling, G. L., & Wilson, J. Q. (1982, March). Broken windows: The police and neighborhood safety. The Atlantic. https://www.theatlantic.com/magazine/archive/1982/03/broken-windows/304465/. Accessed 30 June 2018.

Lamb, H. R. (1984). Deinstitutionalization and the homeless mentally ill. *Psychiatric Services, 35*(9), 899–907.

Langsley, D. G. (1985a). Community psychiatry. In H. I. Kaplan & B. J. Sadock (Eds.), *Comprehensive textbook of psychiatry/IV* (4th ed., pp. 1878–1884). Baltimore: Williams & Wilkins.

Langsley, D. G. (1985b). Prevention in psychiatry: Primary, secondary, and tertiary. In H. I. Kaplan & B. J. Sadock (Eds.), *Comprehensive textbook of psychiatry/IV* (4th ed., pp. 1885–1888). Baltimore: Williams & Wilkins.

McNamee, S. J., & Miller, R. K. (2009). *The meritocracy myth*. Lanham: Rowman & Littlefield.

Mechanic, D. (2008). *Mental health and social policy: Beyond managed care* (5th ed.). Boston: Allyn & Bacon.

Mullaly, B. (2002). *Challenging oppression: A critical social work approach*. Don Mills: Oxford University Press Canada.

Myers, D. G. (2001). *The American paradox: Spiritual hunger in an age of plenty*. New Haven: Yale University Press.

National Association of Social Workers (NASW). (2017). Social work profession. http://www.socialworkers.org/pressroom/features/general/profession.asp. Accessed 8 July 2017.

National Law Center on Homelessness and Poverty. (2016). *Housing not handcuffs: Ending the criminalization of homelessness in U.S. cities*. Washington, D.C: Author.

Piven, F. F., & Cloward, R. A. (1971). *Regulating the poor: The functions of social welfare*. New York: Vintage.

Platt, A. M. (1977). *The child savers: The invention of delinquency*. Chicago: University of Chicago Press.

Rossi, P. H. (1991). *Down and out in America: The origins of homelessness*. Chicago: University of Chicago Press.

Skocpol, T. (1992). *Protecting mothers and soldiers: The political origins of social policy in the United States*. Cambridge: Belknap Harvard.

Snow, D. A., & Anderson, L. (1993). *Down on their luck: A study of homeless street people*. Berkeley: University of California Press.

Soss, J., Fording, R. C., & Schram, S. (2011). *Disciplining the poor: Neoliberal paternalism and the persistent power of race*. Chicago: University of Chicago Press.

Sue, D. W. (2010). *Microaggressions in everyday life: Race, gender, and sexual orientation*. Hoboken: Wiley.

Tsemberis, S. (2011). Housing first: The pathways model to end homelessness for people with mental illness and addiction manual. *European Journal of Homelessness, 5*(2).

Wacquant, L. (2009). *Punishing the poor: The neoliberal government of social insecurity*. Durham: Duke University Press.

Weber, M. (2002). *The Protestant ethic and the "spirit" of capitalism and other writings*. London: Penguin.

Wetherell, M., Taylor, S., & Yates, S. J. (Eds.). (2004). *Discourse theory and practice*. London: Sage.

Zelizer, V. A. R. (1985). *Pricing the priceless child: The changing social value of children*. Princeton: Princeton University Press.

Chapter 7
Community-Based Strategies to Address Homelessness

Diane R. Bessel

Introduction

This chapter examines the varied community-based strategies used to address the complex problem of homelessness in the United States. Characterized by multiple, often competing, perspectives and disagreement about its causes and consequences, the problem of homelessness lacks a simple, single pathway, or solution (Mumford et al. 2010). Instead, it requires actors to work beyond the capacity of any single organization or sector, and across disciplinary boundaries, to develop new and promising approaches (Roberts 2000; Perrault et al. 2011; Thompson 2013).

Over the past 40 years, housing providers, advocates, and municipalities have engaged in collaborative problem-solving in an effort to end homelessness. Often, these activities were required by funders – such as the introduction of the Continuum of Care model and required implementation of local Homeless Management Information Systems (HMIS) by the US Department of Housing and Urban Development (HUD). In other instances, coordinated planning was undertaken as part of a larger advocacy effort, as illustrated by the development of local plans to address chronic homelessness, or sparked by innovation, as with the development of coordinated entry and assessment systems.

The chapter describes how communities have responded to these various challenges, changes, requirements, and evolutions by engaging a wide variety of skills from research and service linkage to planning, policy-making, and evaluation to serve diverse homeless individuals and families. It begins with a brief discussion of

---

Electronic supplementary material: The online version of this chapter (https://doi.org/10.1007/978-3-030-03727-7_7) contains supplementary material, which is available to authorized users.

D. R. Bessel (✉)
Daemen College, Amherst, NY, USA
e-mail: dbessel@daemen.edu

H. Larkin et al. (eds.), *Homelessness Prevention and Intervention in Social Work*, https://doi.org/10.1007/978-3-030-03727-7_7

the initial development of homelessness assistance systems and continues through to present day. The chapter also highlights some of the key strengths and unintended consequences of these efforts while filling a surprising and critical gap in the social work literature regarding their role in addressing the problem of homelessness.

The Development of Homelessness Assistance Systems

Demand for homeless-specific programming (i.e., housing and services) came in direct response to complex changes in the nation's economy (for a comprehensive review of the history of homelessness in the USA, see Baumohl 1996; Kusmer 2002; and Rossi 1989). Beginning in the 1970s, the country entered an economic downturn as deindustrialization and the shift to a service- and information-based economy eliminated many unskilled and semiskilled jobs (Mintz and Kellogg 1988). Rust Belt industrial cities and factory towns were hardest to hit by the changing economy and characterized as "breeding grounds for homelessness" – not only for older workers but also for the children who anticipated following in their parents' footsteps (Kusmer 2002).

The economic recessions of the late 1970s and early 1980s also aggravated conditions that had been developing since the previous decade: dwindling affordable housing supplies for poor and working class families, the decrease in single room occupancy (SRO) housing, declining support for persons with severe mental illness, the growth of single-parent households, and reductions in cash assistance for the unemployed and indigent (Burt et al. 2002; U.S. Department of Housing and Urban Development [HUD] 2002). Continuing labor market difficulties added substantial numbers of people of color as well as single women, women with children, and two-parent families to the group of men who had previously composed most of the population seeking shelter (Mintz and Kellogg 1988).

By the early 1980s, the national homeless population included an estimated 250,000–350,000 persons (U.S. Department of Housing and Urban Development [HUD] 1984).[1] As demand for assistance increased, charitable organizations began offering meals and other supports to those at risk for homelessness and overnight shelter to their homeless clientele. The sheer volume of need and the shifting nature

[1]This estimate is based on the early federal definition of homelessness. Under this definition, an individual is considered homeless if he or she is (1) sleeping in an emergency shelter; (2) sleeping in places not meant for human habitation, such as cars, parks, sidewalks, or abandoned or condemned buildings; (3) spending a short time (30 consecutive days or less) in a hospital or other institution but ordinarily sleeping in the types of places mentioned above; (4) living in transitional/supportive housing but having come from streets or emergency shelters; (5) being evicted within a week from a private dwelling unit and having no subsequent residence identified and lacking the resources and support networks needed to obtain access to housing; or (6) being discharged from an institution and having no subsequent residence identified and lacking the resources and support networks needed to obtain access to housing.

of homelessness generated greater interest in developing solutions to the emerging problem (HUD 2002). In 1983, Congress took its first steps to commit federal resources to address homelessness since the Great Depression, appropriating $100 million to assist homeless and hungry persons through the Emergency Food and Shelter Program (EFSP).

Operating out of the Federal Emergency Management Agency (FEMA), EFSP involved a unique public-private partnership designed to supplement and expand the work of local social service and charitable organizations providing emergency food and housing assistance to people in need. The program provided approved jurisdictions funding for food (i.e., served meals or groceries), lodging in shelters or hotels, rent or mortgage payments, utility bill payments, and equipment (Emergency Food and Shelter Program National Board n.d.).

Funding was made available, on a competitive basis, to any charitable organization or government entity helping hungry and homeless people or those at risk due to economic hardships. Communities replicated the EFSP's design at the local level and took responsibility for advertising the availability of funds, reviewing applications to ensure organizations had resources necessary to provide assistance (e.g., financial capacity, volunteers, staff), and determining how funds would be allocated, with an initial emphasis on improving efficiency and responsiveness.

While EFSP provided much needed funding to address the growing demand for food and shelter, it did little to facilitate the development of organized and comprehensive homelessness assistance systems (Weinreb and Rossi 1995). EFSB's wide eligibility criteria resulted in an increase in providers who worked with a specific population or within a specific geography but had little or no connection to one another. Additionally, providers typically offered very limited assistance to homeless and near-homeless clientele and were not equipped to address their myriad needs beyond provision of food and shelter.

Noting the disorganized and highly fractured nature of homeless service provision, advocates began demanding that the federal governments acknowledge homelessness as a national problem requiring a more comprehensive solution (National Coalition for the Homeless 2006). In response, the US Department of Housing and Urban Development (HUD) made its first attempt to describe the scope of loosely defined shelter systems in 1984, estimating that there were 100,000 shelter beds found in approximately 1900 shelters.

By 1988, national estimates had grown to 275,000 beds in 5,400 shelters (U.S. Department of Housing and Urban Development [HUD] 1989). Concerned about the rising demand for assistance, lack of coordination among homelessness service providers, and the increased amount of federal dollars being allocated to address the problem (including a $325 million increase in EFSP funding from 1984 to 1987), Congress passed the first major federal legislative response to homelessness through the Stewart B. McKinney Homeless Assistance Act of 1987 (renamed the McKinney-Vento Homeless Assistance Act in 2000).

When describing the legislation's purpose, Congress indicated that the problem of homelessness had become severe and, in the absence of more effective efforts, was expected to worsen. The legislation also stated that the causes of homelessness were many and complex and that there was no single, simple solution given the many different subpopulations and reasons for homelessness. The legislation also acknowledged that the federal government had a clear responsibility as well as the capacity to play a more effective and responsible role to meet basic human needs and engender respect for the dignity of people experiencing homelessness (Public Law 100-77; HR 558). Finally, the landmark legislation established the Interagency Council on the Homeless (renamed the Interagency Council on Homelessness in 2004), an independent entity within the executive branch charged with coordinating the federal response to homelessness and maximizing the government's effectiveness in contributing to the end of homelessness.

The legislation also significantly increased federal dollars ($490 million in FY 1987) for expanded homeless housing. This involved authorizing the Emergency Food and Shelter Program (EFSP); establishing the Emergency Shelter Grant (ESG) program to improve existing shelters by providing resources to defray operations, maintenance, repair, and security costs; and developing new housing-related programming, including:

1. Transitional housing programs designed to help homeless families and single persons with disabilities acquire the skills necessary to maintain themselves in conventional housing through the Supported Housing Program (SHP)
2. Permanent housing for homeless persons with disabling conditions that would otherwise preclude their achieving and/or maintaining independent and secure housing using Shelter Plus Care (S+C)
3. Rental subsidy payments for private property owners for units rehabilitated under the Section 8 Moderate Rehabilitation Program to provide housing assistance for low-income persons at 30% of the median income

In addition to housing, the legislation included homelessness prevention, street outreach, and supportive services (i.e., stand-alone services and those attached to shelter and housing programs), as well as the first grants to support primary health and substance abuse services for people experiencing homelessness through the Health Care for the Homeless provision. It also established the Community Mental Health Services Block Grant program for services to homeless individuals with chronic mental illness; education, training, and community services for homeless adults; special provisions for the education of homeless children; access to the federal Food Stamp and Temporary Emergency Food Assistance Programs (TEFAP) for homeless individuals; and special provisions for veterans related to job training and reintegration assistance.

Case Study: Homeless Assistance in Buffalo, New York

While Buffalo was once a booming steel and automobile manufacturing town, New York's economic health plummeted as well-paying, skilled, and semi-skilled jobs were relocated or lost. Since the 1980s, the city has been besieged by high unemployment rates, generally ranging between 5% and 9% (U.S. Bureau of Labor Statistics 2017). Buffalo is currently ranked as the third poorest large city (250,000+) in the country, with a poverty rate of 31.4% (U.S. Census Bureau 2017).

In addition to high rates of unemployment and poverty, Buffalo experienced a substantial growth in its homeless population during the early 1980s. Concern about the community's ability to effectively address the needs of homeless people led a coalition of 35 human service agencies to conduct the area's first study of the homeless population in 1984. At the time, Buffalo's homeless population was estimated at 5250 individuals, including persons experiencing mental illness (30%), substance abuse (28%), victims of domestic violence (13%), and runaway and homeless youth (7%). By 1988, more than 7,500 individuals had experienced homelessness – a 30% increase.

The volume of homeless and near-homeless individuals requiring services increased steadily, as did the number of local organizations providing assistance. More than 75% of these providers received funding through the local Emergency Food and Shelter Board (EFSB).

Early on, the community acknowledged that homelessness services were highly disorganized, with each provider focusing on its own homeless population and clientele. Programs were not working together to address larger issues related to homelessness: educational, vocational, and financial programming; help for clients facing difficulties accessing government benefits; efforts to reduce community stigma and negative views about people experiencing homelessness; and problems connecting clients to transitional and permanent housing following initial crisis experiences.

The Move to HUD'S Continuum of Care Model

The McKinney-Vento Homeless Assistance Act had one additional purpose – to use public resources and programs in a more coordinated manner to meet the urgent needs of the homeless population. For the first 7 years following its passage, however, HUD – the primary funder of homeless housing and services – did not impose any requirements for systemic planning, comprehensiveness, or evaluation at the community level (HUD 2002). Instead, EFSP and ESG funds were awarded to eligible communities based on a need-allocation formula (calculated using recent population, unemployment, and poverty statistics), while McKinney-Vento-funded programs, including SHP and S+C, required individual programs to apply for funds through national competitions.

Organizations seeking funding for homeless-related programs were asked to demonstrate that a need existed for the services they proposed. However, HUD did not insist that they show how their services fit within the larger community or whether proposed programs would employ the most effective or efficient methods (HUD 2002). Instead, the federal government assumed that local communities would establish their own criteria for recommending and establishing needed programming (Interagency Council for the Homeless 1995).

At the time, however, it was not uncommon for local communities to face difficulties tracking what services were available, what was being applied for, and what was in the process of being developed (HUD 2002). While local officials could block homeless housing and service projects from moving forward, they had only limited access to community need data and were likely concerned with the political ramifications of refusing a project – allowing homeless programs and services to continue to develop with little to no oversight.

By 1994, HUD was providing nearly $1.2 billion in funding for homelessness services annually. Investigations of homeless programs in major US cities revealed widespread duplication of services with few resources available to address areas of critical need (including care for high-need populations). Examinations also revealed that efforts to bring an end to homelessness were severely lacking and that communities faced substantial difficulties in their attempts to create effective strategies to do so (Interagency Council on the Homeless 1995).

Recognizing that the existing funding strategy did not compel communities to develop coordinated and comprehensive homelessness assistance systems, HUD adopted a new approach to its funding competition, requiring the submission of a single application for all local funding requests that described how each project addressed specific needs and fit within the homeless assistance system. Individual organization applications for program funding were no longer accepted.

HUD also required communities to determine the best uses of homeless dollars through a local prioritization process. In doing so, HUD stipulated that communities (1) establish a local planning process involving various stakeholders, (2) conduct research on the needs of the local homeless population, (3) prioritize areas of greatest need based on this research, (4) create action plans to address needs, and (5) implement their plans to create a more efficient homeless assistance system. Communities were required to rank proposed housing and service projects based on identified priorities. The entire application was then scored by HUD, and specific projects were funded based on how they were prioritized within the application. Finally, HUD called for the development of a "Continuum of Care" – a term that refers to the comprehensive system designed to help people move people from homelessness (or at imminent risk of homelessness) to housing.

The typical homeless care continuum included prevention programs to keep people from becoming homeless, outreach and assessment activities, emergency shelter (typically 30 days or less), transitional housing (i.e., up to 2 years of specialized housing that includes training and supports to prepare people for independent living), permanent housing (i.e., housing with supportive services for persons with a disability or permanent affordable housing – with or without subsidies), and a range of supportive services including counseling, case management, education and job training, employment supports, access to governmental benefits, and budget assistance (U.S. Department of Housing and Urban Development [HUD] 1996; HUD 2002).

The Continuum of Care model called for the movement of homeless persons through locally determined, organized, and comprehensive service delivery systems to support their return to community living and self-sufficiency (HUD 1996). Within the model, there is an implicit assumption that a homeless person's skills and capabilities can and should be increased through their participation in the continuum. As British sociologist Charles Hoch (2000) described:

> The concept of a continuum of care binds the diverse hierarchy together with an underlying rationale of social improvement. The homeless will reach social independence by traveling through the hierarchical continuum of care. First, take the homeless family from the streets to emergency care. Once stabilized, transfer the family to a transitional shelter to outfit the mother and children to enter conventional labor and housing markets (with or without subsidy). After as much as two years of counseling, education, job training and economic support, the mother, equipped with the tools for autonomy, will find employment and an apartment. (p. 867)

As the quote illustrates, different, though complementary, services are necessary to serve the needs of the homeless while requiring cooperation among community entities within the continuum (Ivery 2004).

The opportunity to secure HUD funding for homeless housing and service programs became a powerful incentive for local communities to work together to develop coordinated and comprehensive homelessness assistance systems that offered an array of services necessary to address the diverse needs of homeless persons (HUD 1996). The move also streamlined HUD's competitive grant-making process and encouraged the development of a coordinated, strategic approach to homeless service planning (HUD 2002; Ivery 2004).

Over time, HUD required increased information about the structure and function of local homeless care continuums. Applicants were asked to document existing housing stock for homeless and formerly homeless persons as well as gaps in existing services as indicated by the size and composition of the homeless population. By increasing these requirements, HUD hoped that communities would be stimulated to move toward greater organization and collaboration while building a more strategic vision of their community's homeless assistance system (HUD 2002). Jurisdictions able to develop proposals based on high levels of collaborative planning efforts and well-articulated use of local data were ultimately more successful in securing funding (HUD 2002). The increased structure and rationality were also expected to improve services for homeless people and increase the likelihood that client needs would be met.

The shift to the Continuum of Care model fundamentally changed how business was done among homeless service providers and created systems developed and regularly examined by local communities (Burt et al. 2002; HUD 2002). Regarding the coordination of homeless assistance, the model resulted in the development of local homeless care continuums and the employment of individuals responsible for engaging key community representatives in research and planning efforts. Thus, continuum participants determined how their homeless assistance systems should look.

Similarly, housing providers determined the best approaches for serving their clientele. HUD did not specify which housing or service models could be funded, nor did it dictate the structure or functions of funded programs. As a result, providers drew heavily upon disciplinary guidelines in developing their programming – employing generally accepted practices and creating systems in-line with their professional obligations and values. HUD, in turn, determined the viability of such programs by providing the lion's share of funding for homeless assistance programming.

The Development of Buffalo's Homeless Continuum

In the early 1990s, a local task force was convened to address the problem of homelessness in Buffalo, New York. Recognizing that solutions to the complex problem of homelessness cut across all causes and conditions, the group began to discuss plans to develop a continuum of housing options and support services for people experiencing homelessness.

The early care continuum included a prevention stage (i.e., supports that targeted at-risk populations to prevent the slide into homelessness), emergency stage (i.e., provision of basic support, including food, clothing, and shelter), transitional stage (i.e., provision of intensive support, including linkages with services, rehabilitation, and independent living skill development), and permanent stage (i.e., on-going and lasting supports made available as a foundation for long-term success).

The task force recommended further study of the homeless population through regular data collection and the development of programming based on client-identified needs. It also called for increased coordination and cooperation efforts and the development of a public-private coordinating body that would foster cooperation and coordination across the homeless service system.

A coalition-based organization was made responsible for coordinating the community's resources to address homelessness and was tasked with the following:

1. Facilitating dialogue and strategic action among government, public, private, and foundation sectors to combat homelessness and its impacts
2. Promoting community awareness and education regarding the issues of homelessness and the conditions leading to it
3. Maintaining a central database of local statistics on the homeless population
4. Providing support for agencies in obtaining funding for homeless projects

(continued)

5. Advocating for changes in housing and social service systems to provide greater opportunities for people who are homeless or at risk
6. Working with service providers and community leaders to maximize services and minimize gaps while maintaining dialogue on local needs

The organization would be responsible for engaging the community in strategic planning around homeless service provision by coordinating the local HUD application and by being involved with the development of consolidated plans as well as EFSP and ESG allocation decisions.

Participants from the mental health, substance abuse, domestic violence, disability, elderly, and military/veteran services fields worked together to identify critical issues and devise strategies to address them. They also developed plans to address disciplinary differences – making it possible for organizations to contribute to the continuum without having their service approaches or philosophies regulated.

HUD's Focus on Data and Results

HUD's adoption of the Continuum of Care model roughly corresponded with national movements to increase efficiency, accountability, and confidence among people accessing assistance from the public and private sector. With these movements came a call for results-oriented management – an organizational practice that incorporates the use of outcomes or results into the administration and operation of human service programming (Center for Applied Management Practices 2003; Sawhill and Williamson 2001).

The results-oriented management approach requires agencies to focus on outcomes – the results or products of their activities – in addition to client and program needs (Center for Applied Management Practices 2003). The method includes four areas of focus: planning (directed toward a specific outcome and not just the operation of the program), organizing (addressing how resources are used to carry out a plan), directing (describing the management function, including staff supervision and training where staff are directed toward producing results), and evaluating (part of the feedback loop to determine how successful the program is in achieving its goals).

The imposition of results-oriented management was shaped profoundly by a desire to reinvent government and transform it from a largely bureaucratic entity to a system that could respond to the ever-changing needs of the people it benefits. Proponents of this approach suggested that government should focus on "steering," or providing guidance and direction through funding and federal programming, while "rowing," or producing goods and services, was best left to the private or nonprofit sectors (Poister 2003; Osborne and Gaebler 1992).

Driven by internal and external pressures, and drawing on some of the ideas coming out of the results-oriented management perspective, Congress passed the Government Performance and Results Act (GPRA) of 1993. The legislation's goals included improving the confidence of American citizens in the capabilities of the federal government to hold agencies accountable, improving federal program effectiveness and public accountability, helping federal managers improve service delivery, improving congressional decision-making, and strengthening the internal management of the federal government (Center for Applied Management Practices 2003).

GPRA required government agencies to report strategic goals for budget expenditures annually to the Office of Management and Budget (OMB) and to track performance on predetermined outcomes (Center for Applied Management Practices 2003). In 2001, OMB began to evaluate all programs outlined in the federal budget based on purpose, strategic planning, management, and accountability to determine whether programs were considered effective, moderately effective, adequate, or ineffective. To demonstrate its effectiveness, HUD reconfigured its programs to show a clear focus on mission and strategy – identifying six strategic goals and eight policy priorities. For homeless assistance systems, the move led to the required implementation of new homelessness data collection systems and the development of strategic plans to end homelessness (Center for Applied Management Practices 2003).

Beginning in 1995, the federal government reported spending more than $1 billion per year on services for people experiencing homelessness (U.S. Department of Housing and Urban Development [HUD] 2001). Despite these expenditures, accurate statistics on the number of people served and the number of people who needed additional support did not exist. The lack of precise, outcome-based data made it extremely difficult to justify existing funding levels and caused a great deal of dissatisfaction among policymakers, funders, and advocates (HUD 2001).

In 2001, Congress directed HUD to provide unduplicated data on the extent of homelessness within each of its service continuum areas (HUD 2001). To comply with this directive, HUD required all homeless continuums to implement a computerized Homeless Management Information System (HMIS) capable of producing an unduplicated count of homeless persons, quantifying the use of services, and aiding in the measurement of the local homeless assistance system's effectiveness. Additionally, it was suggested that HMIS programming should enable housing and service providers to share client- and agency-level information within the community through data-sharing agreements.

Ideally, each HMIS system would include information on all housing programs located in a geographic or continuum area. However, HUD recognized that this may not be possible and required a 70% participation rate within 3 years of initiation to be considered compliant (HUD 2001). To that end, HUD administrators included HMIS-specific scoring elements in its Continuum of Care funding application beginning in 2004. Continuums had less than 2 years to research, design, and implement a community-wide HMIS, with limited technical resources or assistance from HUD.

The push toward HMIS required local homeless care continuums to engage a wide variety of new skills, including, but not limited to, examining federal policy and system requirements, scoping the problem to determine the type of information needed, specifying levels of encryption and data security standards, identifying and engaging key community stakeholders, communicating with vendors, negotiating with organizational actors, performing usability tests to secure end user feedback, designing and implementing project plans, securing project resources, conducting HMIS readiness assessments, creating training materials and protocols, developing

HMIS policies and procedures, documenting project activities, establishing required measures, addressing data quality and reporting issues, and engaging in day-to-day problem-solving.

The Buffalo Area Services Network (BAS-Net)

Work on the Buffalo Area Services Network (BAS-Net), Buffalo's HMIS, began during the fall of 2001. Recognizing the importance of buy-in for the local HMIS, project coordinators sought to include community stakeholders in all aspects of the decision-making and planning process.

In their initial meetings, participants identified the potential of the system for each of the continuum's 48 facilities by highlighting its benefits for homeless clients, housing providers, and the community at large. First, the team identified how the HMIS could streamline the intake and assessment process for clients and reduce the amount of information required at program entrance. Second, participants explained how HMIS could expedite the documentation of client and program outcomes making it possible to easily access aggregated records for use in financial and programmatic reports. Finally, participants emphasized the importance of accurate data collection to develop a clearer understanding of the scope of homelessness and effectiveness of interventions within the community.

Following these initial meetings, participants began to envision what a local HMIS might look like, how it could function, and what would be required to get the program off the ground. They called in a local HMIS expert to discuss design options and started to look at available systems.

After almost a year of deliberation, the committee began community education and outreach activities around HMIS in the summer of 2002. The group hosted special presentations and invited housing and service providers to attend so that they could better understand the project. The primary goal of the meetings was to receive critical feedback before deciding on a technology solution or system strategy.

Following these meetings, participants came back to the table re-energized and committed to developing solutions that would address identified concerns. Community member comments were used in narrowing the list of vendors and in determining the direction for the system. Likewise, provider feedback helped the team to develop and solidify critical HMIS-related policies related to access, customizability, confidentiality and HIPAA compliance, performance measurement, and use of the system as a data repository.

By 2004, 42 of the 48 housing programs were included on BAS-Net. The community decided on a set of key measures, which were collected by all participating agencies and used in grant writing, policy advocacy, and community education activities. These measures are also used to determine the effectiveness and efficiency of each program as well as the overall system. A BAS-Net Advisory Committee was also established to address a wide range of issues and to make recommendations regarding changes to HMIS Policies and Procedures.

Despite the challenging timetable and often overwhelming nature of the task, HMIS proved to be an invaluable tool for homeless clients, service providers, care continuums, communities, and funders (Center for Social Policy 2002). Homeless clients benefited from improved opportunities to receive well-coordinated care, more readily accessible information about the availability of beds and other services, and reductions in the information they were required to share when seeking assistance. Homelessness service providers secured improved internal and external data, which allowed for better client tracking. They were also able to streamline their referral processes and strengthen community partnerships while meeting HUD reporting requirements.

Continuums of care were better able to quantify gaps in the system and to gather information for inclusion in their HUD Continuum of Care and other funding applications. Communities developed a better understanding of the problem of homelessness, including its causes and trends, for use in planning, education, and advocacy activities. For HUD and other funders, HMIS provided opportunities to secure data on homelessness assistance systems and their needs for use in funding- and policy-related decision-making (Center for Social Policy 2002).

In keeping with its emphasis on data and results, HUD joined with the National Alliance to End Homelessness (NAEH) and the newly re-formed US Interagency Council on Homelessness in 2004 to promote the development of 10-year plans to address homelessness. Born out of recognition of the powerful role that effective community planning efforts could play in reducing the number of people experiencing homelessness, the campaign began with extensive outreach to various public, private, and nonprofit organizations to raise awareness about its importance among opinion leaders and to build necessary political will (National Alliance to End Homelessness 2000).

The George W. Bush administration and the US Conference of Mayors quickly adopted the 10-year planning strategy to assist a specific subpopulation of the homeless known as the chronically homeless (initially defined as an unaccompanied homeless individual with a disabling condition who has been homeless for 1 year or longer or four or more times in a 3-year period) – setting a national goal of ending chronic homelessness by 2012. Emphasis was placed on the chronically homeless population based on a groundbreaking study, which found that 10% of the homeless population – the chronically homeless – exhausts half the available resources for the homeless population. This is, in general, due to their continued need for high-cost services, including shelter and emergency medical and police services (Culhane et al. 2002).

By 2006, more than 300 US locations committed to developing their own 10-year plans to end chronic homelessness (Culhane and Metraux 2008; Cunningham et al. 2006). While these plans were specific to the community in which they were developed, they often included common elements such as the following:

1. Placement of greater emphasis on quality data collection and best practice research to better understand local conditions and identify solution-focused approaches to directly address the needs of various homeless subpopulations

2. Engagement of a wide variety of community members, including persons responsible for mainstream and homeless-specific resources from state and local mental health, public health, corrections, probation, veterans affairs, housing, and substance abuse departments; substance treatment providers; labor or employment departments, employment service providers, and employers; homeless assistance providers; nonprofit and for-profit housing developers and operators; public assistance providers; and officials from the governor, mayor, or county executive's offices
3. Efforts to "close the front door to homelessness" through greater use of prevention and anti-poverty programs, such as Temporary Assistance for Needy Families (TANF), Mental Health Block Grants, Social Services Block Grant, Substance Abuse Prevention and Treatment Block Grant, Community Services Block Grants, Community Development Block Grants, State Children's Health Insurance Program, Community Health Centers. Medicaid, Public and Indian Housing, Section 8 Rental Certificate and Voucher Programs, Section 811 Supportive Housing for Persons with Disabilities Program, Supplemental Security Income, Veterans Benefits, Veterans Medical Centers, Veterans Employment Programs, Welfare-to-Work Grants, job training, and Youth Employment and Training Programs
4. Development of innovative solutions to end chronic homelessness that would save money as they reduce use of other public systems. For example, the use of safe havens, permanent or semipermanent living spaces, which offer, but do not require, the use of supportive services or strict sobriety as a condition of stay. Also Housing First approaches that place homeless individuals directly into housing units bypassing or significantly shortening stays in emergency shelters with services offered following housing stabilization. Or early rapid rehousing, a type of Housing First program which provides homeless families short-term rental assistance and services, which end once rental assistance terminates
5. Opportunities to build necessary infrastructure by increasing the supply of safe, adequate, and affordable housing; increasing employment and income opportunities; and improving access to health care for disadvantaged populations while recognizing that attempts to change the homeless assistance system must take place within the context of larger efforts to help poor people through public education and awareness, legislator education, and advocacy

The wide development of 10-year plans resulted in a host of new community collaborations and expanded access to needed resources as well as introducing innovative housing and service models and countless other creative solutions to address the complex problem of homelessness (Cunningham et al. 2006).

PRISM: A Community Solution to Homelessness

In the fall of 2003, Buffalo, New York, began its own 10-year planning process to address chronic or long-term homelessness. Drawing on an exhaustive examination of best practice research, the effort focused on five key areas, Prevention, Resources, Independence through Housing, Services, and Maintenance (PRISM), and encouraged participants to look at homelessness using a new perspective.

Community members felt that it was critically important to ground the planning process in the voices of homeless and low-income people. Toward that end, a survey of more than 1000 at-risk, current, and formerly homeless individuals was completed prior to the start of planning efforts.

Additionally, planners felt that homeless advocates and service providers should play a large role in shaping the community's future direction. These individuals participated in a series of open community forums, which corresponded with each of the five key focus areas. Forums were activity-based and drew on both the expertise and creativity of participants. Challenges associated with the local homeless continuum were illuminated and collaborative problem-solving encouraged.

Concurrently, homeless think tanks (i.e., focus groups with homeless persons) were held at various service locations throughout the community. Think tanks were a valuable mechanism that allowed planners to share results from the survey and engage homeless clients, asking "does this seem true to you?" Think tanks were also used to share national best practices in housing and service provision with those currently experiencing homelessness to determine their interest in them.

Taking into consideration not only the input from the community forums but local data collection, homeless think tanks, consultation with key community players, and national best practices, volunteers developed a final plan, made up of 14 goals and broken into four key sections:

1. Education and Empowerment: Highlighting the need for wider awareness and use of mainstream resources and existing community services
2. Continuum of Care Alignment: Improving Buffalo's existing homeless system by developing and codifying systematic approaches and meeting gaps
3. Community Supports: Identifying safe, adequate, and affordable housing and employment as crucial to preventing homelessness and maintaining housing
4. Systems Change: Building public will to institute policies, programs, and campaigns that will end homelessness

Following the release of the plan, PRISM moved into its implementation and evaluation phases, during which progress on specific identified goals was monitored.

Testing New Collaborations, Resources, and Innovative Strategies

In the years following the initial implementation of 10-year plans to end chronic homelessness, there were ample opportunities to draw on newly formed community collaborations, identified community resources, and innovative housing and service models, including new Housing First and Rapid Rehousing approaches.

In 2008, the USA experienced a widespread economic crisis with the collapse of the subprime mortgage industry and in the wake of the bursting housing bubble (Florida 2009). While the collapse of large financial institutions was prevented by the national bailout of banks, stock markets dropped worldwide (Florida 2009). The crisis played a significant role in the failure of key businesses, declines in consumer wealth (estimated in trillions of US dollars), and a downturn in economic activity. In many communities, the housing market also suffered, resulting in evictions and foreclosures, and people experienced prolonged periods of unemployment (Florida 2009; Immergluck 2009).

To stave off the crisis, Congress passed the American Recovery and Reinvestment Act (ARRA) in 2009 with a primary objective of saving existing jobs and creating new ones as soon as possible. Additionally, ARRA established temporary relief programs for those most affected by the recession, including $1.5 billion for the Homelessness Prevention and Rapid Re-Housing Program (HPRP). HPRP funds were distributed to communities based on the ESG formula.

HPRP charged funded communities with creating partnerships and program models to quickly help more than 1.3 million people across the nation to find or keep their housing (U.S. Department of Housing and Urban Development [HUD] 2017a). To be eligible, individuals or families needed to be at or below 50% of the area median income (AMI) and to demonstrate that they would be homeless "but for" the assistance. HPRP participants met with a case manager to determine their needs and secure financial assistance as well as housing relocation and stabilization services. In addition to efforts included through ARRA, President Obama signed the Homeless Emergency Assistance and Rapid Transition to Housing (HEARTH) Act (Public Law 111-22; S. 896) into law in 2009. The goal of this legislation was to significantly expand homelessness prevention programming and to provide new incentives for the use of rapid rehousing models, especially for homeless families.

HEARTH legislation created substantial changes in the Emergency Shelter Grant program including (1) changing its name to the Emergency Solutions Grant (ESG) to signify its shift to funding homelessness prevention and rehousing efforts as well as emergency shelter; (2) increasing eligible activities to include prevention and rehousing activities (such as short- and midterm rental assistance, housing relocation or stabilization services, and moving costs); (3) expanding eligibility criteria to include people who are at risk of homelessness including people who have earned less than 30% of AMI and move frequently due to economic reasons; live doubled-up;

are facing eviction; live in a hotel, motel, or severely overcrowded housing; or are exiting an institution; and (4) making significant changes in the amount of ESG funding available and how that funding could be used (National Alliance to End Homelessness 2009).

HEARTH also expanded the definition of homelessness – making it possible to use limited HUD Continuum of Care funding (up to 10%) for people who were not previously considered homeless. The new definition included situations where a person is at imminent risk of homelessness or where a family or unaccompanied youth is living unstably. Here, imminent risk included situations in which the person must leave their current housing within 14 days with no other place to go and no other resources or support networks available to assist them in obtaining housing (National Alliance to End Homelessness 2009).

While McKinney-Vento Homeless Assistance was reauthorized through the passage of the HEARTH Act, there were a variety of modifications made to HUD Continuum of Care funding. Most notably, SHP, S+C, and Moderate Rehabilitation programs were consolidated into a single Continuum of Care program, and rehousing services were added as an eligible activity. Thirty percent of all Continuum of Care funding (nationally) was designed for new permanent housing for individuals with a disabling condition or families with an adult member who has a disabling condition. At least 10% of funding was slated for permanent housing activities for homeless families. Finally, HUD was required to provide incentives for use of strategies proven to reduce homelessness, including rapid rehousing and permanent supportive housing for chronically homeless persons (National Alliance to End Homelessness 2009).

Within 18 months of the HEARTH legislation's signing, Congress required HUD to make regulations for implementing the new McKinney-Vento programs known. HUD issued its interim rule in July 2012 focusing on regulatory implementation of the Continuum of Care program, especially as it related to the Continuum of Care planning process. The ruling also called for mandatory use of coordinated entry and assessment, a process designed to organize housing and service program intake, assessment, and referral processes using standardized tools (U.S. Department of Housing and Urban Development [HUD] 2012).

HUD explained that the coordinated entry and assessment system would be used for entrance into emergency shelter, transitional housing, and permanent supportive housing as well as prevention, diversion, and rapid rehousing programming. Once properly implemented, system operators would know the entry criteria for all local programs and would send people who met eligibility criteria to an appropriate program. Operators would also be able to accommodate special needs and consumer preferences, wherever possible (HUD 2012).

Drawing on the experiences of HPRP, local homeless care continuums were obligated to establish and operate a coordinated entry and assessment system that provided an initial comprehensive assessment of the housing and service needs of all homeless individuals and families. The new rule also required all HUD-funded programs (including former Emergency Shelter Grant, now Emergency Solutions Grant awardees, and Continuum of Care awardees) to use the coordinated entry and assessment system developed (HUD 2012).

The coordinated entry and assessment system was required to cover a specified geographic area, to be well-advertised, and to be easily accessed by individuals and families seeking housing or services. A specific policy was required to guide the operation of the coordinated entry and assessment system – detailing how the system would address the unique needs of individuals and families fleeing, or attempting to flee, domestic violence, dating violence, sexual assault, or stalking but who are seeking shelter or services from non-victim service providers. HUD also required that the screening, assessment, and referrals completed by HUD funding recipients (and sub-recipients) were consistent with the written standards established by the local homelessness continuums of care, utilizing a comprehensive and standardized assessment tool (HUD 2012).

Aside from the requirement established by HUD, there were a number of reasons to consider implementation of coordinated entry and assessment, including reducing the burden placed on consumers who are already experiencing a high degree of stress in their lives, improving the speed at which a person or family can be appropriately housed, improving collaboration among service providers, streamlining referrals and ensuring easier access to services, prioritizing and more effectively addressing the needs of hard-to-serve clients, and improving system performance overall.

There were also numerous challenges associated with the design and implementation of coordinated entry and assessment systems, including the lack of available resources to fund its undertaking; capacity challenges especially related to geography; communication barriers; issues of client non-compliance, safety, and liability; external regulation; and other organizational considerations (HUD 2017b). Nevertheless, homeless care continuums across the country have moved forward with their design and implementation (HUD 2017b).

Coordinated Entry and Assessment in Buffalo, New York

More than 45 representatives from 30 organizations as well as county-level departments of social services and mental health participated in a series of workshops to develop the coordinated entry and assessment system in Buffalo, New York.

Prior to beginning their work together, participants established ground rules and a set of guiding principles for coordinated entry and assessment suggesting that efforts should:

- Seek to minimize wait, be easy to use and understand, and focus on positive customer experiences.
- Be based on an objective and standardized assessment conducted by well-trained and well-qualified professionals.

(continued)

- Be client-centered and client-driven with a focus on offering services that fit specific needs.
- Ensure the availability and accessibility of holistic services for all clients.

The overall goal was to develop long-term solutions for people in need rather than short-term fixes. Participants also stressed that specific consideration must be given to hard-to-serve populations, including domestic violence victims, victims of human trafficking, persons with limited English proficiency, persons with disabling conditions (including senior citizens), sex offenders, arsonists, and people with recent felony convictions.

Participants mapped each segment of the care continuum from prevention and diversion through permanent supportive housing – to identify critical gaps that would need to be addressed for coordinated entry and assessment to be successful. They also articulated the importance of using a standardized assessment tool with a scoring mechanism to determine the most appropriate referrals; a well-trained, neutral staff to complete assessments; flexible access to the coordinated entry and assessment system with 24/7 availability; transparency in program criteria; use of up-to-date resource information; and regular evaluation of all aspects of the process.

Participants reviewed the coordinated entry and assessment systems developed in communities across the nation, ultimately opting to develop a hybrid model using an existing hotline to identify individuals in need of assistance and a centralized, professional assessment team housed at the local department of social services.

An initial implementation action plan was developed, and committees formed to complete various activities, including development of the standardized assessment tool, establishment of qualifications and training for the coordinated entry and assessment team, development of policies and procedures for the referral process, and determinations about oversight mechanisms and evaluation strategies for the coordinated entry and assessment system.

Conclusions

Over the past several decades, housing providers, advocates, and municipalities have been repeatedly called upon to develop community-based strategies to address the problem of homelessness. This chapter highlights some of the key strengths and unintended consequences of these community-based efforts. It also suggests a need for additional social work research related to the various functions played by community operatives – including research, service linkage, planning, policy-making, evaluation, and collaborative problem-solving – and the role they play in developing and supporting homelessness assistance systems. Such research would contribute to the knowledge base and help to identify opportunities to build social work practitioners' skills.

Following the economic downturn of the 1970s and 1980s, few homeless-specific resources were available to address the rapidly growing need for assistance among diverse homeless populations. The assistance that was available was highly disorganized, duplicative, and fractured. To address this problem, housing and service providers came together to form comprehensive homelessness assistance systems that included prevention, outreach and assessment, emergency shelter, transitional housing, permanent housing, and a range of supportive services to encourage the return to community living and self-sufficiency.

Homelessness continuums of care have historically been challenged to make difficult decisions – engaging in research and community-wide planning activities to identify critical gaps in services and prioritizing the development of specific housing and services. When funding for these programs was imperiled by the lack of clear evidence demonstrating their effectiveness, community actors stepped into new and difficult roles, developing highly technical and complicated management information systems to benefit homeless clients, service providers, care continuums, communities, and funders alike.

Finally, continuums of care have been instrumental in the development of effective strategies to end homelessness – crossing organizational, sectoral, and disciplinary boundaries to form new collaborations; identifying critical community resources; and implementing effective homeless housing and service models, such as Housing First. Whether undertaken at the request of a funder, as part of a larger advocacy effort, or sparked by opportunities to innovate, communities play a critical role in efforts to solve this complex problem.

References

Baumohl, J. (1996). *Homelessness in America*. Phoenix: The Oryx Press.

Burt, M. R., Aron, L. Y., & Lee, E. (2002). *Helping America's homeless: Emergency shelter or affordable housing?* Washington, D.C.: Urban Institute Press.

Center for Applied Management Practices. (2003) Results-oriented management and accountability satellite training. https://apps.hud.gov/offices/adm/grants/training/LMpresentation.doc. Accessed 11 Oct 2017.

Center for Social Policy. (2002). *Homeless management information systems: Implementation guide*. Boston: John W. McCormack Institute of Public Affairs.

Culhane, D. P., & Metraux, S. (2008). Rearranging the deck chairs or reallocating the lifeboats? Homelessness assistance and its alternatives. *Journal of the American Planning Association, 74*(1), 111–121.

Culhane, D. P., Metraux, S., & Hadly, T. (2002). The impact of supportive housing for homeless people with severe mental illness on the utilization of public health, corrections, and emergency shelter systems: The New York-New York initiative. *Housing Policy Debate, 13*(1), 107–163.

Cunningham, M., Lear, M., Schmitt, E., & Henry, M. (2006). *A new vision: What is in community plans to end homelessness?* Washington, D.C.: National Alliance to End Homelessness.

Emergency Food and Shelter National Board. (n.d.). About us. https://www.efsp.unitedway.org/efsp/website/websiteContents/index.cfm?template=about.cfm. Accessed 11 Oct 2017.

Florida, R. (2009, March). How the crash will reshape America. *Atlantic Monthly*. https://www.theatlantic.com/magazine/archive/2009/03/how-the-crash-will-reshape-america/307293/. Accessed 10 Oct 2017.

Hoch, C. (2000). Sheltering the homeless in the US: Social improvement and the continuum of care. *Housing Studies, 15*, 865–876.

Immergluck, D. (2009). The foreclosure crisis, foreclosed properties, and federal policy: Some implications for housing and community development planning. *Journal of the American Planning Association, 75*(4), 406–423.

Interagency Council on the Homeless. (1995). *Priority home! The federal plan to break the cycle of homelessness*. Washington, D.C.: Author.

Ivery, J. M. (2004). *An examination of factors that influence the motivation for participation in a collaborative partnership of homeless service providers* (Unpublished doctoral dissertation). Virginia Commonwealth University, Virginia.

Kusmer, K. L. (2002). *Down and out, on the road: The homeless in American history*. Oxford, UK: Oxford University Press.

Mintz, S., & Kellogg, S. (1988). *Domestic revolutions: A social history of American family life*. New York: The Free Press.

Mumford, M. D., Zaccaro, S. J., Harding, F. D., Jacobs, T. O., & Fleishman, E. A. (2010). Leadership skills for a changing world: Solving complex social problems. *Leadership Quarterly, 11*, 11–35.

National Alliance to End Homelessness. (2000). *A plan: Not a dream. How to end homelessness in ten years*. Washington, D.C.: National Alliance to End Homelessness.

National Alliance to End Homelessness. (2009). Summary of HEARTH Act. https://endhomelessness.org/resource/summary-of-hearth-act-2/. Accessed 11 Oct 2017.

National Coalition for the Homeless. (2006). Fact sheet on The Stewart B. McKinney Homeless Assistance Act. https://web.archive.org/web/20071203073025/http://www.nationalhomeless.org/publications/facts/McKinney.pdf. Accessed 11 Oct 2017.

Osborne, D., & Gaebler, T. (1992). *Reinventing government: How the entrepreneurial spirit is transforming the public sector*. Reading: Addison-Wesley.

Perrault, E., McClelland, R., Austin, C., & Sieppert, J. (2011). Working together in collaborations: Successful process factors for community collaboration. *Administration in Social Work, 35*(2), 282–298.

Poister, T. H. (2003). *Measuring performance in public and nonprofit organizations*. San Francisco: Jossey-Bass.

Public Law H.R. 100-77; HR 558. (1987). *The Stewart B. McKinney Homeless Assistance Act* of 1987.

Public Law 111-22; S. 896. (2009). Homeless Emergency Assistance and Rapid Transition to Housing Act of 2009.

Roberts, N. C. (2000). Wicked problems and network approaches to resolution. *The International Public Management Review, 1*, 1–19.

Rossi, P. (1989). *Down and out in America: The origins of homelessness*. Chicago: University of Chicago Press.

Sawhill, J. C., & Williamson, D. (2001). Mission impossible? Measuring success in nonprofit organizations. *Nonprofit Management and Leadership, 11*, 371–386.

Thompson, L. (2013). *Creative conspiracy: The new rules of breakthrough collaboration*. Boston: Harvard Business Review Press.

United States Bureau of Labor Statistics. (2017). Unemployment data Buffalo city New York. https://www.google.com/publicdata/explore?ds=z1ebjpgk2654c1_&met_y=unemployment_rate&idim=city:CT3611000000000:CT3663000000000&fdim_y=seasonality:U&hl=en&dl=en. Accessed 11 Oct 2017.

United States Census Bureau. (2017). Quick facts: Buffalo city, New York. https://www.census.gov/quickfacts/fact/table/buffalocitynewyork/PST045216. Accessed 10 Oct 2017.

United States Department of Housing and Urban Development [HUD]. (1984). *A report to the secretary on the homeless and emergency shelters*. Washington, D.C.: Author.

United States Department of Housing and Urban Development [HUD]. (1989). *A report on the 1988 National Survey of shelters for the homeless*. Washington, D.C.: Author.

United States Department of Housing and Urban Development [HUD]. (1996). *Guide to Continuum of Care planning and implementation*. Washington, D.C.: Author.

United States Department of Housing and Urban Development [HUD]. (2001). *Report to Congress: HUD's strategy for homeless data collection, analysis, and reporting*. Washington, D.C.: Author.

United States Department of Housing and Urban Development [HUD]. (2002). *Evaluation of Continuums of Care for homeless people*. Washington, D.C.: Author.

United States Department of Housing and Urban Development [HUD]. (2012). Homeless Emergency Assistance and Rapid Transition to Housing (HEARTH): CoC program interim rule. https://www.hudexchange.info/resource/2033/hearth-coc-program-interim-rule/. Accessed 11 Oct 2017.

United States Department of Housing and Urban Development [HUD]. (2017a). HPRP promising practices and success stories. https://www.hudexchange.info/programs/hprp/hprp-promising-practices-and-success-stories/. Accessed 11 Oct 2017.

United States Department of Housing and Urban Development [HUD]. (2017b). Coordinated entry core elements guidebook. https://www.hudexchange.info/resources/documents/Coordinated-Entry-Core-Elements.pdf. Accessed 11 Oct 2017.

Weinreb, L., & Rossi, P. H. (1995). The American homeless family shelter system. *Social Service Review, 37*, 86–107.

Chapter 8
Homelessness in Los Angeles and New York City: A Tale of Two Cities

Benjamin F. Henwood and Deborah K. Padgett

Introduction

Each year, the Department of Housing and Urban Development (HUD) produces an Annual Homeless Assessment Report (AHAR) to Congress that estimates the size of the country's homeless population based on a point-in-time (PIT) count conducted by local jurisdictions. In 2016, it was estimated that 549,928 people experienced homelessness on a single night, with 32% unsheltered or sleeping rough. Of this number, almost 121,000 were children (22% of the total), 35,686 were unaccompanied youth ages 18–24 (7% of the total), and over one-third were experiencing homelessness as part of a family (US Department of Housing and Urban Development [HUD] 2016). While there may be concerns about the accuracy of these estimates, undercounts are more likely than overcounts of the numbers of homeless persons in the USA.

Since 2010, the overall trend in the number of homeless Americans has been declining. Still, in certain high-cost cities, including the two largest in the USA – New York City (NYC) and Los Angeles (LA) – there are record high numbers of people experiencing homelessness. In fact, 20% of the overall homeless population in the USA can be found in these two cities (HUD 2016), where the number of low-income renters far outstrips the number of affordable units by over 500,000 (Joint Center for Housing Studies 2017).

Electronic supplementary material: The online version of this chapter (https://doi.org/10.1007/978-3-030-03727-7_8) contains supplementary material, which is available to authorized users.

B. F. Henwood (✉)
University of Southern California, Los Angeles, CA, USA
e-mail: bhenwood@usc.edu

D. K. Padgett
New York University, New York, NY, USA
e-mail: dkp1@nyu.edu

H. Larkin et al. (eds.), *Homelessness Prevention and Intervention in Social Work*, https://doi.org/10.1007/978-3-030-03727-7_8

Although NYC and LA have much in common, including large homeless populations and significant income inequality (Berube 2014), there has been a significant divergence in how each city has approached the homelessness crisis that was first recognized in the 1980s (Padgett et al. 2015). With a strong state-city agreement to fund housing and shelters and a right-to-shelter legal mandate that requires the city to provide temporary shelter, NYC followed an assertive and multifaceted approach. In contrast, in LA where the warmer climate may contribute to a higher number of homeless people willing to sleep outdoors, there was a narrower focus of relying on faith-based organizations to provide shelter and concentrating the homeless population in a circumscribed Skid Row. These differences are reflected in the proportion of people who are sheltered versus unsheltered in each location. In 2016, three out of four people experiencing homelessness (a total of 34,189 people) were unsheltered in LA, whereas nearly all people experiencing homelessness (a total of 70,685 people) in NYC were sheltered (HUD 2016).

In this chapter, we describe this country's response to a homelessness crisis that began in the early 1980s and explain how the rise of Housing First, an evidence-based approach to ending homelessness that gained national prominence in the early 2000s, changed the national conversation from managing to ending homelessness (Padgett et al. 2015). Using this as background, we then describe how two US cities – NYC and LA – approached homelessness in vastly different ways, a reflection of each city's unique history, evolving social priorities, and civic values. We specifically examine how these differences played out and consider how addressing such local variation is critical to future efforts to end homelessness.

Responding to the Homelessness Crisis

A large governmental response to the homelessness crisis in the 1980s set the stage for explosive growth in the 1990s of a vast array of homeless services that would become the "homelessness services industrial complex" (Padgett et al. 2015). This patchwork of national, state, and local programs was influenced by three sequential and overlapping approaches – charitable, rights-based, and business model (Padgett et al. 2015). The charitable approach is rooted in traditional faith-based charities, such as rescue missions, that were places to dry out, get a meal, and hear a sermon. Included in this lineage are much larger but still charity-driven philanthropic organizations that are generally secular and more broadly defined in purpose. The rights-based approach reflects a manifestation of human rights activism that puts advocacy first by raising public consciousness and arguing for the human right to housing, which is no small effort (Byrne and Culhane 2011). The business model approach, which represented public-private partnerships infused with business practices, arose as homeless organizations expanded in size and scale and as private donors and businesses became more influential. Although profits were not the goal, homeless organizations could presumably benefit from business practices, such as monitoring productivity, maintaining quality assurance, and focusing on results. This also made the public-private partnerships go more smoothly since both sides shared the same language.

The system that emerged from these three approaches blended temporary housing and services into a staircase, with shelters at the bottom, permanent housing at the top, and treatment adherence being central to movement up the staircase (see Fig. 8.1). The steps immediately above emergency shelters consisted of various forms of transitional housing, ranging from dormitory-style community residences to single-room occupancy (SRO) buildings to congregate apartments (toward the middle steps). These low and middle steps of the staircase – temporary, supervised, and rule-driven (e.g., mandating curfews, abstinence, and medication compliance) – absorbed the overwhelming majority of homeless individuals willing to come in off the street. A very small minority made their way (through good behavior and lucky timing) to the coveted top step. As a consequence, many homeless people became caught up in the "institutional circuit" of going from streets to jails to hospitals to shelters (Hopper et al. 1997) for years at a time.

Housing First (HF), which originated in NYC in 1992 with the establishment of Pathways to Housing, Inc. by Dr. Sam Tsemberis, rose out of and posed a direct challenge to the staircase approach by offering immediate access to permanent housing to homeless adults with serious mental illness. In other words, the individual is able to leap to the top step without preconditions other than agreeing to case management home visits and maintaining the apartment according to the lease agreement expected of any tenant. As such, HF represented a paradigm shift for homeless services by replacing a well-established "housing readiness" assessment with the idea that all people are deserving of housing.

Positioning access to permanent housing as the first – rather than last – step not only reversed the staircase order, it also sent a message of respect and dignity that encouraged clients to engage in support services tailored to their needs. The basic principle of consumer choice in HF differs fundamentally from "treatment-first" or staircase services in two ways: (1) taking psychiatric medications is not a requirement

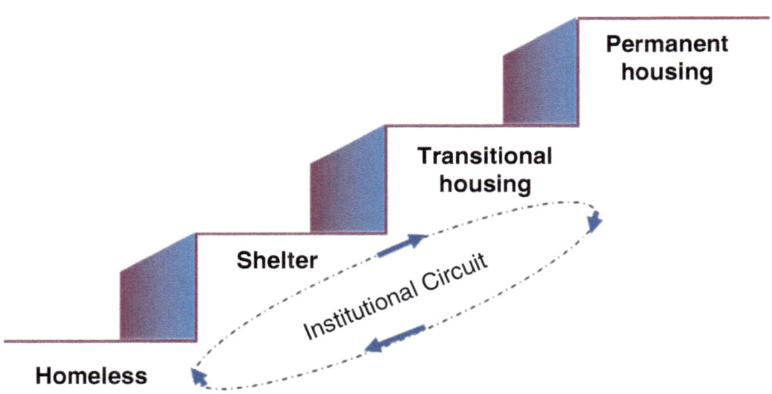

Fig. 8.1 A staircase approach to housing and services

(although HF psychiatrists are central to its team approach); and (2) HF programs practice harm reduction with respect to use of alcohol and drugs. In this context, harm reduction means that consumers do not lose their housing if still using substances (even though substance abuse specialists are a central part of HF service provision). Put another way, housing is both an intervention (and the gateway to engagement into services) and a human right.

As a direct challenge to the status quo, HF has had a pronounced effect in shaping funding and policies for homeless services throughout the USA. An extensive body of research in the USA and abroad shows that HF produces robust positive outcomes, including housing stability, cost savings, and reductions in drug and alcohol use (Padgett et al. 2015). By 2007, HF was strongly endorsed by HUD in its directives to local jurisdictions seeking federal funding. It was also adopted by the US Department of Veterans Affairs in a cooperative initiative known as the HUD-VASH (Veterans Affairs Supportive Housing) program. HUD-VASH has reduced veteran homelessness by nearly 50% since its implementation (HUD 2016). However, as we discuss in the next section, the accumulating evidence of HF's success that led to its adoption in many cities (and countries), including Los Angeles, did little to change the policies of its city of origin.

Homelessness in New York City: A Concerted Civic Response

NYC was the epicenter of the US homelessness crisis in the 1980s, a crisis that persisted despite fluctuations in the US economy and the city's burgeoning efforts to stem the tide. After a near-disastrous economic downturn in the 1970s, NYC began a period of economic recovery in which rising property values, increasing income inequality, and an aging affordable housing stock placed its economically vulnerable citizens in a precarious state of housing insecurity.

By the late 1980s, the appearance of people sleeping rough was becoming commonplace. Visible amidst million-dollar condos and gleaming office buildings, homeless men and women were no longer confined to the Lower East Side's Bowery district as in earlier years (Hopper 2002). Labeled vagrants and bag ladies, they filled city and private shelters and slept rough in doorways, in parks, and on the subways. The problematic behaviors of those in the throes of psychosis, addiction, or both were frequently the subject of media reports portraying the homeless as dangerous and deranged. Though constituting only one-third of the homeless population, persons with serious mental illness were stereotypically singled out as a public nuisance despite their status as victims of systemic neglect (Susser et al. 1989).

NYC in the early 1990s experienced growing calls for law and order spurred by sensational media reports of crime and public disorder. The election of Mayor Rudolph Giuliani in 1993 ushered in a new era of law enforcement rooted in the "broken windows" theory of policing, whereby minor "quality-of-life" offenses are vigorously prosecuted as threats to public order and a deterrent to more serious crimes. Under the leadership of NYC Police Chief William Bratton, enforcement of this policy intensified the criminalization of street homeless persons. By virtue of living outdoors, acts of daily living, such as urination, sleeping in doorways, and drinking alcohol, rendered these men and women liable to citations, fines, and arrests (Blasi 2007).

From Charity to State-City Cooperation in Public Funding

As in the rest of the nation, NYC's faith-based charities were among the first to come forward. Churches and synagogues drew on volunteers and donations to offer soup kitchens, clothing drives, and small night shelters on their premises (usually in the basement). However, the scope of the problem, along with a long-standing civic commitment to publicly funded services, led to an unprecedented level of state-city cooperation to alleviate it.

The groundbreaking New York/New York (NY/NY) Agreement enacted in 1990 was based upon state-city cooperation in allocating funds for 3615 apartments to house mentally ill homeless adults (Houghton 2001). Allocated through its Office of Mental Health, this funding was the state's first foray into housing provision and an acknowledgment that recovery from serious mental illness entails more than psychiatric treatment. For its part, NYC issued municipal bonds to build supportive housing units and fund rental vouchers for existing units (Houghton 2001). The concept of supportive housing pioneered in New York State entailed subsidized rent (to make housing affordable) along with support services typically located within the building where clients lived. Still in existence at this writing, the NY/NY Agreements have grown in funding and scope; the last iteration (NY/NY III) enacted in 2005 promised 9000 units of supportive housing (Supportive Housing Network of New York 2006).

From the beginning, the NY/NY Agreements relied on contracting with private nonprofit organizations to render services for formerly homeless adults living in dormitory-style settings or shared apartments in buildings occupied by other vulnerable groups, such as the elderly or persons with AIDS. Although NIMBY (not in my backyard) responses led to concentrations of such residences in NYC's more tolerant (or less empowered) neighborhoods, the expansion of supportive housing for psychiatrically disabled New Yorkers grew rapidly in the 1990s. Yet, the supply could not meet the growing demand, nor did it address the needs of people without serious mental illness, such as families and single adults down on their luck but not disabled. For these individuals, the city's shelter system was their primary destination.

Advocacy and the Right-to-Shelter Court Ruling

Early on, NYC was a home to strong advocacy groups seeking rights as well as services for the homeless. The Partnership for the Homeless – founded by activist attorney Peter Smith in 1982 – was a group of faith-based organizations that combined charitable efforts with advocacy. The Coalition for the Homeless, founded in 1981, effectively used litigation to bring attention to the city's homeless people and spur action on their behalf. The Coalition's co-founder, attorney Robert Hayes, was instrumental in bringing about the landmark Callahan v. Carey decision in 1981, a court-ordered consent decree that made NYC the nation's leader in guaranteeing a legal right to shelter. This decree led to a near-tripling of shelter beds in the city (Houghton 2001). As the years progressed and homelessness did not abate, the right to shelter became the fallback explanation for the city's policies favoring shelters over permanent housing. City officials argued, with little evidence, that access to housing (rather than a shelter bed) was a perverse incentive that might draw non-homeless families into the system and overwhelm its capacity.

The Rise of a Homeless Services Industry and Housing First

Growing levels of federal, state, and local funding helped shape the evolution of a homeless services industry in NYC in which nonprofit organizations competed for multi-million-dollar contracts to work with the city's shelters, hospitals, and jails to ensure homeless persons had access to emergency shelter and services. As such, the industry depended on a vast number of employees – outreach workers, shelter staff, security guards, cooks, drivers, case managers, janitors, administrators, executive directors, etc. As mentioned earlier, permanent supportive housing for persons with psychiatric disabilities was made possible by the NY/NY Agreement, but providers were far more likely to offer transitional housing in keeping with the presumed need for treatment compliance and supervision amidst congregate living. Homeless families were placed in group shelters and cluster housing (aging and often dilapidated hotels and buildings rented at above-market rates from private landlords).

The beginning of HF took place in 1992, a few years into the city's homelessness crisis. HF founder Sam Tsemberis worked closely with attorneys, psychiatrists, and social workers to ensure that Pathways to Housing, Inc. gained a foothold in the city's emerging homeless industry. Relying on assertive community treatment (ACT) teams and close working relationships with private landlords, Pathways provided immediate access to scatter-site apartments and supportive services for homeless single adults with serious mental illness.

Unique in its consumer choice approach, Pathways took advantage of the same funding streams that staircase programs depended on and grew to serve over 300 tenants annually (Padgett et al. 2015). Despite its growth, Pathways remained small compared to the expansive multifaceted staircase programs dominating the landscape of homeless services in the city, such as Bowery Residents' Committee, Common Ground, Project Renewal, and The Bridge, Inc. In contrast to this small local role, the national impact of HF expanded rapidly after 2006, and it became widely adopted by many cities across the USA and Canada (Padgett et al. 2015).

High Levels of Public Funding, Low Levels of Progress

At this writing, NYC's Department of Homeless Services has an annual budget of over one billion dollars of which virtually all goes to shelters. This funding by far exceeds what is spent in any other jurisdiction (city, county, or state) in the USA. There are a couple disconcerting footnotes to this observation. First, in 2016, the city experienced its largest homeless count in history – over 68,000 in number. Second, the original Pathways to Housing, Inc. closed in 2014 due to poor management decisions and inadequate funding to cover shortfalls amidst shrinking Medicaid reimbursements. In part due to its small size, Pathways lacked the funding stability to survive in a highly competitive staircase-driven service environment.

NYC's homeless service sector, while nonprofit in designation, adopted a business model approach to sustaining an industry that employed thousands ranging from low-paid case managers to highly compensated executives (some salaries rivaling those earned in the for-profit sector). These organizations grew to be large bureaucracies with heavy administrative and labor costs, their sustenance comprised of NY/NY funds as well as government programs, including Medicaid and federal McKinney-Vento funds.

Relatively high levels of public funding for homeless services have been maintained despite recent cuts in federal funding from the US Department of Housing and Urban Development (HUD) due to the city's heavy reliance on shelters over permanent housing (Nahmias 2016). Despite decreases nationally in 2016, the spike in homeless numbers in NYC was a dismaying reminder that the problem appears to be impervious to status quo solutions. In response to renewed public outcry, Mayor Bill De Blasio released a policy statement in early 2017 promising to build 90 new shelters and renovate 30 additional shelters, with the city's police department providing security (City of New York 2017). Although the need for affordable housing is prominently mentioned in the statement, the action items are distinctly familiar – HF is not mentioned in its 128 pages. Mayor De Blasio, NYC's most progressive leader in recent memory, projected a hoped-for but modest 4% decrease in homelessness over 10 years, relying on shelters as the means to this end.

Summarizing NYC's response to homelessness, the charitable approach was supplanted early on by relatively generous public funding and rights-based guarantees. Nurtured by public funding from national and local sources, a burgeoning industry emerged that united public officials and nonprofit programs in a massive common enterprise. Fundamental to this growth were civic values favoring government action on behalf of the poor and vigorous advocacy and litigation to ensure that such action did not falter.

The national shift toward HF and permanent housing has left NYC in a unique position as the most generous yet among the least innovative homeless service providers in the nation. To be sure, the city has experienced population growth and sharp income disparities alongside shrinking stocks of affordable housing. Although the supply-demand ratio of affordable housing is indeed a serious problem, several countervailing forces favor status quo over evidence-proven solutions. Homeless advocates point with pride to the city's right-to-shelter mandate as unparalleled nationally in its scope (having no restrictions based on weather or season). Meanwhile, city officials cite the shelter mandate as justification for diverting funds from permanent housing solutions to shelter building and upkeep (under threat of litigation if shelter beds are not readily available). A seemingly intractable bind emerges with this emphasis on building new shelters as it has reinvigorated NIMBY reactions from local community leaders.

Also favoring the status quo is an assortment of stakeholders, such as landlords who reap profits from the city's renting of run-down buildings and shelters and nonprofit agencies upon whom thousands depend for jobs including some top executives who receive corporate-level salaries. These programs are verbally supportive of permanent supportive housing, if for no other reason than it is a priority for federal funding and has achieved international prominence. However, despite its distinction as the original home of HF, NYC does not have a faithful enactment of a HF program at this writing. Hybrid approaches, such as tying permanent housing to treatment requirements or allowing more lenient supervision in congregate housing, abound in the meantime.

The city is home to several large philanthropies, and some, such as the Robin Hood Foundation, are focused on ending poverty and homelessness. However worthy, wealthy donations cannot provide housing for the poor, as creating affordable housing is a structural change dependent on political will as well as public and private funding. Compared to other cities, NYC does not lack for funding, and its progressive leaders have in recent years made valiant efforts to change course. However, the city has deeply entrenched special interest groups who have little to gain from structural changes favoring lower-income residents. In this environment, the city continues to manage, rather than end, homelessness.

Homelessness in Los Angeles: Containment and Charity

Between 2016 and 2017, homelessness increased by 20% in LA from approximately 28,000 to 34,000 people experiencing homelessness on a given night (LAHSA 2017a). Much of the increase reflects broad-scale housing insecurity, with only 25% of all households in LA having sufficient income to afford the median monthly home payment (Joint Center for Housing Studies 2017). Of those who are homeless, only 26%, or almost 9,000 people, stay in shelters, leaving the vast majority residing on the streets, in tents, in makeshift shelters, or living out of vehicles. The visibility of street homelessness in LA is nowhere more apparent than in Skid Row, where approximately 5000 homeless men and women occupy the streets and sidewalks. There is no greater concentration of homeless adults in America than is found in this 50-square block area in downtown LA. Still, most people who experience homelessness in Los Angeles can be found outside of Skid Row, and other densely concentrated areas of homelessness exist in Venice and Hollywood. Without a legal mandate to provide shelter, as is the case in NYC, and favorable weather that prevents front-page stories about people freezing to death on the streets, shelter beds remain limited so that the vast majority of people experiencing homelessness in LA are unsheltered. In short, homelessness is increasingly visible throughout LA, which has resulted in public outcry and requests from public officials that the Governor of California declare a state of emergency (Sewell 2016) – an emergency that was decades in the making.

Policy of Containment

The current condition of Skid Row better resembles a refugee camp than the center of one of America's great cities. On any given day, the streets of Skid Row are lined with makeshift shelters and tents – and bodies – of people who are experiencing homelessness. Today's Skid Row grew out of explicit policy in the 1970s and 1980s that was officially described in city planning documents as a "containment policy," which referred to concentrating services for the poorest people in one area of the city (Keil 1998). This policy created a "service-dependent ghetto" that continues today and runs contrary to decentralization efforts of homelessness and poverty that occurred in most other major urban areas, including NYC (Goetz 1992; Wolch and Dear 1993).

In Skid Row, faith-based missions have a long history as key partners in homeless services that became even more important as homelessness in Skid Row continued to rise in the late 1980s and 1990s. In fact, Skid Row offers a rare example of an area that embraced faith-based missions (including the Midnight Mission, Open Door Skid Row Ministry, Los Angeles Mission and Union Rescue Mission) as key partners in homeless services, not only in the past (as many cities have done) but continuing into the present (as few cities have done). Although missions have been the recipients of significant funding as homeless shelters, their position within a linear staircase model has left them vulnerable given the federal policy shift toward HF.

Today, missions still serve a vital role in providing shelter but now have other neighboring organizations that provide permanent supportive housing (PSH). Some programs, such as SRO Housing Corporation, come from a tradition rooted in a treatment-first approach, while others, including Downtown Women's Center and Skid Row Housing Trust (SRHT), have long been advocates of HF. These organizations work within the Skid Row area to provide apartment buildings so that people maintain their residency in Skid Row as they transition from homelessness to housing. This approach continues to concentrate disadvantage but also recognizes Skid Row as a legitimate community unto itself – regardless of how ill-conceived the development of the community may have been. In this process, SRHT has pioneered high-end architectural design within single-site PSH programs both inside and outside of Skid Row. In fact, SRHT has used award-winning architects and developed LEED-certified buildings that are resource-efficient (they use less water and energy and reduce greenhouse gas emissions), which are more typical of wealthy real estate development than homelessness service organizations.

Ironically, the Skid Row containment policy represented a compromise between homeless advocates and wealthy investors in that it helped to maintain low-income housing (mostly through single-room occupancy hotels, or SROs) and provide services to the poor and disabled in one area of downtown while allowing investors to develop other portions of the downtown area (Reese et al. 2010). Selective policing or enforcement of certain laws in certain areas helped ensure that people experiencing homelessness stayed within the containment area of Skid Row (Berk and MacDonald 2010). Yet, as the numbers of homeless people continued to rise throughout the 1980s, containment proved a short-term fix that had disastrous results, including concentrated disadvantage and higher crime.

In 2006, LA's Safer Cities Initiative was implemented under Police Chief William Bratton and introduced 50 additional police officers in Skid Row who were tasked with reducing crime and punishing people living on the streets, often for minor infractions. Bratton pioneered this approach to crime, often referred to as "broken windows" policing, in his former position as NYC's Police Chief. This approach, which essentially made it a crime to be homeless, was largely ineffective and ultimately made later efforts at decentralization more difficult (Blasi 2007; Culhane 2010; Reese et al. 2010).

Dispersed Homelessness in Los Angeles

The large concentration of homelessness in Skid Row caused by the city's containment policy did not keep homelessness from being a problem in other parts of LA. Areas including Venice Beach and Hollywood also have dense concentrations of homeless people – many of whom are youth and young adults (Rice et al. 2007). And homeless encampments can be found in underpasses and on the streets throughout LA, populated by those who refuse to go to Skid Row. While some claim that most people experiencing homelessness come to LA from other places because it is a more favorable environment – what has been called a magnet effect – survey research has consistently found that the vast majority of people experiencing homelessness in LA are either from LA or were stably housed in LA before becoming homeless (LAHSA 2017a).

While plans to address homelessness beyond earlier containment policies had been lacking in LA throughout the 1980s, the Los Angeles Homeless Services Authority (LAHSA) was developed in 1993 to better coordinate and administer federal funds for homelessness as a result of a legal battle to address the severe shortage of shelters (Reese et al. 2010). In 2016, LAHSA administered nearly $105 million from HUD in renewed and new grants to prevent and end homelessness, which contrasts with the $1.2 billion budget spent by NYC on homeless services.

Despite LA's history of misguided policies that led to the development of Skid Row, recent efforts are notable for increased coordination across city and county offices to address homelessness. For example, public and private funders came together as part of the Home for Good campaign to create a more coordinated approach to funding permanent supportive housing (PSH) for chronically homeless people through the creation of the Funders Collaborative. Launched in 2010, the Home for Good initiative, which explicitly embraces a housing-first approach, has grown into a countywide effort that represents over 200 cross-sector partners working collaboratively on systems and solutions to end homelessness. Based on these efforts, LA now leads the nation in rates of housing homeless individuals; in 2016, 14,214 homeless individuals in LA moved into permanent housing. The pace of providing such housing is also increasing and is up 61% in the past 2 years (8802 people received housing in 2014, and 10,917 people received housing in 2015) (LAHSA 2017b).

Still, in part because new people are becoming homeless, the homeless population continues to rise in LA – a 20% increase in 2016. It is perhaps because the visible, unsheltered homelessness crisis has become ubiquitous across LA that the Home for Good campaign was able to appeal to the general public and secure more resources dedicated to addressing homelessness. In the fall of 2016, voters approved a measure by a required 2/3 majority for a $1.2 billion bond to build new units of permanent supportive housing for people who have experienced homelessness over the next 10 years. This was followed by a second measure in the spring of 2017 that increased the sales tax to generate over $350 million annually for services and programs designed to prevent and end homelessness (LAHSA 2017a). Increasing expenditures on homelessness through a self-imposed tax is indicative of the seriousness of LA's growing crisis. Given a decades-long policy of containment that relied on faith-based services, resolving this crisis will require continued political will and funding to make Skid Row a thing of the past.

Homelessness Policies in Twenty-First-Century America: A Tale of Two Cities Revisited

As described in the previous sections, NYC and LA approached homelessness in markedly different ways, which reflects each city's unique history. NYC responded early and generously based on civic values and relied on secular nonprofit organizations that grew into a multi-billion-dollar industry, whereas LA tried to contain the problem and relied heavily on a charity-based approach through the missions in Skid Row. LA's containment policy represents an overall anomaly in this country, with NYC doing what most other places did – decentralize homeless services and resources. NYC's emphasis on rights-based guarantees, along with continued advocacy for congregate living, led to a dominance of shelters over permanent housing, whereas LA's response left most people unsheltered.

Despite these differences, both NYC and LA have shared aspects in their response to homelessness. For example, both places attempted to criminalize homelessness under broken windows policing (under the same police chief's leadership), and both were influenced by NIMBY pressure that ensured higher-income and less tolerant neighborhoods were more likely to avoid having homeless services. Most salient for today's homelessness crisis is that both places have high housing costs, which can largely explain why both have failed to stem the tide of homelessness as of 2016 as compared to the rest of the USA. Recent research has confirmed a strong relationship between rising rents and increased homelessness in large metro areas, including NYC, LA, Washington, D.C., and Seattle. In fact, Glynn and Fox (2017) showed that a 5% average rent increase in NYC or LA would lead to between 2000 and 3000 more people falling into homelessness. Contributing to housing costs is an undersupply of affordable housing in both cities. In NYC, there has been an absolute shrinkage in available housing due to an aging housing stock, while LA is creating newer housing stock within the context of there never having been enough.

Today, NYC continues to spend billions of dollars on homeless services, yet the homeless population continues to rise. Ironically, LA's lack of investment may allow it to leapfrog shelter dependence and avoid creating a homeless industry outside of Skid Row by investing new resources in solutions to homelessness, such as HF. This will take increased investment in housing and services, as has been recently approved in LA, but it also requires a trained workforce for which social work should play a leading role. There is also a need for the development of a pipeline of workers who have training and a mindset that homelessness can be ended, which points to a pivotal role for social work education.

Yet, homelessness is ultimately not a problem that can be addressed only by the homelessness service sector. That is, rising structural inequality will continue to ensure a tragic flow of people onto the streets of major cities, such as LA and NYC, as long as housing affordability remains out of reach and there are limited public benefits to assist all those in need. As housing affordability continues to get worse, increased prevention of homelessness is needed, which will need to be embraced along with effective downstream approaches, such as HF.

HF is not a panacea, but it offers a path to housing stability and an end to homelessness that has been proven in many US cities and throughout Canada (Henwood et al. 2015; Padgett et al. 2015). Moving forward, it will be important to understand how local civic values and previous efforts to address homelessness continue to play a role as NYC, LA, and other areas grapple with how best to address homelessness.

References

Berk, R., & MacDonald, J. (2010). Policing the homeless. *Criminology & Public Policy, 9*(4), 813–840.

Berube, A. (2014). All cities are not created unequal. *Brookings Institution, 20*. https://www.brookings.edu/research/all-cities-are-not-created-unequal/

Blasi, G. (2007). *Policing our way out of homelessness: The first year of the safer cities initiative on skid row*. Los Angeles: USC Center for Sustainable Cities.

Byrne, T., & Culhane, D. P. (2011). The right to housing: An effective means for addressing homelessness? *University of Pennsylvania Journal of Law and Social Change, 14*(3), 379–390.

City of New York. (2017). Turning the tide on homelessness in New York City. https://www1.nyc.gov/site/dhs/about/tide.page. Accessed 30 June 2018.

Culhane, D. P. (2010). Tackling homelessness in Los Angeles' Skid Row. *Criminology and Public Policy, 9*(4), 851–857.

Glynn, C., & Fox, E. B. (2017). Dynamics of homelessness in urban America. https://arxiv.org/pdf/1707.09380.pdf. Accessed 30 June 2018.

Goetz, E. (1992). Land use and homeless policy in Los Angeles. *International Journal of Urban and Regional Research, 16*(4), 540–554.

Henwood, B. F., Wenzel, S., Mangano, P. F., Hombs, M., Padgett, D., Byrne, T., Rice, E., Butts, S., & Uretsky, M. (2015). *The grand challenge of ending homelessness* (Grand Challenges for Social Work Initiative Working Paper No. 10). Cleveland: American Academy of Social Work and Social Welfare.

Hopper, K. (2002). *Reckoning with homelessness*. Cornell: Cornell University Press.

Hopper, K., Jost, J., Hay, T., Welber, S., & Haugland, G. (1997). Homelessness, severe mental illness, and the institutional circuit. *Psychiatric Services, 48*(5), 659–665.

Houghton, T. (2001). *A description and history of the New York/New York Agreement to house homeless mentally ill individuals*. Ithaca: Corporation for Supportive Housing.

Joint Center for Housing Studies at Harvard University. (2017). *The state of the nation's housing 2017*. Boston: Author.

Keil, R. (1998). *Los Angeles*. New York: Wiley Press.

Los Angeles Homeless Services Authority (LAHSA). (2017a). Data and reports. https://www.lahsa.org/homeless-count/reports. Accessed 30 June 2018.

Los Angeles Homeless Services Authority (LAHSA). (2017b). 2017 Greater Los Angeles homeless count results. https://www.lahsa.org/documents?id=1873-2017-greater-los-angeles-homeless-count-presentation-los-angeles-county-and-continuum-of-care.pdf. Accessed 30 June 2018.

Nahmias, L. (2016). HUD slashes funding for some New York City homeless shelters. https://www.politico.com/states/new-york/city-hall/story/2016/05/hud-slashes-funding-for-some-new-york-city-homeless-shelters-101531. Accessed 30 June 2018

Padgett, D. K., Henwood, B. F., & Tsemberis, S. (2015). *Housing first: Ending homelessness, transforming systems, and changing lives*. New York: Oxford University Press.

Reese, E., Deverteuil, G., & Thach, L. (2010). 'Weak-center' gentrification and the contradictions of containment: Deconcentrating poverty in downtown Los Angeles. *International Journal of Urban and Regional Research, 34*(2), 310–327.

Rice, E., Milburn, N. G., & Rotheram-Borus, M. J. (2007). Pro-social and problematic social network influences on HIV/AIDS risk behaviours among newly homeless youth in Los Angeles. *AIDS Care, 19*(5), 697–704.

Sewell, A. (2016, June). Gov. Jerry Brown again refuses to declare a state of emergency on homelessness. LA Times. http://www.latimes.com/local/lanow/la-me-ln-governor-homelessness-emergency-20160616-snap-story.html. Accessed 30 June 2018.

Supportive Housing Network of New York. (2006). An extraordinary achievement, an enormous challenge: Implementing the New York/New York III Agreement. https://shnny.org/uploads/Implementing_the_NY-NY_III_Agreement.pdf. Accessed 30 June 2018.

Susser, E., Struening, E. L., & Conover, S. (1989). Psychiatric problems in homeless men: Lifetime psychosis, substance use, and current distress in new arrivals at New York City shelters. *Archives of General Psychiatry, 46*(9), 845–850.

U.S. Department of Housing and Urban Development. (2016). The 2016 annual homeless assessment report (AHAR) to congress part 1: Point-in-time estimates of homelessness. https://www.hudexchange.info/resources/documents/2016-AHAR-Part-1.pdf. Accessed 30 June 2018.

Wolch, J., & Dear, M. (1993). *Malign neglect: Homelessness in an American city*. San Francisco: Jossey-Bass.

Chapter 9
The Criminalization of Homelessness

Amanda Aykanian and Sondra J. Fogel

Each day, thousands of people in the USA find themselves without a home because of personal struggles (e.g., mental health issues and substance abuse), interpersonal issues (e.g., domestic violence and family conflict), and systemic obstacles (e.g., poverty and rising housing costs). Further, homelessness in the USA affects people of all races, ethnicities, ages, and genders. Therefore, developing effective interventions and policy solutions to promote housing security is a challenging undertaking. While many communities have made great strides in reducing the number of people who experience homelessness each year, others have struggled to do so. When homelessness rates rise, and the demand for shelter and supports outweighs the supply, communities may find it difficult to develop adequate and appropriate solutions. Limited resources, restricted budgets, and a lack of political and public support can also present barriers to implementing best practices for ending homelessness. When compounded by victim blaming and hostility from the broader community, policymakers may resort to strategies that lack long-term impact. It is here, at the crossroads of meeting the needs of people experiencing homelessness and appeasing the concerns of residents and other stakeholders, that the *criminalization of homelessness* can result.

This chapter first presents an overview of criminalization and the historical origins of anti-homeless policies. Second, it illustrates the influential factors and common arguments used to justify such policies. Third, it demonstrates how

Electronic supplementary material: The online version of this chapter (https://doi.org/10.1007/978-3-030-03727-7_9) contains supplementary material, which is available to authorized users.

A. Aykanian (✉)
University at Albany, Albany, NY, USA

S. J. Fogel
University of South Florida, Tampa, FL, USA
e-mail: sfogel@usf.edu

H. Larkin et al. (eds.), *Homelessness Prevention and Intervention in Social Work*, https://doi.org/10.1007/978-3-030-03727-7_9

criminalization approaches do little to end homelessness or promote housing stability. Finally, it presents alternatives to criminalization and recommendations for what social workers can do to prevent and end the use of anti-homeless policies.

Anti-homeless Policies

Conversations about homelessness, crime, and policing often include unavoidable behaviors (e.g., sleeping and urination) and seemingly harmless acts (e.g., sitting or lying down on sidewalks). This tendency results from the fact that people experiencing homelessness often have limited access to facilities for life-sustaining activities, such as places for sleeping, eating, using the bathroom, and tending to personal hygiene. This situation is especially common in communities that lack homeless shelters or drop-in centers and in communities where the demand for such services outstrips the supply. As a result, such behaviors are often conducted in public spaces, which may be met with complaints and concerns from community members and business owners.

When the existence of homeless people causes fear or tension in a community, criminalizing their behavior is one way to reduce their presence or to restrict where and what they can do (Amster 2003; Covin 2012). In the words of Randall Amster (2003), "If you want to eliminate a particular social class or subculture or deviant group, locate some behavior that is largely peculiar to that group and make it illegal (p. 200)." Therefore, policies that criminalize homelessness, also known as anti-homeless policies, go beyond punishing behaviors commonly understood to be illegal, such as prostitution or illicit drug use (National Law Center on Homelessness and Poverty 2016). Criminalizing homelessness involves making illegal the more mundane activities or behaviors associated with homelessness and poverty, regardless of whether those behaviors would typically be considered crimes.

Anti-homeless policies result in homeless people being ticketed or arrested for acts that the average citizen could do with little concern. Behaviors targeted by such policies include, for example, public intoxication, loitering, begging or panhandling, personal hygiene, sleeping outside or in cars, and sitting or lying down in public spaces. While violating anti-homeless laws typically results in monetary fines or simply being forced out of a community (e.g., being driven or put on a bus to a new location), misdemeanor charges and convictions can also result (National Law Center on Homelessness and Poverty 2016).

While homelessness itself is an experience that affects a wide range of people, including single adults, families, children, and young adults, anti-homeless policies most often target those homeless individuals likely to be seen or encountered in public spaces. This includes people sleeping outdoors (e.g., in parks, on sidewalks, or in cars), people who lack an interest in or access to day or night shelter, panhandlers on street corners or outside businesses, homeless people passing time in public spaces, and individuals participating in street economy activities like prostitution or squeegeeing car windshields. More recently, laws have been used to target groups providing food or other goods to homeless people, such as churches that hand out lunch bags in parks (National Law Center on Homelessness and Poverty 2016).

The Origins of Anti-homeless Policies

The criminalization of homelessness, and the negative public perceptions that often accompany it, can be traced to colonial America. This was a time when able-bodied people, who did not conform to established community norms, were often punished. America's approach for providing public social supports was grounded in the Elizabethan Poor Laws of England, which reflected the social and cultural mores of an economically depressed England. These laws instituted the practice of letting local government decide who was worthy of care and the type of social care to be offered (Trattner 1989). With government bodies left to determine eligibility and worthiness of supports, it is perhaps not surprising that, in the early decades of this nation, those who were "vagrants refusing to work could be committed to a house of correction; whipped, branded, or put in pillories and stoned and even put to death" (Trattner 1989, p. 10).

As America developed, some individuals that were without a home and unable to work—such as widows, children, elders, and the disabled—often were provided for by community members, religious groups, or the limited social care governmental programs. Meanwhile, by the 1850s, those who were homeless and seen as a community problem were frequently put in overnight spaces, known as tramp rooms, in police stations (Kusmer 2002, p. 14). It was here that the night would be spent indoors on a floor away from the rest of the community and under supervision.

From our earliest beginnings as a nation, homelessness was associated with beggars, transients, and a general disconnection from the local community (Wong 2008). Early public attitudes toward the homeless varied, with rural areas being kinder than emerging urban centers where the thrust of industrialization reinforced social norms of the importance of work and self-control (Kusmer 2002). It was the early Charity Organization Societies (COS) that initially took the lead to intervene. It was the COS that innovated wayfarers' lodges for homeless men and women as an alternative to the police station tramp rooms, in exchange for some type of labor or work effort (Kusmer 2002). In addition, there were simultaneous efforts by those doing charity work to close the tramp rooms, opining that the required demonstration of a work ethic and work product would hold as evidence of the ability to reform vagrants.

Unfortunately, the stance of the COS and other charity workers regarding the homeless reinforced stereotypical perceptions—of laziness and lack of motivation to work—espoused by those who created tramp rooms. Over time, those who administered wayfarers' lodges and religious groups that ran shelters (e.g., the Salvation Army), as well as state legislators, introduced work farms as an alternative to tramp rooms for those deemed to be vagrants and social nonconformists (Kusmer 2002).

While these efforts may have offered shelter to homeless men and women, they reflected the public consensus that those who failed to contribute to the community in a meaningful way were deviants and in need of reform. By the turn of the twentieth century, criminalizing those who refused to accept the ostensibly good intentions of the early charity professionals and other social reformers began in earnest. Today, the criminalization of homelessness is used in cities across the country and continues to increase with each passing year. Because the homeless population in the USA is diverse, a number of groups are affected by criminalization efforts, including teens living on the streets after being forced out of their homes, families sleeping in cars following an eviction, chronically homeless adults who have struggled to gain stability in traditional housing and service settings, and homeless travelers or transients passing through communities.

Why Communities Implement Anti-homeless Policies

The primary goal of anti-homeless policies differs drastically from the goals of other homeless-specific interventions, such as permanent supportive housing. Anti-homeless policies are intended to reduce the presence of homeless people in specific locations or in an entire community. These policies are not designed to improve the circumstances that contribute to homelessness or to provide better assistance to those who find themselves homeless. Instead, criminalizing homelessness is a response to public space being occupied by homeless people and the fear that they pose a direct and imminent threat to the safety and well-being of the community (Amster 2003; Foscarinis 1999). In this way, homeless people have come to be recognized as a symbol of disorder, creating tension between them and the broader community. "Off-putting" is how Bill de Blasio, the mayor of New York City, described panhandlers when discussing his wish that the behavior was illegal (Jorgensen 2017).

Impact of Public Sentiment

The popularity of anti-homeless policies may reflect overarching changes in public opinion toward homeless people or homelessness in general. When homelessness began gaining attention as a social problem in the USA, public sentiment was more sympathetic and tolerant. However, as the problem persisted, and people were faced with a visual reminder of poverty and destitution in their community, this sentiment shifted (Smith 1996). Although the criminalization of homelessness is happening in many parts of the world, a survey comparing the USA and Germany found that Americans had less compassion for and less concern about the rights of people experiencing homelessness (Tompsett et al. 2003).

As Smith 1996 suggests, the extreme marginalization and social exclusion of homeless people have pushed them into a category of "unworthy poor." Negative shifts in opinions about homelessness or poverty do not necessarily happen consistently across population groups or classes, and changing public sentiment does not always have a direct policy impact. However, when opinions change within socially elite groups that have the ability to influence policymaking, it can have significant effects (Blasi 1994). This process was illustrated in a recent debate about plans to build a new winter homeless shelter in Saratoga Springs, New York. Business owners and community members sued the city over the shelter, which would be built next to an existing shelter. One business owner said, "To parade homeless in that neighborhood is not a smart thing to do. They are not clean, they are not well-managed, and they don't have to identify themselves" (Liberatore 2017).

Perceived Threats to Commerce and Quality of Life

A common reason for enacting anti-homeless laws is reducing the presence of homeless people in business or tourism districts and the fear that these areas will attract more homeless people. Communities want their spaces to draw shoppers and attract new business. It is often believed that the presence of homeless people will deter customers, negatively affect business success, and reduce the community's economic capital (Mitchell 1997). For example, in 2013, city councilors in Columbia, South Carolina, voted to criminalize homelessness, due to concerns that the city had become a magnet for homeless people. Homelessness was described as a risk to business (Goldberg 2013), which illustrates how these policies are rationalized as being protective of the economic security of a community.

Anti-homeless laws are often justified as strategies to improve the quality of life for community members. In fact, improving quality of life has been an explicit goal of policing strategies in New York City for years in which homeless people have been specifically targeted, as well as behaviors associated with homelessness, such as panhandling (Vitale 2008). The belief seems to be that reducing the presence of homeless people will restore or maintain the aesthetic integrity of public space and will attract people to the area for patronage and leisure. However, improving the quality of life for community members is often done at the cost of quality of life for homeless people, which sends a clear message that homeless people are not considered part of the broader community (Foscarinis 1999).

Perceived Threats to Public Safety

Many communities consider homelessness to be a direct threat to public safety. Because public responses to people experiencing homelessness are largely based on fear and a misunderstanding of the complex causes of homelessness, the police are often the primary means of intervention (Fitzpatrick and Myrstol 2011; McNamara et al. 2013). For example, the Safer City policing initiative in Los Angeles' Skid Row was implemented to reduce crime thought to be associated with the high concentration of homelessness in the city (Berk and MacDonald 2010; Culhane 2010). Similarly, as part of New York City's Quality of Life Campaign, the city redirected its police department's focus to restoring public order, through aggressive and punitive policing efforts that targeted the homeless and other marginalized groups (Vitale 2008). The use of homelessness-focused policing strategies has contributed to homeless individuals being overrepresented in correctional facilities (Kushel et al. 2005).

Experts suggest that linking behaviors like sleeping in parks or on sidewalks to public safety threats is an unconvincing argument that lacks empirical support (Foscarinis 1999). However, many communities view homelessness as associated with social disorder, urban decay, and crime, and it is not unusual to rationalize firm responses to homelessness as attempts to increase safety. Homeless individuals, however, are generally not arrested for violent crimes or other felonies (Fitzpatrick and Myrstol 2011; Martell et al. 1995; Snow et al. 1989)—despite public perceptions to the contrary. Rather, it is social incivilities, such as public intoxication, loitering, aggressive panhandling, public urination, drug use, prostitution, and criminal actions toward other homeless individuals, that are most often the reason for homeless individuals being arrested (Berk and MacDonald 2010).

Often lost in the conversation about homelessness and crime is that homeless people are commonly victims rather than perpetrators (Meinbresse et al. 2014; Wachholz 2005). The National Coalition for the Homeless (2014) reported increasing violence against the homeless beginning in 2008. In fact, people experiencing homelessness are disproportionately victimized compared to individuals who are housed (Garland et al. 2010). Crimes committed against homeless individuals include assault and robbery, as well as rape and sexual victimization, which are particularly common among homeless women. Sadly, some of the more violent crimes against homeless individuals have been fatal. Between 1999 and 2013 (the latest data available), there were 1437 violent crimes against homeless people, and 375 of the victims died as a result (National Coalition for the Homeless 2014). It is important to note when considering the crime data that these numbers are likely an undercount of the actual victimization that occurs. Many violent attacks are likely not reported to authorities for any number of reasons, including the victims themselves potentially being targeted for future harassment.

Perceived Need to Manage the Homeless Population

When homelessness is associated with crime, declining quality of life, and economic downturn, laws that criminalize homelessness function as a means of control or management that target people of a certain status. Restricting where people are physically allowed to be, what they can do in public, and limiting their ability to conduct basic acts of living are all examples of limiting the rights and liberties of people who are homeless. Further, while homeless people may not be perceived as dangerous by police, they may be viewed as individuals who interfere with the rights or lives of other community members. Police are often called to surveil and follow, remove from an area, ticket, or arrest homeless individuals for activities that bother business owners or other community members, such as panhandling or sleeping on park benches.

When certain classes of people are perceived to be bothersome, offensive, or threatening signs of social disorder, society tends to view them as something to be controlled, managed, or abolished (Irwin 1985). The police and criminal justice system have become common mechanisms for controlling homeless people and other marginalized groups, especially those with high service needs (Fitzpatrick and Myrstol 2011; McGuire and Rosenheck 2004). This approach is especially prevalent for homeless individuals with co-occurring mental health and substance use issues, who are overrepresented in correctional facilities and are incarcerated longer than other groups (McNiel et al. 2005). It has also been argued that incarceration, especially in jails, is used as a way of controlling or detaining people whose behavior society deems unacceptable, who are socially detached, and who society would prefer not to think about or see (Irwin 1985).

Arguments Against Anti-homeless Policies

Unclear Impact and Costly Implementation

Although a major rationale for anti-homeless policies is concerns about public safety, there is insufficient evidence supporting the premise that criminalizing homelessness reduces crime. The Safer City Initiative in Los Angeles, for example, was intended to reduce nuisance, property, and violent crime in Skid Row, because it was believed that these crimes resulted from the high concentration of homelessness in that neighborhood (Berk and MacDonald 2010; Culhane 2010). However, in their evaluation of the program's impact, Berk and MacDonald (2010) found only a modest reduction in crime. Crime remained quite high, which suggests that most of the crime in the area was not attributable to homeless people. Further, there was no evidence of crime rising in neighboring communities. In other words, policing efforts to disperse homeless people out of Skid Row did not result in increased crime rates in surrounding communities. The authors also point out that since homeless people are often victims of crime, a reduction in victims, rather than criminals, may have contributed to the reduction in crime (Berk and MacDonald 2010).

Even if an anti-homeless policy has a positive impact on crime rates or perceived public safety, there remain questions about how sustainable implementation is for communities. The costs associated with increased policing, arrests, and incarceration can be overwhelming. In addition to having only a slight impact on crime, the

Safer City Initiative in Skid Row is one example of potentially unsustainable policy. Due to high implementation costs associated with policing efforts and administrative processing, the initiative is inherently time-limited (Culhane 2010). Similarly, one county in Florida spent over 5 million dollars—roughly $15,000 per person, per year—arresting and incarcerating 37 chronically homeless individuals a total of 1250 times over a 9-year period (Impact Homelessness 2014).

Negative and Unintended Consequences

Attempting life-sustaining activities in public spaces, perceived dangerousness, and involvement in petty crimes increase the likeliness that homeless people will be arrested rather than being offered other assistance (Garland et al. 2010). Although little research has assessed the true impact of anti-homeless laws, it is well established that contact with the criminal justice system can result in challenges to achieving and maintaining economic and housing stability. These barriers are particularly problematic for people experiencing or at high risk of homelessness (Metraux et al. 2010). It is also likely that the risk for experiencing homelessness after incarceration may vary by group. For example, when Fries et al. (2014) asked a sample of detainees where they would most likely live following their release from jail, women were more likely than men to anticipate post-jail homelessness.

Following a period of incarceration, homeless individuals can have significant difficulty securing safe and stable housing because of their criminal record and likely co-occurring biopsychosocial disorders. For example, a criminal record can be a significant barrier to accessing housing, especially government-subsidized housing vouchers or units. Landlords can use criminal background checks as a basis for selecting tenants, and public housing authorities and federal housing programs have the autonomy to determine their own eligibility criteria related to criminal history. Additionally, police sweeps of sidewalks, parks, and homeless encampments often result in the loss or destruction of personal belongings, including identification documents, which can create an obstacle to housing, as well as employment and voting (National Law Center on Homelessness and Poverty 2016).

In addition to being costly to communities, laws that criminalize homelessness have significant economic impacts on the people they target. Even in the face of federal guidance to the contrary, communities continue to use tactics that criminalize homelessness and poverty, placing undue burden on the most economically vulnerable. This issue was the topic of an article in the *Brown Political Review* in which the author, Gabriel Zimmerman, illustrated Rhode Island's ongoing efforts to criminalize poverty and homelessness and the extreme economic impact on the state's poorest individuals. As Zimmerman noted, the fees associated with criminalization tactics and court proceedings can be insurmountable. Perhaps most alarming is that prohibitive ticket fees and bail, legal, and court costs can result in debt-related incarceration when a person is simply unable to pay (Zimmerman 2017). What starts as a monetary fee may escalate into a misdemeanor criminal charge. Thus, while the initial cost for a crime may seem minor, the ultimate punishment can be devastating.

Depending on the community and type of violation, punishments for breaking anti-homeless laws vary. In some cases, the punishment is an arrest, which can lead to incarceration. If employed, spending time in jail may mean missing work and could jeopardize a person's job and income, while extended incarceration can also cause public benefits to lapse. More commonly, violating an anti-homeless law is punished with a citation and accompanying fee. For many homeless people, paying a fee is impossible due to a lack of adequate income. However, not paying a fee will typically result in the fee being increased and may even lead to an eventual arrest warrant. Further, there are often fees associated with different aspects of the criminal justice process, which can quickly compound—especially if a person chooses to fight a charge. Further, drawn-out legal challenges come with additional costs and the need to miss more work (National Law Center on Homelessness and Poverty 2016). As a result, homeless individuals may forego their right to challenge a charge due to the economic impact of the process.

Legal Arguments

Legal advocates, such as the National Law Center on Homelessness and Poverty, have contested anti-homeless policies on multiple grounds. The strongest and most successful legal arguments against the criminalization of homelessness address their inherently flawed assumptions and the ways many policies violate the constitutional rights of homeless people.

Flawed Logic

The threat of arrest or incarceration is often used to deter undesired behaviors. However, any model that relies on the use of an incentive or disincentive assumes that humans are in control of their own behavior and able to rationally choose how to act. It has been argued that some of the behaviors that anti-homeless policies target are often unavoidable and are not done by choice (Foscarinis 1999). For example, in communities where the number of homeless individuals exceeds the number of shelter beds, sleeping in public spaces becomes largely unavoidable. Similarly, when faced with the absence of public restrooms or hygiene facilities, urinating outside often becomes a homeless person's only option. In these situations, it could be said that a person had no effective choice in committing the act or that the act was done out of necessity. It could also be argued that if a normally law-abiding person were put in the same circumstance, they would behave in the same way. Thus, criminalizing homelessness is considered a faulty incentive model (Smith 1994).

Constitutional and Other Legal Challenges

Anti-homeless policies have been criticized on a variety of constitutional bases (National Law Center on Homelessness and Poverty 2016). Laws against panhandling have been challenged under the First (Freedom of Religion, Speech, and Press) and Fourteenth Amendments (Rights of Citizenship); laws against sleeping or camping in public have been challenged under the Eighth (Excessive Bail, Fines, and Punishments Forbidden) and Fourteenth Amendments; and, seizing or destroying personal belongings has been challenged under the Fourth Amendment (Protection from Unreasonable Searches and Seizures) (Smith 1994).

Successful challenges to laws that criminalize homelessness have become more common in recent years. For example, since 2015, laws banning or restricting panhandling have been struck down by courts in Colorado, Florida, Illinois, Maine, and Massachusetts for violating the First Amendment (National Law Center on Homelessness and Poverty 2016). Other types of laws have also been struck down. For example, Miami, Florida, had a policy of arresting homeless people for sleeping, eating, or congregating in public, and police would often destroy or confiscate people's personal belongings. A district court determined that restricting essential activities, such as sleeping, without providing an alternative, violates a person's right to travel and due process (under the Fourteenth Amendment) and their right to be free from cruel and unusual punishment (under the Eighth Amendment) (Smith 1994).

Legal challenges have also been successful when a law was too vague or ambiguous, when a behavior was criminalized without providing an alternative (e.g., restricting sleeping in public without providing adequate shelter), or when a law lacked a compelling government benefit (Smith 1994). In addition to arguing constitutional violations, some have challenged efforts to criminalize homelessness based on the position that the law criminalizes the entire experience of being homeless. For example, sleeping in public is often unavoidable when a city lacks adequate shelter for its homeless population. In this way, the behavior is both involuntary and a direct result of being homeless. Thus, by criminalizing acts necessitated by the homeless experience, anti-homeless policies effectively criminalize the status of being homeless. The Columbia, South Carolina, city council vote to criminalize homelessness, described earlier, was a status-based policy. The plan was to simply give all homeless people encountered by police, regardless of their behavior, a choice: go to a shelter, get arrested, or leave Columbia (Goldberg 2013). Challenges to status-based criminalization are less common than constitutional challenges but have had some success (Smith 1996). In fact, following immediate backlash from police, city employees, and homeless advocates, the Columbia city council rescinded its decision (Goldberg 2013).

The Federal Government's Position

In recent years, the United States Interagency Council on Homelessness (USICH), the Department of Justice (DOJ), the Department of Housing and Urban Development (HUD), and the Department of Education (DOE) have taken clear stances against the criminalization of homelessness. In 2010, USICH and DOJ held an interagency summit to develop constructive alternatives to criminalization. Summit attendees represented multiple stakeholder groups, including federal and local governments, police departments, continuums of care, and people experiencing homelessness. USICH then published the report, "Searching Out Solutions: Constructive Alternatives to the Criminalization of Homelessness," which includes guidance for creating comprehensive systems of care, collaborating with law enforcement and human service providers, and developing new justice system strategies (United States Interagency Council on Homelessness 2012). USICH has also issued guidance for how communities can connect people living in homeless encampments with needed services and housing, rather than focusing on closing encampments or forcing people to relocate (United States Interagency Council on Homelessness 2012, 2015).

Under the Obama Administration, DOJ took a stance against criminalizing homelessness and called the practice unconstitutional. In 2015, DOJ issued a statement of interest in a federal case challenging a ban on sleeping in public in Boise, Idaho. The agency concurred with the plaintiffs, a group of homeless individuals who had been convicted of violating the ban, that the ban was unconstitutional because the number of shelter beds available could not accommodate the number of homeless people in the city (United States Department of Justice 2015). In 2016, the department submitted a letter of support for a bill in Seattle, Washington, that protects the constitutional rights of people living in public spaces by preventing the city from removing people from encampments. Also, in 2016, the department directed courts to put an end to policies that jail individuals unable to afford fines and to stop practices geared toward maximizing revenue rather than public safety (Apuzzo 2016).

Recognizing police departments' role in preventing criminalization and developing effective community responses to homelessness, DOJ's Office of Community Oriented Policing Services dedicated an entire issue of its Community Policing Dispatch newsletter to ending homelessness. Developed in collaboration with USICH, HUD, the Department of Health and Human Services, and the National Law Center on Homelessness and Poverty, the newsletter encouraged alternatives to criminalization, offered strategies for involving law enforcement in response systems, and highlighted resources to effectively engaging with individuals experiencing homelessness (Community Policing Dispatch 2015).

HUD is the primary federal funding source for homeless services and housing, and the agency solicits applications from communities for funding every year. The application is a competitive process and submissions are scored on a points system. In 2016, HUD began incentivizing the prevention of criminalization in its funding application process by awarding points on applications for conducting activities to ensure homelessness is not criminalized. Acceptable activities include community education strategies targeting policymakers, law enforcement, and local businesses (U.S. Department of Housing and Urban Development 2016).

Homeless youth are subject to the same laws and restrictions targeting homeless adults while also being affected by policies that specifically apply to them, such as curfews and truancy laws. Recognizing that the enforcement of criminalization ordinances, status offense laws, and school-based policy can uniquely impact homeless youth, the DOE included guidance in the Every Student Succeeds Act directing schools to work with local lawmakers to ensure that the enforcement of such laws does not hinder homeless children's ability to attend school (U.S. Department of Education 2015).

The federal government's position on any issue can vary with changes in presidents and administrations. Major federal stances on the criminalization of homelessness took place under the Obama Administration. At the time of this writing, the Trump Administration has not issued a formal position on the criminalization of homelessness or specific anti-homeless policies. However, President Trump and his DOJ have made strides to significantly overhaul police reform efforts put in place under the Obama Administration (Charles 2017). These changes include a tougher stance on crime and less of a focus on police-community relationship building, which could result in increased efforts to target crimes associated with homelessness. Additionally, deep proposed budget cuts to HUD's housing subsidies and other assistance are likely to contribute to an increase in homelessness (Booker 2018; Thrush 2018). Together, these two policy trends suggest that neither homelessness nor its criminalization will end soon.

Alternatives to Anti-homeless Policies and Opportunities for Social Workers

Social workers are uniquely positioned to lead efforts to prevent the criminalization of homelessness and to support communities in developing alternative solutions. In addition to developing and evaluating programs and services necessary to strengthen the homeless service system, social workers can conduct advocacy activities, collaborate with community partners, develop cross-sector partnerships, and raise awareness through education (Aykanian and Lee 2016). Following is a discussion of opportunities for social workers to help prevent and end the criminalization of homelessness, coupled with examples of solutions from across the USA to illustrate constructive alternatives to anti-homeless policies.

Preventing Homelessness and Strengthening the Service System

A primary solution to ending the criminalization of homelessness is implementing robust homelessness prevention and intervention programs that create low-barrier access to needed services and housing. A high rate of homelessness is a symptom of enduring poverty, a lack of affordable housing, inadequate policy and prevention strategies, and a service system that cannot keep pace with needs. When facing these challenges, it is likely that communities will be more inclined to consider criminalization to be a viable option, especially if coupled with public opinion reflecting annoyance with or fear of homeless people.

Homelessness experts, advocacy organizations, and the federal government support approaches that prioritize low-barrier access to permanent housing with necessary supports. The evidence-supported interventions discussed elsewhere in this textbook (e.g., Housing First and Critical Time Intervention) are examples of appropriate strategies for promoting housing stability. The National Alliance to End Homelessness advocates for system models that make emergency shelters highly accessible and housing focused. They encourage communities to think about shelters as key components of the homelessness response system, rather than simply a place to sleep in emergency situations. The Navigation Center in San Francisco aligns with this position in its shelter by not instituting curfews or requiring sobriety (National Law Center on Homelessness and Poverty 2016). Increasing access to and connections with services can also be done through less conventional ways. For example, public libraries are common places of respite and sources of information for people experiencing homelessness. Recognizing this, many libraries now employ social workers to help connect homeless patrons to resources and services.

In addition to designing and implementing effective programs, policy advocacy is a vital tool for gaining needed political support to ensure that the service system is adequately funded and unhindered by problematic policy. As advocates, social workers can encourage policy approaches that increase access to affordable and permanent housing to ensure that homelessness, when it does occur, is brief and rare. Some specific advocacy priorities might include (1) strengthening housing protections by ensuring that people are not unjustly evicted; (2) increasing access to affordable housing through universal protections, expanding rental subsidy programs, and zoning plans that encourage the creation of affordable housing units; and (3) strengthening service systems through data-driven and evidence-based policy and programming decisions (National Law Center on Homelessness and Poverty 2016).

Developing Innovative Partnerships

Collaborative partnerships, especially with entities outside the traditional service system, can be useful for developing strategic responses to homelessness and preventing a reliance on criminalization tactics. In many cases, successfully preventing criminalization may mean engaging partners from sectors that have not traditionally been involved in the homeless service system, such as public libraries and hospitals. In fact, some communities have had significant success working with two groups most often associated with the adoption, rather than prevention, of anti-homeless policies—the police and the business community.

Compassionate and Collaborative Use of Police

The police have a dual role—protecting citizens and, by necessity, intervening in the lives of other citizens (McNamara et al. 2013)—which can result in ambivalence or tension between them and their community's homeless population. On one hand, the police may be called to break up homeless encampments or shew away panhandlers from a downtown area. On the other hand, they are often responsible for the safety of homeless individuals during times of natural disaster, victimization, and other emergencies (Fogel 2016). These conflicting experiences of intimidation and rescue may cause homeless people to distrust law enforcement officials or to be reluctant to engage with them.

Like social service providers, religious groups, and medical professionals, the police have frequent contact with people experiencing homelessness. Some law enforcement officials have begun to recognize that this contact creates opportunities for the provision of supports not often associated with typical community policing (McNamara et al. 2013). For example, police departments across the country are implementing compassionate strategies for working with homeless people that focus on making service connections. In 2015, the San Antonio Police Department formed the Homeless Outreach Positive Encounters (HOPE) team. This decision came after nearly a decade of issuing more than 6000 citations annually to people for violating anti-homeless laws—for sitting or lying on sidewalks, public urination, camping in public, and panhandling—while the number of homeless people in the city continued to increase. HOPE is an eight-officer team dedicated to using outreach to forge relationships with the city's homeless as a first step to helping people connect with available services (Zielinski 2017).

Community resources currently devoted to the criminalization of homelessness would be better spent if redirected into appropriate prevention and diversion services. There is little consensus on how best to balance humane and just treatment of people experiencing homelessness with appeasing the surrounding community's concerns about safety, crime, or curbside aesthetics. However, there are ways to improve the relationship between the police and people experiencing homelessness, such as increasing police training on homelessness and establishing a police liaison or special unit to work with homeless services and other providers (McNamara et al. 2013).

Social workers can be useful partners for police departments interested in rethinking their role in a community's response to homelessness and their approach to interacting with people experiencing homelessness. In Monroe, Washington, the police sergeant and a social worker teamed up to conduct outreach and serve as a point of contact for homeless people in need of service connections or resources (Sullivan 2017). Other communities have adopted similar strategies to integrating social workers within the police department for outreach and referral to services. Collaborating in this way is just one example of what a partnership between police and social workers might look like. Social workers can also help develop police department policies, provide trainings to officers, and facilitate the relationship between the police and the homeless service system (Aykanian and Lee 2016; McNamara et al. 2013).

Partnerships with the Business Community

Business owners are often in a position of instigating the creation of anti-homeless policies, justified based on the perception that the presence of homeless people is a threat to business (Amster 2008). Social workers could develop strategies to educate the business community about causes of, solutions to, and the local context surrounding homelessness (Aykanian and Lee 2016). Local business owners, business improvement districts, and chambers of commerce can also be engaged as collaborative partners in a community's homelessness response. For example, Washington, D.C.'s downtown business improvement district dedicates a sizeable portion of its budget to homelessness-related services. The group partners with property owners, business owners, city government, and service providers to employ a street outreach team to engage homeless individuals and connect them to services and housing supports (http://www.downtowndc.org/programs/homeless-services).

Advocating for Daytime Respites, Public Hygiene Facilities, and Public Storage

Many of the behaviors targeted by anti-homeless laws, such as loitering and storing personal belongings in public, are ones that could be avoided with the creation of alternative solutions. Social workers can advocate for needed resources and facilities designated for activities often criminalized when conducted in public. For example, after agreeing to stop enforcing a law that prohibited homeless people from storing their personal belongings on public property (e.g., setting it down on sidewalks), Pomona, California, agreed to build lockers so that individuals would have a safe alternative for storing their things (Smith 2016). To curb public urination violations, communities in Oregon, Virginia, California, and Massachusetts have built free-standing public bathrooms that, while not exclusively for homeless people, provide an option for those without access otherwise (Oliver 2017).

Day shelters are also valuable resources for people experiencing homelessness and can be used for things like eating, resting, showering, and doing laundry. Strong partnerships with the business community and faith-based groups can make securing space for such facilities less challenging. For example, the Washington, D.C. business improvement district mentioned earlier created a day shelter where homeless people can go in between overnight shelter hours to spend the day, do laundry, shower, and eat (National Law Center on Homelessness and Poverty 2006). They also piloted a drop-in center for homeless teens and young adults in collaboration with a church and service organization. The drop-in center is a place for homeless youth to rest, socialize, eat, and access service referrals (Giambrone 2016).

Protecting the Rights of Homeless People

The United Nations Human Rights Committee condemned the criminalization of homelessness, noting that it "raises concerns of discrimination and cruel, inhuman, or degrading treatment" (U.N. Human Rights Committee 2014). Social workers can promote the recognition and protection of homeless people's basic rights through legal advocacy to support challenges to unconstitutional laws and to protect homeless people's right to vote (Aykanian and Lee 2016). Organizations like the National Coalition for the Homeless and the National Alliance to End Homelessness often promote campaigns for issues related to basic rights protections that social workers can align with and draw inspiration from. Such advocacy can also extend to protecting homeless individuals from victimization. As Levin (2015) notes, "Targeted violence against the homeless further isolates and degrades them individually and communally while diminishing their collective sense of security" (p. 1726). Currently, homelessness is not protected in federal hate crime legislation. However, advocates are pressing for homelessness to be included as a protected status group in state hate crime laws. A hate crime is a "discriminatory criminal act(s) committed because of an individual's actual or perceived membership in a particular socially identifiable status group" (Levin 2015, p. 1716).

Some states have established a Homeless Bill of Rights to formally protect the civil and human rights of people experiencing homelessness, which includes protections against criminalization, constitutional violations, and discriminatory housing and service practices. Rhode Island was the first state to establish a Homeless Bill of Rights, and their bill protects people experiencing homelessness from discriminatory policing and educates homeless people about what the police can and cannot do to them (Rankin 2015). Additionally, Illinois created a bill of rights to protect homeless people from discrimination from employment, medical services, transportation, and voting. These bills are more likely to have social impacts than immediate legal ones but are a powerful statement of what a community perceives as fair and just treatment for its most vulnerable citizens.

Advocating for Improved Legal Systems and Discharge Planning

Social workers can educate policymakers, departments of correction, and courts about innovative models and help to identify system change opportunities. There are several ways to improve the legal system to both prevent homelessness and reduce the potential harms of criminalization efforts. First, there is a need for laws that guarantee access to legal counsel in eviction cases. Having legal counsel can prevent eviction, but legal aid organizations are often overburdened by the demand for services (National Law Center on Homelessness and Poverty 2016). Second, court systems, especially those in cities with high rates of homelessness, can learn from innovative homeless court programs (HCPs) being implemented across the country. For example, the first HCP began in 1989 in San Diego County, California. The HCP, among other things, holds court sessions in shelters for misdemeanor cases to circumvent challenges homeless people may face getting to court. The program also allows rehabilitative efforts, such as attending job training or educational programs, to count for fines and community service requirements, which can prevent debt-related incarceration (Binder 2002; http://www.homelesscourtprogram.com/). According to the National Center for State Courts, ten states have established such programs: South Carolina, California, Texas, Arizona, New Mexico, Missouri, Utah, Washington, Colorado, and Michigan (Lopez 2017).

Finally, in circumstances when a person is incarcerated after violating an anti-homeless policy, or any other law, strong discharge planning can help mitigate the effects of criminal justice involvement. Discharge planning is another area where social workers can partner with jails, prisons, police departments, and courts to ensure that people leaving incarceration have access to needed services and case management for successful reentry. The National Law Center on Homelessness and Poverty (2016) advocates starting the discharge planning process when a person is still incarcerated and suggests the process include homelessness risk assessment, establishing connections to community-based services, and planning for ongoing legal needs as individuals reenter society and need to access housing, employment, and benefits.

Community Education and Awareness Building

Since public opinion is often a main driver of anti-homeless policies, there are many opportunities for social workers to help shift attitudes through community education and awareness building. In addition to individual social workers and provider agencies, schools of social work are well-positioned for these kinds of activities. For example, Binghamton University's School of Social Work hosted a public screening of the film, *Tiny: The Life of Erin Blackwell*, which chronicles the main character's experiences with homelessness, poverty, addiction, and parenting over the course of 20 years. The film was followed by a panel of professors and local homelessness experts who answered community member questions and discussed solutions (Cole 2017).

Conclusion

In the last decade or so, the USA has made significant strides in reducing homelessness nationally while also increasing its reliance on criminalization tactics. Although common in municipalities across the country, anti-homeless policies have been widely regarded by homeless advocates as legally problematic and counterproductive to the mission of ending homelessness. In other words, anti-homeless policies are a reaction to perceived problems that homelessness causes rather than a solution to homelessness or its common causes. From a social justice perspective, the criminalization of homelessness deserves attention because it targets those most vulnerable to social and economic injustices. Further, it shows how public perceptions can influence local authorities in ways that limit the rights of those less fortunate. With these factors in mind, eliminating and preventing the criminalization of homelessness fit squarely within the roles and responsibilities of the social work profession.

References

Amster, R. (2003). Patterns of exclusion: Sanitizing space, criminalizing homelessness. *Social Justice, 30*(1), 195–221.

Amster, R. (2008). *Lost in space: The criminalization, globalization, and urban ecology of homelessness*. El Paso: LFB Scholarly Publishing.

Apuzzo, M. (2016, March 14). Justice Dept. condemns profit-minded court policies targeting the poor. https://www.nytimes.com/2016/03/15/us/politics/justice-dept-condemns-profit-minded-court-policies-targeting-the-poor.html. Accessed 30 June 2018.

Aykanian, A., & Lee, W. (2016). Social work's role in ending the criminalization of homelessness: Opportunities for action. *Social Work, 61*(2), 183–185.

Berk, R., & MacDonald, J. (2010). Policing the homeless: An evaluation of efforts to reduce homeless-related crime. *Criminology and Public Policy, 9*(4), 813–840.

Binder, S. R. (2002). *The homeless court program: Taking the court to the streets*. Washington, D.C.: American Bar Association Commission of Homelessness and Poverty.

Blasi, G. (1994). And we are not seen: Ideological and political barriers to understanding homelessness. *American Behavioral Scientist, 37*(4), 563–586.

Booker, B. (2018). White house budget calls for deep cuts to HUD. NPR. https://www.npr.org/2018/02/13/585255697/white-house-budget-calls-for-deep-cuts-to-hud. Accessed 20 May 2018.

Charles, J. B. (2017). Justice Department ends era of pushing police reform. Governing the States and Localities. http://www.governing.com/topics/public-justice-safety/lc-sessions-justice-police-reforms-trump-doj-milwaukee.html. Accessed 20 May 2018.

Cole, M. (2017, May 2). Binghamton University hosts film screening and panel discussion to raise awareness about homelessness. National Center for Excellence in Homeless Services. https://nationalcenterforexcellenceinhomelessservices.wordpress.com/2017/05/02/binghamton-university-hosts-film-screening-and-panel-discussion-to-raise-awareness-about-homelessness/. Accessed 30 June 2018.

Community Policing Dispatch. (2015). [e-newsletter issue]. The E-Newsletter of the COPS Office, 8(12). U.S. Department of Justice. https://cops.usdoj.gov/html/dispatch/12-2015/index.asp. Accessed 20 May 2018.

Covin, L. (2012). Homelessness, poverty, and incarceration: The criminalization of despair. *Journal of Forensic Psychology Practice, 12*(5), 439–456.

Culhane, D. P. (2010). Tackling homelessness in Los Angeles' Skid Row: The role of policing strategies and the spatial deconcentration of homelessness. *Criminology and Public Policy, 9*(4), 851–857.

Fitzpatrick, K. M., & Myrstol, B. (2011). The jailing of America's homeless: Evaluating the Rabble Management Thesis. *Crime and Delinquency, 57*(2), 271–297.

Fogel, S. J. (2016). Reducing vulnerability for those who are homeless during natural disasters. *Journal of Poverty, 21*(3), 208–226.

Foscarinis, M. (1999). Out of sight – Out of mind?: The continuing trend toward criminalization of homelessness. *Georgetown Journal on Poverty, Law and Policy, 6*(2), 145.

Fries, L., Fedock, G., & Kubiak, S. P. (2014). Role of gender, substance use, and serious mental illness in anticipated postjail homelessness. *Social Work Research, 38*(2), 107–116.

Garland, T. S., Richards, T., & Cooney, M. (2010). Victims hidden in plain sight: The reality of victimization among the homeless. *Criminal Justice Studies, 23*(4), 285–301.

Giambrone, A. (2016, September 8). A new space for homeless youth quietly opened in a church downtown. Washington City Paper. http://www.washingtoncitypaper.com/news/housing-complex/article/20833081/a-new-space-for-homeless-youth-quietly-opened-in-a-church-downtown. Accessed 20 May 2018.

Goldberg, E. (2013, September 9). Columbia, South Carolina rescinds decision to criminalize homelessness. Huffington Post. http://www.huffingtonpost.com/2013/09/04/columbia-criminalizing-homelessness_n_3866273.html. Accessed 20 May 2018.

Impact Homelessness. (2014). *Insider's briefing: The state of chronic homelessness in Osceola County*. Orlando: Author.

Irwin, J. (1985). *The jail: Managing the underclass in American society*. Berkley/Los Angeles: University of California Press.

Jorgensen, J. (2017, July 7). Mayor de Blasio says he wishes panhandling 'didn't exist' in New York City because 'it's off-putting'. New York Daily News. http://www.nydailynews.com/new-york/de-blasio-wishes-panhandling-didn-exist-nyc-article-1.3308982. Accessed 20 May 2018.

Kusmer, K. L. (2002). *Down and out, on the road: The homeless in American history*. New York: Oxford University Press.

Kushel, M. B., Hahn, J. A., Evans, J. L., Bangsberg, D. R., & Moss, A. R. (2005). Resolving doors: Imprisonment among the homeless and marginally housed population. *American Journal of Public Health, 95*(10), 1747–1752.

Levin, B. (2015). Reassessing laws on hate violence against the homeless. *American Behavioral Scientist, 59*(13), 1715–1728.

Liberatore, W. (2017, July 17). Residents sue Spa City over Code Blue shelter. Times Union. http://www.timesunion.com/local/article/Residents-sue-city-over-Code-Blue-shelter-11292328.php. Accessed 20 May 2018.

Lopez, C. (2017, May). Homeless courts. National Center for State Courts. http://www.ncsc.org/sitecore/content/microsites/trends/home/Monthly-Trends-Articles/2017/Homeless-Courts.aspx. Accessed 20 May 2018.

Martell, D. A., Rosner, R., & Harmon, R. B. (1995). Base-rate estimates of criminal behavior by homeless mentally ill persons in New York City. *Psychiatric Services, 46*(6), 596–601.

McGuire, J. F., & Rosenheck, R. A. (2004). Criminal history as a prognostic indicator in the treatment of homeless people with severe mental illness. *Psychiatric Services, 55*(1), 42–48.

McNamara, R. H., Crawford, C., & Burns, R. (2013). Policing the homeless: Policy, practice, and perceptions. *Policing: An International Journal of Police Strategies and Management, 36*(2), 357–374.

McNiel, D. E., Binder, R. L., & Robinson, J. C. (2005). Incarceration associated with homelessness, mental disorder, and co-occurring substance abuse. *Psychiatric Services, 56*(7), 840–846.

Meinbresse, M., Brinkley-Rubinstein, L., Grassette, A., Benson, J., Hamilton, R., Malott, M., & Jenkins, D. (2014). Exploring the experiences of violence among individuals who are homeless using a consumer-led approach. *Violence and Victims, 29*(1), 122–136.

Metraux, S., Byrne, T., & Culhane, D. P. (2010). Institutional discharges and subsequent shelter use among unaccompanied adults in New York City. *Journal of Community Psychology, 38*(1), 28–38.

Mitchell, D. (1997). The annihilation of space by law: The roots and implications of anti-homeless laws in the United States. *Antipode, 29*(3), 303–335.

National Coalition for the Homeless. (2014). *Vulnerable to hate: A survey of hate crimes and violence committed against homeless people in 2013*. Washington, D.C.: Author.
National Law Center on Homelessness and Poverty. (2006). *A dream denied: The criminalization of homelessness in U.S. cities*. Washington, D.C: Author.
National Law Center on Homelessness and Poverty. (2016). *Housing not handcuffs: Ending the criminalization of homelessness in U.S. cities*. Washington, D.C: Author.
Oliver, N. (2017, June 10). For its first free-standing, modern public bathroom, Richmond looks to Portland ultra-durable model. Richmond Times-Dispatch. http://www.richmond.com/news/local/city-of-richmond/for-its-first-free-standing-modern-public-restroom-richmond-looks/article_dc2741f6-f1a9-5abf-8fc3-ddcf268fe1ab.html. Accessed 20 May 2018.
Rankin, S. (2015). A homeless bill of rights (revolution). *Seton Hall Law Review, 45*(2), 383–444.
Smith, D. (1994). A theoretical and legal challenge to homeless criminalization as public policy. *Yale Law and Policy Review, 12*(2), 487–517.
Smith, J. (1996). Arresting the homeless for sleeping public: A paradigm for expanding the Robinson Doctrine. *Columbia Journal of Law and Social Problems, 29*(2), 293–335.
Smith, D. (2016, September 11). Pomona settles lawsuit over confiscation of homeless people's property. Los Angeles Times. http://www.latimes.com/local/lanow/la-me-ln-pomona-homeless-settlement-20160911-snap-story.html. Accessed 20 May 2018.
Snow, D. A., Baker, S. G., & Anderson, L. (1989). Criminality and homeless men: An empirical assessment. *Social Problems, 36*(5), 532–549.
Sullivan, K. (2017). Embedded social worker addressing homelessness: Delgado teams of up with Monroe police sergeant. Monroe Monitor. https://monroemonitor.com/Content/News/News/Article/Embedded-social-worker-addressing-homelessness/26/337/10603. Accessed 20 May 2018.
Thrush, G. (2018). HUD floats a plan intended to reduce reliance on housing assistance. New York Times. https://www.nytimes.com/2018/04/25/us/hud-housing-assistance.html. Accessed 20 May 2018.
Tompsett, C. J., Toro, P. A., Guzicki, M., Schlienz, N., Blume, M., & Lombardo, S. (2003). Homelessness in the U.S. and Germany: A cross-national analysis. *Journal of Community and Applied Social Psychology, 13*(3), 240–257.
Trattner, W. I. (1989). *From poor law to welfare state*. New York: The Free Press.
U.N. Human Rights Committee. (2014). Concluding observations on the fourth report of the United States of America. National Law Center on Homelessness and Poverty. https://www.nlchp.org/INT_CCPR_COC_USA_16838_E.pdf. Accessed 20 May 2018.
U.S. Department of Education. (2015). Every student succeeds act. https://www2.ed.gov/policy/elsec/leg/essa/index.html. Accessed 20 May 2018.
U.S. Department of Housing and Urban Development. (2016). Notice of funding availability (NOFA) for the fiscal year (FY) 2016 continuum of care program competition. https://www.hudexchange.info/resources/documents/FY-2016-CoC-Program-NOFA.pdf. Accessed 20 May 2018.
U.S. Department of Justice. (2015). Justice Department files brief to address the criminalization of homelessness. https://www.justice.gov/opa/pr/justice-department-files-brief-address-criminalization-homelessness. Accessed 20 May 2018.
U.S. Interagency Council on Homelessness. (2012). Searching out solutions: Constructive solutions to the criminalization of homelessness. https://www.usich.gov/tools-for-action/searching-out-solutions. Accessed 20 May 2018.
U.S. Interagency Council on Homelessness. (2015). Ending homelessness for people living in encampments: Advancing the dialogue. https://www.usich.gov/tools-for-action/ending-homelessness-for-people-in-encampments. Accessed 20 May 2018.
Vitale, A. S. (2008). *How the quality of life campaign transformed New York politics*. New York: NYU Press.
Wachholz, S. (2005). Hate crimes against the homeless: Warning-out New England style. *Sociology and Social Welfare, 32*(4), 141–163.

Wong, I. (2008). Homelessness. In T. Mizrahi & L. E. Davis (Eds.), *Encyclopedia of social work* (20th ed., pp. 377–383). Washington, D.C.: National Association of Social Workers.

Zielinski, A. (2017, May 16). What's behind SAPD's shifting approach to homelessness. San Antonio Current. https://www.sacurrent.com/the-daily/archives/2017/05/16/whats-behind-sapds-shifting-approach-to-homelessness. Accessed 20 May 2018.

Zimmerman, G. (2017, April 17). Nickels and dimes: The criminalization of Rhode Island's poor. Brown Political Review. http://www.brownpoliticalreview.org/2017/04/nickels-dimes-criminalization-rhode-islands-poor/. Accessed 20 May 2018.

Chapter 10
Pay-for-Success Financing: Innovation in Funding Supportive Housing Initiatives

Calvin L. Streeter, Maya Williams, and Ann Howard

Introduction

The pay-for-success (PFS) model, sometimes called social impact bonds, has gained momentum in recent years as an innovative way to bring private investments to support efforts designed to reduce social problems. Stagnant funding for the nonprofit sector and years of sluggish progress toward solving seemingly intractable social problems have led some to hope that PFS financing will spark social innovation by attracting new capital to support program delivery, improve government accountability, and increase rigor in performance measurement (Baldini 2016). PFS financing shifts the risk associated with funding social service innovations from taxpayers to investors who finance programs. These investors receive repayment from the government, or other end-payor, only if a predetermined performance metric, or outcome, is achieved. By using rigorous third-party evaluators to measure a program's success, PFS encourages the use of evidence-informed practices that can deliver measurable results that produce real impacts in people's lives.

PFS programs provide the up-front working capital needed to implement interventions that are proven to produce positive results, generate significant public

---

Electronic supplementary material: The online version of this chapter (https://doi.org/10.1007/978-3-030-03727-7_10) contains supplementary material, which is available to authorized users.

C. L. Streeter (✉)
University of Texas at Austin, Austin, TX, USA
e-mail: cstreeter@utexas.edu

M. Williams
Washington University, St. Louis, MO, USA
e-mail: maya.williams@wustl.edu

A. Howard
Ending Community Homelessness Coalition, Austin, TX, USA
e-mail: annhoward@austinecho.org

H. Larkin et al. (eds.), *Homelessness Prevention and Intervention in Social Work*, https://doi.org/10.1007/978-3-030-03727-7_10

value relative to the cost of the current system of services, and save the government money over time. The savings generated (or sometimes the avoided costs) from the successful implementation of the intervention can be used to repay the investors their principal, and sometimes a modest return, or can be reinvested back into the project, providing additional resources to further scale the project. Philanthropic investors prefer this model instead of a one-time gift to support a program, as they have the option of reinvesting their resources in this or other projects more than once.

This chapter outlines the basic principles of PFS financing and explores some of the challenges and opportunities learned from early PFS initiatives. It provides an overview of several current projects from across the USA that focus on affordable housing and programs designed to end homelessness.

Background

After several years of planning, the first PFS project was launched in 2010 in the United Kingdom as a 6-year pilot designed to reduce recidivism from a prison in Peterborough (Barajas et al. 2014). Between 2010 and 2015, an intervention called One Service tested the hypothesis that offering comprehensive and individualized support services to prisoners would reduce the likelihood of them returning to prison while providing opportunities to build a new life on the outside (Social Finance 2014).

The PFS funding vehicle was developed on the premise that societal costs associated with high recidivism rates created a unique opportunity to monetize social impact and develop a novel mechanism for financing social innovation. It also allowed government and other stakeholders to rethink how public funds are allocated and administered for social service interventions. If recidivism rates could be decreased, the associated costs to society (i.e., taxpayers) would also be reduced. While existing evidence suggested the program should work, it was unknown whether recidivism would in fact be reduced by this intervention. Impact investors were willing to take a chance by funding this innovative project with the expectation that positive results would produce cost savings for the government. The government would then use those savings to return their investment with a small rate of return. Evaluation of the first cohort of 1000 inmates found the program had reduced recidivism in the intervention group by 8.4% relative to a comparable national baseline (Social Finance 2014). While this reduction was below the 10% decrease needed to trigger immediate repayment to investors, the performance indicated that investors were on track to receive a return on investment in 2016 if the reduction remained above 7.5% (Ganguly 2014).

Before these results were known, enthusiasm for PFS's innovative potential spread quickly to other parts of the world as impact investors and government officials began to explore how this novel financing strategy could be used to address other difficult social problems and needs, like ending homelessness, preventing teen pregnancy, eliminating health disparities, and improving workforce development. When Barack Obama was elected president in 2008, a group called America Forward recommended that his transition team create a "social innovation fund." The Obama administration embraced the idea and in 2009 established the first-ever Social Innovation Fund administered by the Corporation for National and Community Service, designed to mobilize private sector partners who would support PFS projects (Office of Social Innovation and Civic Participation 2017). Since its inception, the Social Innovation Fund has leveraged $340 million in federal investment to attract $672 million in nonfederal sources resulting in more than $1 billion invested in growing effective programs. The Obama administration laid the groundwork for PFS, paving the way for its expansion under the Trump administration, which has declared its intent to expand public-private partnerships across all sectors of the government (Social Innovation Fund 2017).

What Is Pay-for-Success Financing?

According to Bal (2018), PFS is about "measurably improving the lives of people most in need by driving government resources toward more effective programs" (p. 2). PFS projects begin with a social problem or challenge the government aims to resolve. Central to any PFS project are the people and communities in need who would benefit from access to more effective services. Through PFS, stakeholders from the public, private, and social sectors come together to design and invest in better programs.

PFS sits at the intersection of three powerful movements (see Fig. 10.1; Bal 2018, p. 3). First, there is a growing demand that resources be directed toward programs that demonstrate positive results based on rigorous evaluation. Effort is good but only if it produces results. Increasingly, funders are imposing performance requirements that demand improved outcomes, not just level of effort, in meeting the needs of society's most vulnerable.

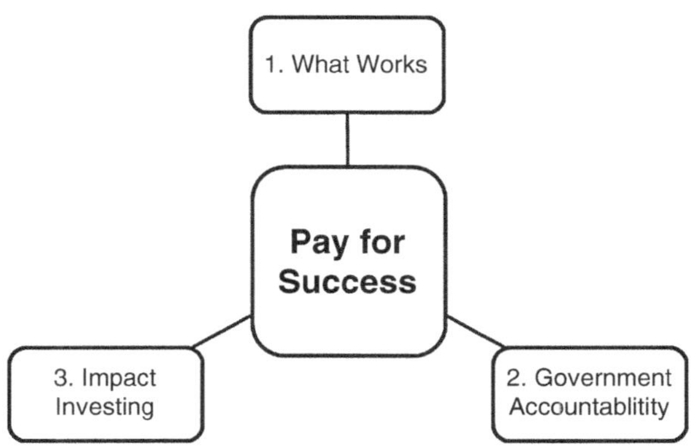

Fig. 10.1 PFS sits at the intersection of three powerful movements

Second, there is increased demand for government accountability. According to Greiling and Halachmi (2013), "accountability has to do with appropriateness of actions and adherence to obligation (p. 387)." Despite recent legislation to increase the amount and scope of government accountability, public perception of the government's responsiveness, efficiency, and effectiveness remains low. Citizens are increasingly using social media and other forms of pressure to demand that elected officials address the most pressing social problems and, at the same time, be good stewards of taxpayer dollars.

Third, a growing number of individuals and corporations are shifting away from traditional models of philanthropy for supporting the nonprofit sector to what has become known as impact investing. Impact investing refers to investments with the intention of generating measurable social and environmental impacts alongside a financial return (Greene 2015). Impact investing falls somewhere between traditional investing, where the focus is on maximizing return on investment, and philanthropy. Impact investments have typically focused on for-profit companies whose mission includes producing some social good. However, increasingly, impact investing has shifted to include the nonprofit sector.

Central to the concept of PFS are public-private partnerships that fund effective social service programs through performance-based contracts. Under the PFS model, impact is measured, and the government makes payments based on results, not activities. If, based on a rigorous evaluation by an independent third party, the program achieves predetermined and agreed-upon outcomes, the government repays the original investment, sometimes with a small return. However, if the expected results are not achieved, the government pays nothing. This focus on paying for positive social impact, rather than services performed, helps reinforce the focus on producing positive social impact and provides a mechanism for the government to ensure it only pays for what works (Corporation for Supportive Housing 2014a, 2014b).

Performance-based contracting is not itself an innovation; such contracts are common in infrastructure development projects. For example, the Department of Defense has procured services from contractors using performance-based contracting for decades. In addition, many local and state governments use performance clauses in their procurement of social services, such as bonuses for contractors delivering job training programs based on the number of clients who obtain and retain employment. What makes PFS financing different is that the model is not simply focused on creating incentives for contractors to produce better outcomes. It also seeks to overcome a set of barriers that hinder the pace of social change, such as political constraints that inhibit the government from investing in prevention efforts, the inability of nonprofit organizations to access the capital needed to expand their operations, and insufficient capacity to develop rapid and rigorous evidence to support what works (Azemati et al. 2013).

How Does Pay-for-Success Work?

PFS can involve many stakeholders working together through a complex set of relationships. According to the Corporation for Supportive Housing (2014a), a typical PFS housing initiative would include an *end-payor*, which could include state or local governments, hospitals, or universities. The end-payor agrees to repay the investors if the intervention achieves the predetermined performance metrics. An *intermediary* identifies and coordinates the partners and oversees the initiative for the long term. This includes identifying *investors*, such as institutional and philanthropic investors, who provide up-front capital to implement the intervention. Housing and service providers work closely with the target population to ensure their needs are being met. And an *independent evaluator* conducts a rigorous evaluation to determine if the agreed-upon metrics have been met. If the evaluation determines that the metrics have been met, the end-payor reimburses the investors with a small return on investment (Corporation for Supportive Housing 2014a, 2014b). In effect, the PFS collaboration provides the up-front financial resources, technical assistance, and community capacity needed to deliver the intervention, and the government, or other end-payor, agrees to reimburse investors after success has been documented by the evaluation.

The Corporation for Supportive Housing (2014a) uses the diagram in Fig. 10.2 to illustrate how PFS works. In this model, the government selects a desired

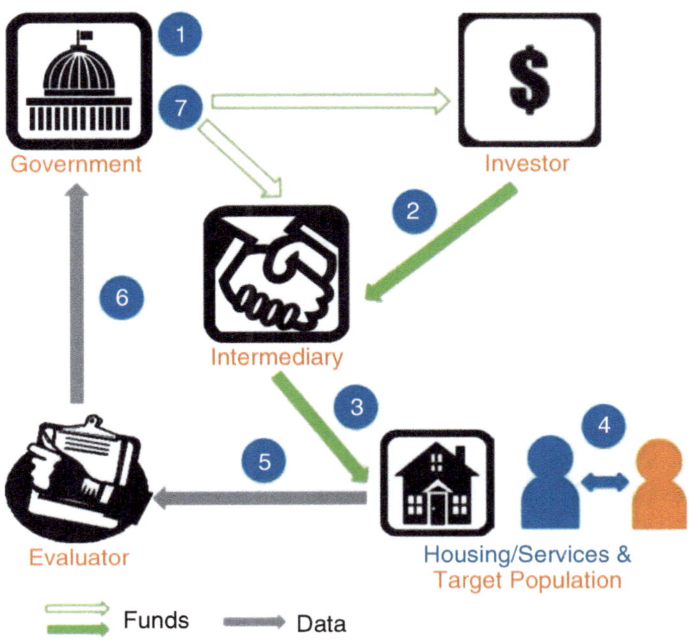

Fig. 10.2 How does pay-for-success work? (Corporation for Supportive Housing 2014a)

intervention, contracts with an intermediary to structure the initiative, and identifies impact investors who provide the up-front capital needed to finance the project. The intermediary gives service providers the working capital needed to implement the intervention, and the service providers deliver the rental assistance and other support services to the target population. The intermediary develops processes to collect the outcome and cost data needed to evaluate the agreed-upon metrics, which is provided to the third-party evaluator. The evaluator applies rigorous evaluation methods and uses the data to determine whether the agreed-upon metrics have been achieved. Based on the evaluation, a decision is made whether and to what degree the investors are entitled to repayment of their investment.

Of course, the actual partnerships and processes are more complex than this. The government must identify an intermediary and make a compelling case for why the intervention is needed and how it will produce the desired social impacts in order to attract investors. There must also be a contractual agreement about what metrics will be used to assess whether the project goals were met and if reimbursement will be made. Once the contract between the end-payor(s) and investor(s) is in place, the intermediary must work closely with service providers to ensure the intervention is being implemented with fidelity and that the providers are adhering to the rigorous evaluation methods designed by the evaluator. The evaluation needs to produce a valid and reliable assessment of the intervention that does not disrupt the ongoing intervention with a vulnerable target population. To learn more about the impact of the intervention, some projects evaluate additional metrics beyond the ones agreed to trigger repayment. To be effective, all stakeholders need to be satisfied that the intervention was implemented as intended and that the evaluation was as rigorous and definitive as possible.

Pay-for-Success Housing Initiatives

Over the last 20 years, the evidence has clearly demonstrated that supportive housing is an effective intervention to improve housing stability, reduce the use of expensive crisis care, and improve outcomes for even the most vulnerable individuals with complex needs (Rog et al. 2014; SAMSHA 2010). In communities throughout the USA, there are individuals who frequently cycle in and out of high-cost crisis services like emergency rooms, jails, detox centers, and homeless shelters. Supportive housing has been shown to significantly reduce the costs associated with those types of crisis services by housing people and then providing the support services needed to maintain them in housing long term (Corporation for Supportive Housing 2014a, b).

Since PFS initiatives are built on the premise that the cost of the intervention will be significantly less than the services as usual model, supportive housing programs are uniquely suited to this type of social impact investing. Several projects are underway across the USA that are designed to use PFS financing to address the needs of people experiencing homelessness or housing insecurity. Below is a brief description of five of those PFS initiatives.

Massachusetts

Massachusetts has more than 1500 chronically homeless individuals who require myriad costly public and emergency services, such as hospitalization, temporary shelter, and high-cost Medicaid benefits (Garvey 2015). Claiming to be the first PFS initiative in the nation addressing chronic homelessness, the Home and Healthy for Good (HHG) program was implemented in 2014 by the Massachusetts Housing and Shelter Alliance (MHSA) for the Commonwealth of Massachusetts. The goal of this 6-year initiative is to provide low-threshold, permanent supportive housing to those who would otherwise rely on costly emergency resources, enabling them to address their often-complex health issues more effectively than they would on the streets or in shelters. This PFS initiative provides 500 units of stable supportive housing to 800 chronically homeless individuals. With $3.5 million in flexible funding, the program incorporates evidence-based practices to build long-term housing and provide supportive services, including access to preventative and primary healthcare (Nonprofit Finance Fund 2017a). If successful, the HHG program will have measurably improved life outcomes for this population, in addition to realizing cost savings for the State of Massachusetts.

The independent evaluator for this initiative is the Root Cause Institute, a Boston-based organization whose mission is to use data to drive performance in nonprofits, foundations, and governments. Using a validated data methodology of provider performance and Medicaid data, Root Cause tracks healthcare usage, number of nights spent in shelters, number of days incarcerated, and length of time in stable housing. The Commonwealth of Massachusetts repays investors with initial payment triggered by 40% housing stability for 12 months. Full repayment of principal is triggered by 80% housing stability for 12 months, and the full repayment plus maximum return on investment is triggered by 94% housing stability for 12 months (Nonprofit Finance Fund 2017a).

Santa Clara County, California

In August of 2015, Santa Clara County received support from Third Sector Capital Partners and launched Project Welcome Home, California's first PFS initiative. It is estimated that more than 2200 chronically homeless individuals live in Santa Clara County (Urban Institute 2017a). This 6-year project received $6.9 million in funding to provide community-based clinical services and permanent supportive housing to 150–200 chronically homeless individuals who are frequent users of the county's emergency rooms, acute mental health facilities, and jail (Mitchell 2015). The lead service provider for the project is Abode Services, a Bay Area housing service provider with a track record of effective and high-quality programming.

The University of California San Francisco (UCSF) School of Medicine is the independent evaluator for the project and is assessing whether provision of permanent supportive housing significantly improves clients' health while decreasing their use of costly county services. A randomized control trial (RCT) is being used to track whether the combination of services implemented by Abode produces measurable improvement in health and social service utilization for these chronically homeless adults. The project's target impact is for more than 80% of participants to achieve 12 months of continuous stable housing. Santa Clara County makes success payments to investors when participants achieve specific tenancy milestones. UCSF will determine success payments based on the number of months of continuous stable tenancy achieved by participants over the 6-year project. At the target level of impact, the amount of success payments would fully repay all investors their principal and base annual interest. At higher levels of impact, additional success payments will be made, subject to a maximum of $8 million in total success payments (Third Sector Capital Partners 2017a).

Denver, Colorado

The cost of providing safety-net services to 250 of Denver's chronically homeless adults is approximately $7 million per year. That includes the cost of 14,000 days in jail, 2200 visits to detox facilities, 1500 arrests, and 500 emergency room visits (Urban Institute 2017b). In 2016, a PFS effort called the Housing to Health Initiative was launched to provide permanent supportive housing to help keep Denver's homeless population out of the criminal justice system while providing stable housing for those in need. Through a 5-year, $8.7 million social impact bond, this project scales Housing First and a modified Assertive Community Treatment (ACT) model – a multidisciplinary team-based approach with assertive outreach that delivers supportive services, including case management, crisis intervention, substance use counseling, mental health treatment, peer support, skills building, and connection to primary care. Services are designed to address barriers to housing stability, manage mental illness, reduce interaction with the criminal justice system, and improve health outcomes. The project targets 250 individuals who frequently use the city's emergency services, including police, jail, courts, and emergency rooms (Corporation for Supportive Housing 2017a).

The Urban Institute is the independent evaluator for the Housing to Health initiative. It will conduct a process evaluation and a randomized control trial study to assess program outcomes (Cunningham et al. 2016). The outcome evaluation is designed to determine if participants retain housing and whether supportive housing increases housing stability and decreases the use of high-cost public services, such as jail, detox, homeless shelters, and hospitals. It also examines the question of whether outcomes differ for participants housed in scattered-site housing or single-site (also known as congregate) housing (Corporation for Supportive Housing 2017a). The primary triggers for repayment to investors are housing stability and reductions in jail days. Initial payment is triggered by 12 months of housing stability and a 20% reduction in jail days. Full payment of principle is triggered by 83% housing stability for 12 months and a 30% reduction in jail days. Maximum repayment is triggered by 100% housing stability for 12 months and a 65% reduction in jail days, up to a maximum of $11.42 million (Nonprofit Finance Fund 2017b).

Salt Lake County, Utah

In 2016, Salt Lake County, Utah, launched two simultaneous PFS projects to address two complex and intertwined issues, homelessness and criminal justice reform (Third Sector Capital Partners 2017b). The criminal justice project, called Recovery, Engagement, Assessment, Career, and Housing (REACH), is designed to improve outcomes for individuals with moderate to severe substance use disorders and a number of other co-occurring criminogenic characteristics by providing holistic support and treatment using the risk-need-responsivity (RNR) model and Moral Reconation Therapy. The homelessness project, Homes Not Jails, aims to scale-up comprehensive rapid rehousing and wraparound supportive services in order to improve housing stability, reduce the number of days spent in the county jail, increase economic stability, and improve behavioral health (Salt Lake County, 2016b).

The two projects have secured investments of $11.5 million and will serve more than 500 of Salt Lake County's most vulnerable and costly residents (Salt Lake County 2016a). Homes Not Jails builds on the Housing First model to provide 315 individuals with a range of housing assistance and support services, including rental assistance, intensive case management, behavioral health treatment, and employment counseling. REACH will serve approximately 225 formerly incarcerated adult males who are at high risk of reoffending.

The independent evaluator for these projects is the Utah Criminal Justice Center (UCJC) in the College of Social Work at the University of Utah (Salt Lake County 2016a). Each program will be evaluated using a randomized control trial design. For the REACH programs, repayment will be triggered by four measures: a 35% reduction in days incarcerated over 4 years, a 35% reduction in statewide arrests over 4 years, a 25% improvement in quarters employed over 2 years, and a 66% successful program engagement of 200 hours within 6 months of enrollment. Salt Lake County will pay a maximum of $5.95 million in success payments for REACH.

For Homes Not Jails, payments will be triggered by a 30% reduction in time spent in shelter or jail over 2 years, 80% successful graduation from the program within 1 year of enrollment, 100% improvement in substance use treatment engagement over 2 years, and 100% improvement in mental health treatment engagement over 2 years. The county will repay a maximum of $5.55 million for Homes Not Jails (Salt Lake County 2016b).

Cuyahoga County, Ohio

Homeless families face many challenges, including the inability to provide safe and stable living environments for their children. As a result, children who are placed in out-of-home foster care because of homelessness remain in the child welfare system for significantly longer than children whose families have housing. Extended stays in foster care can negatively impact children's educational attainment and future employment status (Doyle 2007; Younes and Harp 2007). To address this cycle of poor outcomes, in 2015, Cuyahoga County launched the first county-level PFS project targeting homelessness and child welfare. Through FrontLine's Critical Time Intervention, Child Parent Psychotherapy, and Trauma Adapted Family Connections, the project aims to reduce the length of stay in foster care and achieve housing permanency and/or family reunification. The intensive treatment will take place over 5 years and serve 135 families. If successful, vulnerable families will be able to reconnect to the community, settle into safe housing, and rebuild a healthy relationship with their children (Third Sector Community Partners 2016).

The independent evaluator for this project is the Center on Urban Poverty and Community Development in the Mandel School of Applied Social Sciences at Case Western Reserve University. The evaluation assesses program effectiveness in helping stabilize families through housing supports and increased levels of public assistance utilization to decrease the level of involvement with child welfare and contacts with case management services over time. Success payments will begin in the first quarter of 2021, 21 quarters after the program's initial launch. Payments will be based on the reduction in the combined number of out-of-home placement days for children in the treatment group versus the control group. Cuyahoga County will pay $75 per reduced foster care day, which represents the current combined average cost of foster care and related placement services. The program's target impact is a 25% reduction in out-of-home placement days for the treated population. At that level of impact, all funders would be repaid their principal investment and base annual interest. At higher levels of impact, investors will receive up to $1 million in additional success payments based on increased savings to the County (Corporation for Supportive Housing 2017b).

Austin, Texas

In March 2015, the Ending Community Homelessness Coalition (ECHO) in Austin, Texas, was one of six grantees selected for a technical assistance grant to assess the feasibility of a PFS initiative focused on creating supportive housing for the city's most vulnerable people experiencing homelessness (Corporation for Supportive Housing 2015). As a community, Austin has a record of working on many fronts to end homelessness. Permanent supportive housing (PSH) is Austin's key strategy to address chronic homelessness for individuals who cannot otherwise access and maintain housing. The Austin City Council initially adopted this strategy in 2010 with a focus on closing a 1900 unit gap for supportive housing. The initial goal of establishing 350 PSH units for individuals experiencing chronic homelessness was achieved in 2014. Based on the success of the initial effort, the City Council renewed its commitment by setting a new goal to create 400 PSH units by the end of 2018, with at least 200 units implemented using the Housing First model (City of Austin 2017).

To be viable, any PFS intervention needs to substantially reduce costs over the existing status quo system, and the cost of the intervention should be less than the combined cost savings and added value to the end-payor. As part of its PFS feasibility study, ECHO and its partners, Social Finance, Inc. and the Corporation for Supportive Housing, were able to document that persons experiencing long histories of homelessness, and who had chronic disabilities and health conditions, are disproportionate users of high-cost public services that provide only short-term respite for their health and basic needs.

According to the cost-benefit analysis, the average cost of the status quo system before supportive housing totaled $101,218 per person per year, whereas system costs after the supportive housing intervention were estimated to average $23,059 per person per year. This showed that, on average, the supportive housing costs were $78,159 lower per person per year than the status quo system (Corporation for Supportive Housing 2016a). Costs per person for the PFS supportive housing intervention were estimated at $28,557, resulting in a projected cost avoidance for the systems of $49,602 – the estimated cost avoidance from the supportive housing intervention ($78,158) minus the estimated cost of the supportive housing intervention ($28,557) (Corporation for Supportive Housing 2016a). The preliminary financial model and framework for this initiative showed that a PFS investment of $17 million over 5 years would produce an expected total net cost avoidance, after success payments, of $42.8 million.

Based on this analysis, ECHO and the City of Austin launched a 6-year PFS-funded PSH project. This initiative does not fund actual housing costs; rather, it provides flexible and comprehensive supportive housing services using an intensive case management approach called Assertive Community Treatment (ACT) to house 250 homeless individuals whose cumulative criminal justice, healthcare, shelter, and emergency medical services place them among the most expensive users of public services. It is anticipated that, during the project, 250 units of housing will be identified through other commitments by the City of Austin to produce affordable housing units, as well as scatter-site units made affordable through several other subsidy sources, such as housing authority vouchers, Medicaid 1115 Waiver-funded supportive housing, and a partnership with United Healthcare to locate Medicaid clients needing housing (Corporation for Supportive Housing 2016a).

While the potential cost savings as outlined by the cost-benefit analysis may serve as the foundation for PFS repayment, success metrics and payment triggers do not have to be based solely on cost avoidance or savings. Some cost reductions can be difficult to document directly and may occur across systems or over time beyond when the PFS contract is completed. Moreover, as suggested by Moore and Khagram

(2004), public value, which is the less tangible benefits to society (e.g., fairness, justice, and equity) that may result from such projects, may be hard to document with traditional metrics. On the other hand, for some communities, these will prove significant in getting the project over the finish line. In Austin, by 2017, business owners, elected officials, and advocates all agreed that the city needed to address homelessness as a top priority. ECHO drafted an Action Plan to End Homelessness that included implementing the PFS funding model to help scale-up PSH. Determined to demonstrate commitment to ending homelessness, on September 14, 2017, the City Council dedicated $1.2 million toward their role as end-payor without commitment of other community partners in healthcare or criminal justice. The promise of ending homelessness for 250 people, who may trouble the business community in downtown Austin, and of leveraging private investment helped the Council endorse the PFS project by voting to fund it.

During the feasibility study, success payments for this project were discussed in relation to three key metrics (Corporation for Supportive Housing 2016a).

1. *Stable housing*. Considerable research has shown that supportive housing has a positive impact on housing retention, even among tenants with long histories of homelessness and the most severe psychiatric, substance use, and health challenges. The goal is to keep at least 80% of project participants housed for at least 12 months.
2. *Reduced criminal justice involvement*. Reductions in the usage of the public safety and criminal justice systems, such as police interactions, jail days, and arrest rates by members of the target population. Exact targets for these reductions would be determined in partnership with the project end-payors during transaction structuring.
3. *Reductions in emergency room usage, emergency medical services, and inpatient costs*. The assumption is that a reduction in inappropriate usage of the emergency and inpatient resources by members of the target population and promoting the usage of appropriate preventive or primary care services will contribute to project success.

Conclusion

Homelessness is a complex social problem that sits at the intersection of many interrelated problems, such as a lack of affordable housing, poverty, addiction, mental illness, access to affordable healthcare, unemployment, and stagnant wages. Existing social services are often so overwhelmed by demand for their services that they are unable to address the underlying causes of homelessness. Governments too often lack the resources and long-term commitment required to invest in preventive approaches that could improve lives and change the conditions that contribute to homelessness. This chapter has presented PFS financing as a new funding approach to mobilize private resources through impact investing to support the development of innovative solutions that will produce measurable impacts.

The Corporation for Supportive Housing (CSH) and Social Finance are leaders in promoting PFS investment to expand the use of supportive housing targeted at the most vulnerable populations. CSH and Social Finance are positioned to support governments and social impact investors in structuring PFS financing options to address the need for more supportive housing.

PFS combines a novel financing model with strong community partnerships to promote innovative programs. While this is a strength of the approach, anyone who has worked on either innovation or partnership initiatives knows that they take time and considerable effort. How much time? CSH (2016b) estimates at least 6–12 months are needed for a feasibility study that leaves communities with all the pieces in place to structure a PFS transaction. The actual partnerships and processes required by a successful PFS initiative can be very complex and involve many stakeholders, each with their own set of interests. This front-end commitment to assessing the feasibility of PFS is well worth the effort as the project roles out. The feasibility assessment is a period when trust is built among the stakeholders, common interests are identified, and agreements are clearly articulated regarding investment repayment.

References

Azemati, H., Belinsky, M., Gillette, R., Liebman, J., Sellman, A., & Wyse, A. (2013). Social impact bonds: Lessons learned so far. *Community Development Investment Review, 22*, 23–33.

Baldini, N. S. (2016). Pay for success: Financing research-informed practice. *Cascade, 89. Fall 2015.* http://www.payforsuccess.org/resource/pay-success-financing-research-informed-practice. Accessed 30 June 2018.

Barajas, A., Burt, K., Johnson, P., Licona, J., Parker, W., Sturtevant, L., Quincey, V., Barajas, L., Harper, T., Larsen, E., Nije, C. O., Reid, K., Tokunaga, M., & Yeh, C. (2014). Social impact bonds: A new tool for social financing. Princeton University. https://wws.princeton.edu/sites/default/files/content/Social%20Impact%20Bonds%202014%20Final%20Report.pdf. Accessed 30 June 2018.

Bal, N. K. (2018). Reinventing Our Communities: Strategies for Outcomes Based Financing. Social Finance, October 2018. https://www.philadelphiafed.org/-/media/community-development/events/2018/reinventing-our-communities/presentations/navjeet-bal.pdf?la=en. Accessed 14 January 2019.

City of Austin. (2017). A roof over Austin: Permanent supportive housing initiative. http://www.austintexas.gov/department/permanent-supportive-housing-initiative. Accessed 30 June 2018.

Corporation for Supportive Housing. (2014a). Social impact investments: A tool for scaling supportive housing. http://www.csh.org/wp-content/uploads/2014/05/SocialImpactInvestment_SHConcept1.pdf. Accessed 30 June 2018.

Corporation for Supportive Housing. (2014b). CSH recognized as national pay for success leaders. http://www.csh.org/2014/10/csh-recognized-as-national-pay-for-success-leader/. Accessed 30 June 2018.

Corporation for Supportive Housing. (2015). CSH announces grants to advance pay for success investments [Press Release]. http://www.csh.org/wp-content/uploads/2015/03/ECHO.pdf. Accessed 30 June 2018.

Corporation for Supportive Housing. (2016a). Social innovation fund pay for success feasibility report: ECHO Austin/Travis County. http://www.austinecho.org/wp-content/uploads/2016/11/ECHO-Pay-for-Success-Feasibility-Report.pdf. Accessed 30 June 2018.

Corporation for Supportive Housing. (2016b). Are you ready for PFS? http://www.csh.org/2016/09/are-you-ready-for-pfs/. Accessed 30 June 2018.

Corporation for Supportive Housing. (2017a). Fact sheet: Denver social impact bond program to address homelessness. http://www.csh.org/wp-content/uploads/2011/12/Denver-SIB-FactSheet.pdf. Accessed 30 June 2018.

Corporation for Supportive Housing (2017b). Fact sheet: The Cuyahoga Partnering for Family Success Program. http://www.thirdsectorcap.org/wp-content/uploads/2015/12/Cuyahoga_PFS_Fact-Sheet_UPDATED-NOV-2015_FINAL.pdf. Accessed 30 June 2018.

Cunningham, M., Pergamit, M., Gillespie, S., Hanson, D., & Kooragayala, S. (2016). *Denver supportive housing social impact bond initiative: Evaluation and research design*. Washington, D.C.: Urban Institute.

Doyle, J. J. (2007). *Child protection and child outcomes: Measuring the effects of foster care*. Cambridge, MA: MIT Sloan School of Management & NBER.

Ganguly, B. (2014). The success of the Peterborough social impact bond. The Rockefeller Foundation. https://www.rockefellerfoundation.org/blog/success-peterborough-social-impact/. Accessed 30 June 2018.

Garvey, M. (2015). Massachusetts chronic individual homelessness pay for success initiative. Institute for Child Success. http://pfs.instituteforchildsuccess.org/wp-content/uploads/2015/11/summary_of_pay_for_success_social_impact_bonds_Massachusetts_homelessness.pdf. Accessed 30 June 2018.

Greene, S. (2015). *A short guide to impact investing*. Washington, D.C.: The Case Foundation.

Greiling, D., & Halachmi, A. (2013). Accountability and organizational learning in the public sector. *Public Performance & Management Review, 35*(3), 380–406.

Mitchell, G. (2015). County of Santa Clara launches California's first "pay for success" project. Santa Clara County, Office of Public Affairs. https://www.sccgov.org/sites/opa/nr/Pages/ProjectWelcomeHome.aspx. Accessed 30 June 2018.

Moore, M., & Khagram, D. (2004). *On creating public value: What business might learn from government about strategic management* [Corporate Social Responsibility Initiative Working Paper No. 3]. Cambridge, MA: John F. Kennedy School of Government, Harvard University.

Nonprofit Finance Fund. (2017a). Massachusetts Chronic Homelessness Pay for Success Initiative: project update. http://www.payforsuccess.org/project/massachusetts-chronic-homelessness-pay-success-initiative. Accessed 30 June 2018.

Nonprofit Finance Fund. (2017b). Denver housing to health initiative: Project update. http://www.payforsuccess.org/project/denver-housing-health-initiative. Accessed 30 June 2018.

Office of Social Innovation and Civic Participation. (2017). Pay for success: An opportunity to find and scale what works. The White House, Office of Social Innovation and Civic Participations. https://obamawhitehouse.archives.gov/administration/eop/sicp/initiatives/pay-for-success. Accessed 30 June 2018.

Rog, D. J., Marshall, T., Dougherty, R. H., George, P., Daniels, A. S., Ghose, S. S., & Delphin-Rittmon, M. E. (2014). Permanent supportive housing: Assessing the evidence. *Psychiatric Services, 65*(3), 287–294.

Salt Lake County. (2016a). Salt Lake County launches two pay for success projects [Press Release]. http://www.thirdsectorcap.org/wp-content/uploads/2016/12/SLCo-Press-Release.pdf. Accessed 30 June 2018.

Salt Lake County. (2016b). Fact Sheet: Salt Lake County Pay for Success Initiative [Press Release]. http://www.thirdsectorcap.org/wp-content/uploads/2016/12/161216_SLCo-Fact-Sheet-FINAL.pdf. Accessed 30 June 2018.

Social Finance. (n.d.). What is pay for success? http://socialfinance.org/what-is-pay-for-success/. Accessed 30 June 2018.

Social Finance. (2014). Peterborough social impact bond reduces reoffending by 8.4%: Investors on course for payment in 2016 [Press Release]. https://assets.rockefellerfoundation.org/app/uploads/20150316202925/Peterborough-Social-Impact-Bond-Reduces-Reoffending-by-8.4-percent.pdf. Accessed 30 June 2018.

Social Innovation Fund. (2017). Social innovation fund fact sheet. Corporation for National and Community Service. https://www.nationalservice.gov/newsroom/marketing/fact-sheets/social-innovation-fund. Accessed 30 June 2018.

Substance Abuse and Mental Health Services Administration. (2010). *Permanent supportive housing: The evidence* [HHS Pub. No. SMA-10-4509]. Rockville, MD: Center for Mental Health Services, Substance Abuse and Mental Health Services Administration, U.S. Department of Health and Human Services.

Third Sector Capital Partners. (2016). Developing the Cuyahoga Partnering for Family Success Program: Partner perspectives and lessons learned. http://www.enterprisecommunity.org/sites/default/files/media-library/where-we-work/ohio/pfs-cuyahoga-partnering-lessons-learned-report.pdf. Accessed 30 June 2018.

Third Sector Capital Partners. (2017a). Project Welcome Home fact sheet. http://www.thirdsectorcap.org/wp-content/uploads/2015/08/150811_SCC-CH-PFS_Fact-Sheet.pdf. Accessed 30 June 2018.

Third Sector Capital Partners. (2017b). Salt Lake County Pay for Success Initiative. http://www.thirdsectorcap.org/salt-lake-county/. Accessed 30 June 2018.

Urban Institute. (2017a). Project Welcome Home. http://pfs.urban.org/pfs-project-fact-sheets/content/project-welcome-home. Accessed 30 June 2018.

Urban Institute. (2017b). Denver's Social Impact Bond Program. http://pfs.urban.org/pfs-project-fact-sheets/content/denver-social-impact-bond-program. Accessed 30 June 2018.

Younes, M. N., & Harp, M. (2007). Addressing the impact of foster care on biological children and their families. *Child Welfare, 86*(4), 21–40.

Part III
Homelessness Services Delivery

Chapter 11
Critical Time Intervention

Carolyn Hanesworth and Daniel Herman

Introduction

Critical Time Intervention (CTI) is an empirically supported case management model that prevents homelessness and fosters recovery among vulnerable people during periods of significant transition. During such periods, which may include the move from hospitals, jails, and prisons to the community as well as the transition from homelessness to housing, people often have difficulty re-establishing connections with needed supports. CTI works in two main ways: (1) by providing direct emotional and practical assistance during the critical time of transition and (2) by strengthening individuals' ties to services and ongoing social supports. Despite its time-limited approach, CTI exerts a long-term impact by effectively building enduring connections to sources of support that remain in place after the intervention ends. Originally developed over 20 years ago, CTI has since been subjected to numerous tests of its impact, including several randomized trials. CTI is now widely used in homelessness services systems, and interest continues to grow in how the model might be effectively applied in other social service and health sectors. This chapter begins by describing the background and rationale for CTI and its key components. It then briefly summarizes evidence for its effectiveness and discusses

---

Electronic supplementary material: The online version of this chapter (https://doi.org/10.1007/978-3-030-03727-7_11) contains supplementary material, which is available to authorized users.

C. Hanesworth (✉)
Mercy College, Dobbs Ferry, NY, USA
e-mail: chanesworth@mercy.edu

D. Herman
Hunter College, City University of New York, New York City, NY, USA
e-mail: dhe0014@hunter.cuny.edu

H. Larkin et al. (eds.), *Homelessness Prevention and Intervention in Social Work*, https://doi.org/10.1007/978-3-030-03727-7_11

recent efforts to apply the model in the context of Rapid Re-Housing, an emerging policy approach that reorients homelessness services away from a reliance on emergency shelter and toward immediate housing placement.

Background and Rationale

CTI grew from the experience of mental health personnel working at two New York City men's shelters during the early 1980s (Valencia et al. 1997). Over time, this team developed comprehensive treatment programs providing assertive on-site outreach, psychiatric medication, rehabilitation groups, entitlement counseling, and case management to men who were chronically homeless and diagnosed with severe mental disorders. The growing availability of transitional and permanent housing programs in the community made it possible for the shelter-based team to place many of their clients into housing following a significant period of shelter-based treatment. To the dismay of the workers (and their clients), many of those placed into housing quickly became homeless again—akin to the so-called *revolving door* phenomenon observed in other service sectors. Despite the efforts of case managers to implement solid discharge plans, the team hypothesized that many men still did not have the help they needed to overcome the natural discontinuity in support they experienced during the transition period.

Transition periods, including the transition from homelessness to housing, are inherently risky for several reasons. First, clients, many of whom have significant needs and limited ability to advocate for themselves, are typically expected to navigate rigid, complex, and fragmented service systems that are often not eager to accommodate them. Second, during these transitions, clients often abruptly lose supportive relationships they may have developed with important people in their lives, including service providers and other clients. Finally, a transition period can also be a difficult time in the relationship between the client and his or her social network, including family members and new service providers, who may not be aware of how best to provide needed support.

To respond to these concerns, the team at the men's shelter devised CTI as a new approach explicitly designed to enhance continuity of support during the *critical time* of transition from shelter to community. The team also hoped that a time-limited intervention provided during this critical period would have lasting benefits by helping to strengthen a network of community supports that would persist beyond the period of the intervention itself.

Description of the Model

The broad design of CTI resembles many case management models in using trained social workers or other social services personnel (referred to as a CTI worker) to actively engage service recipients, assess client needs, and effectively link clients to services and supports. However, it differs from traditional models in several important ways. First, as just described, CTI is delivered during a significant period of transition. Often, but not always, this period follows discharge from a shelter, hospital, or other institution. Second, CTI is designed to be time-limited and involves decreasing the intensity of contact between the worker and the client over time. This approach helps promote the goal of quickly and effectively connecting the client to supports that will be in place when the CTI worker withdraws. Third, the intervention itself is divided into three specific phases, each lasting roughly 3 months that guide the activities of the worker: (1) Transition, (2) Tryout, and (3) Transfer of Care. Each phase has somewhat different goals, but all activities should contribute to connecting clients to ongoing supports. Finally, CTI is highly focused. Although clients served typically have many unmet needs and priorities, CTI workers focus only on priority areas that are seen to be directly relevant to reducing the client's near-term risk of becoming homeless.

The CTI model is intended to be flexible. It can be applied with various populations, including single adults, families, and youth, and in either rural or urban areas. Regardless of the population served, the core principles are the same, as are the main activities carried out by the worker in each of the intervention's three phases. How CTI is implemented in various contexts will differ primarily by the specific priority areas that are seen as critical for the relevant population and transition.

Core Principles

Strengths Based

The CTI worker should ground their approach in a strengths-based assessment of the client in their environment. The work centers on leveraging the person's or family's inner resources, while connecting and maintaining external resources. Within this frame, the worker honors the client's right to self-determination by empowering them to make important decisions about themselves and/or their family while employing a shared decision-making approach. In all cases, the worker engages the client as a partner and collaborator.

Individualized

Clients are extremely diverse and vary in strengths and challenges across a broad continuum. For instance, some may be capable of successfully transitioning to permanent housing with little intervention needed beyond basic financial assistance. Others have more serious challenges associated with mental illness, addiction, domestic violence, or persistent barriers to employment. Thus, CTI workers adjust their approach based on the client's presentation of need.

Culturally Sensitive

The CTI worker adheres to values that respect the diverse worldviews, perspectives, and experiences of clients. Clients may have deeply held views about treatment programs, managing money, family relationships, and other important issues that influence their decisions and may be inconsistent with what the worker views as constructive. These issues should be approached with sensitivity and care, with the goal of maximizing the client's self-determination to the greatest degree possible.

Recovery Oriented

Borrowing from the principles of recovery-oriented mental health care, CTI workers strive to instill hope, healing, empowerment, and connection into their work with clients. Through careful listening and attention, the CTI worker acts in partnership with the client, who is viewed as the expert on their own life. Interactions are warm, respectful, and sensitive to the client's right to determine the outcome of their work together. Finally, workers aim to continuously convey the message that all clients can progress toward their personal goals despite life's challenges.

Transparent

Clients have a right to know the exact nature, purpose, and extent of the services they are receiving, including the duration of assistance that will be provided. Transparency maximizes the likelihood of developing an open and productive relationship between worker and client and encourages clients to share important information. Workers achieve this by clearly explaining the time-limited, phase-based design of CTI, as well as the roles and responsibilities of both client and worker during the intervention period.

Trauma Informed

Substantial research demonstrates that many people who become homeless have been exposed to one or more severe traumatic stressors in either childhood, adulthood, or both. This may lead to a variety of adverse health and mental health impacts that can compromise clients' capacities in multiple life domains. Trauma-informed care incorporates the recognition of these impacts into case management practices by emphasizing safety and promoting opportunities for clients to rebuild a sense of control and empowerment. Establishing trust between workers and clients is central to trauma-informed care and is promoted by the values noted above, including transparency, cultural sensitivity, shared decision-making, and recovery-oriented strategies to promote safety and autonomy.

The Phases of CTI

Like all case management or care coordination models, CTI relies primarily on mobilizing and organizing existing services and supports. CTI does not create additional housing, income, treatment, or other resources on its own but seeks to maximize access to and the impact of existing resources. Through a set of three timed phases that begin when the transition occurs, CTI aims to provide direct assistance while effectively linking vulnerable individuals to needed services and supports that will persist after the intervention ends. The intensity of direct contact between worker and client should gradually reduce over time. This supports the goal of a slow transfer of responsibility for providing support from the CTI worker to other resources in the community. The first phase is high intensity to ensure that adequate resources are identified and strong connections are made. The middle and final phases reduce in intensity, which encourages both worker and client to test out the viability and effectiveness of resources that are expected to endure after the case management relationship ends. Ideally, the three phases of CTI are preceded by a pre-CTI period in which the worker begins to establish a relationship with the client. Typically, this period takes the form of at least one face-to-face contact between worker and client.

CTI is sensitive to the changing needs that clients have during the transitional period from institutional to community living. Very different challenges characterize the three phases. Therefore, assessment is viewed as an ongoing process in which the worker continues to evaluate client needs and capacities as well as the strengths and gaps in community resources and supports.

Phase One: Transition to the Community

As the transition begins, CTI workers focus their initial work on building an effective relationship with the client while making a preliminary assessment of key priority areas for intervention. Special attention is given to factors precipitating housing loss in the past, as well as current needs and difficulties. Since the intervention is time-limited, services must be prioritized; some will need immediate attention, while others can be addressed later. During this phase, workers have a high level of contact with the client via regular phone calls and in-person visits to the new residence to evaluate the client's adjustment to community living.

The main tasks during this phase are to make an accurate assessment of client needs and strengths, as well as the availability and capacity of needed supports, and to begin the process of effectively linking clients to appropriate resources. Solid linkages are crucial to the success of the intervention, because these are the people and agencies that will gradually assume the primary role of supporting the individual once the CTI period ends. The process of forming effective linkages to community providers can be illustrated with a relay race metaphor. Although there is a delineated area in which the baton must be passed in any relay, the process is best

Table 11.1 Primary worker activities prioritized in each phase of CTI

Phases	Pre-CTI	Phase One: Transition	Phase Two: Tryout	Phase Three: Transfer
Purpose	Establish preliminary connection with client	Provide direct assistance and implement transition plan	Facilitate and test client's problem-solving skills	Terminate CTI services with support network safely in place
Worker activities	Meet with client at least once before transition occurs	Make home visits Assess client strengths and needs Assess capacities of support system Accompany clients to community providers Meet with informal and formal supports Supplement role of supports when necessary Mediate conflicts between client and supports	Observe operation of support network Help to modify network as necessary Intervene when a crisis arises	Reaffirm ongoing roles of support network members Hold meeting to symbolize transfer of care

accomplished when the runner receiving the baton gets a running start. The runner passing the baton then must run with the receiver until the grip on the baton is secure. For a while, both runners share a hold of the baton. This is a metaphor for the shared responsibility for the client's well-being that especially marks the latter part of Phase One and sets the stage for Phase Two (Table 11.1).

Phase Two: Tryout

This stage is devoted to testing and adjusting the systems of support that have been established. Ideally, the worker steps back somewhat, reducing the level of direct contact with the client in order to monitor the effectiveness of the support system. The worker continues to pay attention to the priorities that have been selected as the key areas of focus for the particular individual. Some areas will need to be targeted for more intensive work, especially those that have triggered a housing crisis in the past.

Sometimes, it is not the client but the actual support systems that need more time to run smoothly. Challenges often arise that require mediation and resolution. In this stage, the CTI worker continues to refine the needs assessment. The basics should already be in place, but the worker can observe where there are holes in the system and where the client needs more or less support or services. CTI workers also assess the viability of linkages in this phase, including their success in responding to and meeting the needs of the client.

When problems arise between a client and new community providers, a CTI worker might schedule a meeting with all parties to try to resolve the difficulty. The goal is to allow the client to maximize their strengths and capabilities and to be available to help in areas where the client, or their support system, are not functioning smoothly on their own.

Phase Three: Transfer

Ideally, the elements of the support system are in place and running successfully during this phase, and the worker has reduced their primary activities to monitoring its functioning. The worker also should initiate a review of the work that the client and worker have done together. They look at where the client was in the beginning of the intervention, where the client moved to during the intervention period, and what possibilities lay ahead in the future.

The most salient issue psychologically during this phase is often dealing with the end of the relationship between client and worker. Separation issues may emerge as termination can evoke feelings related to past losses and underlying feelings of anger and abandonment. Clients may also be tempted to sabotage progress as a means of maintaining or increasing contact with the worker. In these cases, the worker lets the client know that they are available to witness progress and need not only be called upon in times of trouble.

Since the CTI relationship ends in this phase, it is vital that all links to community providers are secure. Last-minute fine-tunings may be needed, but ideally everything should be in place for the client's network of long-term support. Toward the end of this period, the CTI worker, client, and various key supports should meet to discuss the transfer of care and go over the client's long-term goals. These key supports might include family members and a therapist, or counselor, especially if the client lives in a residence with supportive services.

Movement Through Phases

Unlike some other phased models, the schedule of movement between CTI phases is based solely on time, not on progress toward goals. This is an important distinction and may feel counterintuitive when workers are first exposed to the model. The rationale is that a firm timetable encourages a highly focused effort that is aimed toward achieving a limited number of realistic goals. It also intends to explicitly direct workers' efforts toward connecting clients with supports that will continue once the intervention ends. Although in some rare cases, the intervention may be extended beyond its planned duration, almost all CTI interventions should closely follow the original timetable for phase transitions and termination.

Assessment of External Resources

Some of the main tasks for a CTI worker are to identify resources, link the client to those resources, and then monitor the effectiveness and strength of the linkages. To do so, a worker must continuously update their knowledge of formal community resources, such as human service organizations, as well as informal supports that may include family, a spiritual community, and neighbors. Emphasis should be placed on the fit between client needs and the capacity of the environment to meet those needs. In communities without robust formal resources, CTI workers rely more heavily on informal supports while also working to bring these supports to their communities through coalition building and advocacy.

The CTI Team

CTI employs a team approach with two key roles: the *CTI worker*, sometimes referred to as the CTI specialist or case manager, and the *CTI supervisor*. For some clients, including those moving into permanent supportive housing, a housing case manager may be assigned by the housing program. In these settings, the CTI worker will act in a complementary function to the case manager. For clients receiving other types of housing assistance, such as Rapid Re-Housing, the CTI worker may function as the sole case manager.

The CTI Worker

The role of the CTI worker is to promote a smooth transition from homelessness, or from a discharging institution, into housing and to secure connections in the community that serve to reduce the risk of recurrent homelessness and other adverse outcomes. Since each client and each situation is different, CTI workers must have basic skills in interviewing, engagement, and assessment to accurately determine, with the client, the best plan for long-term success. Effective CTI workers function as trusted allies and advocates, and they possess a keen eye for detail and timely follow-up. The ideal CTI worker is a person with a background in human services who understands the personal challenges and systemic barriers associated with poverty and the experience of residential instability and who applies an open, flexible, and optimistic approach to the work. They are adept at interdisciplinary team work, comfortable working in the community rather than the office, effective at reaching out and building alliances with other providers, and endowed with a strong ethical sense and respect for the dignity and worth of the client. The CTI worker's effectiveness may be enhanced by formal professional education but mainly requires the capacity for effective relationship building, empathy, and support.

The CTI Supervisor

The CTI supervisor oversees services delivered by the team's CTI workers. Through involvement and practice with people affected by homelessness, the supervisor demonstrates proficiency in guiding the worker's activities during all phases of the intervention. The supervisor ensures that workers' practice is consistent with the phase-specific activities and foci of the CTI model and that clients' progress is carefully monitored to ensure that phase transition dates are observed. The supervisor also ensures that model-specific case planning and recording documents are being completed correctly and are up to date for all workers.

The supervisor should encourage open communication and demonstrate a willingness to support, as well as instruct, supervisees. CTI workers are often faced with difficult dilemmas, as they are frequently helping vulnerable people negotiate environments with limited resources. Both workers and supervisors must remember that the measure of success in CTI is the creation of an ongoing support system that can help clients weather inevitable crises and life challenges. In communities where supports and needed resources are limited or nonexistent, supervisors can take steps to address these gaps at the macro level by engaging with community coalitions that can address these needs.

Documentation

Fidelity to the model is enhanced using case planning and recording tools that explicitly support CTI's focused, phased approach. These include the *Phase Plan Form* and the *Caseload Tracking Form* (see www.criticaltime.org for copies of these tools and other helpful information). The Phase Plan Form is used to identify the specific priority focus areas to be addressed during each phase. For example, if a person enters Phase One and is struggling with depression, the goal of securing mental health care becomes prioritized for attention during this phase. Focus areas should be limited to two or three per phase and directly related to increasing stability in housing. At the end of each phase, the worker and client review and record progress made in the specific area. This plan can be modified as needed but serves to guide and focus the work.

The Caseload Tracking Form assists supervisors and workers in their efforts to keep track of where clients are in the course of the intervention. During supervisory meetings, staff should review cases that are new, those that are facing crises, those ready to transition to a new phase, and those that are nearing termination. Since phase transitions are determined by time and not by client readiness or goal completion, this form ensures that clients move into the next phase on time. As noted above, extensions may be warranted in unusual circumstances, but such extensions should be evaluated and approved by the CTI supervisor.

Evidence

CTI has been studied extensively since its introduction, with several studies focusing on populations experiencing homelessness. We briefly review some of the key findings of these studies below.

The model was initially studied as one of several federally funded research demonstration projects focusing on homelessness and mental illness carried out during the early 1990s. Led by Dr. Ezra Susser, Elie Valencia, and Sarah Conover, this was a randomized trial in which 96 homeless men with diagnosed psychotic disorders being referred into community housing were randomly assigned to receive usual discharge planning or discharge planning plus 9 months of CTI delivered by shelter-based case managers. All men were followed for 18 months to assess housing status and a number of secondary outcomes. The extended follow-up period was used in order to test whether any observed impact of the intervention would endure once the intervention ended. Those assigned to the CTI condition were three times less likely to become homeless again over the follow-up period (Susser et al. 1997). Notably, the positive impact of CTI persisted past the end of the 9-month period of active intervention, providing support for the hypothesis that the intervention successfully enhanced enduring supports in the community.

A second randomized trial tested CTI in preventing homelessness for persons with psychotic disorders following discharge from large publicly operated psychiatric hospitals. One hundred and fifty men and women, all of whom had been homeless prior to their current admission, were randomly assigned to receive discharge planning and follow-up services typically provided by the hospital or standard services plus a 9-month CTI intervention. This trial differed somewhat from the first study since many subjects were not placed into housing at the point of discharge; in fact, many left the hospital with no clear housing option identified. Both groups were followed for 18 months to assess housing status and other outcomes. A positive effect of the intervention was again observed; the risk of homelessness among subjects assigned to CTI was five times lower than among subjects assigned to usual services (Herman et al. 2011). A secondary analysis also showed a significant reduction in the risk of rehospitalization associated with assignment to the CTI condition (Tomita and Herman 2012). Another analysis showed that persons assigned to the CTI condition who received more contacts with the CTI worker before discharge (i.e., during the pre-CTI period) were significantly less likely to become homeless than those who received little contact with the CTI worker before discharge from the hospital (Herman et al. 2011).

Another randomized trial examined the impact of CTI on homeless families. In this study, an adapted version of the model called Family CTI, or FCTI, was tested with 200 newly homeless families in which the mothers had diagnosed substance use or mental health problems. As in the studies described earlier, the FCTI intervention lasted for 9 months and followed the basic CTI three-phase model aiming to provide time-limited direct support while connecting families with services and supports as they left shelter for housing in the community. Families were randomly assigned to receive either FCTI provided by workers trained and supervised in the model or usual care services delivered by caseworkers employed by the county. FCTI workers had caseloads of approximately 12 families, while the usual care caseloads were roughly twice as large. The conditions also differed with respect to housing access. Families assigned to the FCTI condition received access to a permanent housing subsidy as soon as possible, while those assigned to the comparison condition received housing only after being judged housing ready by their caseworker. Families in both conditions were followed by trained interviewers for a total of 24 months following entry into the study. Children from each participating family were selected using a procedure designed to adequately represent different age groups, yielding a sample of 311 children (Samuels et al. 2015; Shinn et al. 2015).

The primary outcomes in this study were multiple measures of mental health and psychological functioning of both mothers and their children. Mothers' mental distress was assessed at baseline and during follow-up via the Brief Symptom Inventory, a multi-item self-report symptom scale. Children's mental health was measured with multiple indicators, including the Child Behavioral Checklist. Results showed that mothers exhibiting high levels of psychological distress while in the shelter system experienced significant reductions in symptoms over time when provided with access to permanent housing, regardless of which condition they had been assigned. Assignment to the FCTI condition was associated with quicker placement into housing and increased connection to services, but this did not lead to improved maternal mental health beyond the impact associated with the receipt of housing itself (Samuels et al. 2015). Among children, the overall trend in both groups was toward improved mental health over time. However, findings demonstrated a positive impact of assignment to FCTI in several domains, including reductions in internalizing and externalizing problems for preschool children and externalizing problems for adolescents. FCTI was also associated with declines in self-reported trouble in school for children between the ages of 6 and 16 (Shinn et al. 2015).

Rapid Rehousing and CTI

Rapid Re-Housing (RRH) is an intervention that provides temporary financial assistance in combination with case management services aimed at moving families and individuals experiencing homelessness quickly out of shelter and into permanent housing. The broad objective is to reduce local systems' reliance on shelter and transitional housing and redirect resources toward homelessness prevention and housing retention. The US Interagency Council on Homelessness and the US Department of Housing and Urban Development both identify RRH as a key strategy for meeting the national goal of ending homelessness (USICH 2015). The National Alliance to End Homelessness identifies three core components of RRH: housing identification, rental and move-in financial assistance, and case management (NAEH 2016). CTI has been identified as a promising case management model by RRH providers across the United States, and efforts are underway to formally adapt the model and create best practices for implementation in this context (NAEH 2016).

Adapting Critical Time Intervention for Rapid Re-Housing (CTI-RRH)

The main differences between the original CTI model and CTI-RRH are the target population and the fact that the case management services are offered in combination with a time-limited rental subsidy. While the original CTI model targeted chronically homeless single adults with behavioral health challenges, CTI-RRH serves families and single adults who do not necessarily have mental illness and may not have experienced chronic homelessness. While persons served by the original CTI programs often had access to permanent supportive housing (or, by virtue of a disability, had access to entitlement income sufficient to cover their rent), CTI-RRH typically targets individuals or families who will be responsible for their own rental payments over the long term. Therefore, the case management goals emphasize economic recovery.

Key Aspects of CTI-RRH

CTI-RRH addresses the unique *timing* and the *nature* of challenges experienced by RRH recipients by providing highly focused case management services during the period of transition from homelessness to housing and effectively linking clients to supports that will help to sustain resources and assistance after RRH support ends. The model is intended to be flexible; it can be applied to all populations receiving RRH, including single adults, families, and youth, and in either rural or urban areas. Its core values are the same as traditional CTI, as are the main activities in each phase of the intervention. The primary differences between how CTI-RRH will be implemented in different contexts pertain to the key focus areas identified as critical in the context of each individual's or family's housing plan as well as variability in available community resources. As in the original model, special attention is given to identifying the reasons why housing was initially lost, so that supports can be implemented to reduce future risk.

CTI-RRH is proposed as a 6-month model composed of the following three phases, each approximately 2 months long, which begin when the individual or family moves into housing. Phase One (Transition) aims to engage clients and build an effective relationship, conduct a thorough assessment, develop a housing stability plan that leverages client strengths and community resources, and begin to link clients to needed services and supports. Phase Two (Tryout) focuses on adjusting, maintaining, and strengthening supportive connections as well as the client's capacity to make use of them. Phase Three (Transfer) concludes the CTI worker's role by ensuring the client's connection and capacity to access needed supports and plan for future challenges on their own. As in the original model, the amount of contact between worker and client decreases as the client moves through the phases of CTI-RRH, promoting a gradual transition to community supports.

The Importance of the Pre-CTI Period in RRH

As noted, Phase One of CTI-RRH starts when the client or family initially moves into housing. The preceding activities—including housing search, placement, and move-in—are seen as occurring during a pre-CTI period. This period typically focuses on supporting clients to locate suitable housing near supports and resources and is ideally delivered by a housing specialist with expertise in locating suitable housing and managing the housing application process. Regardless of which worker is responsible for assisting with the housing placement process, the CTI case manager will begin Phase One activities when housing has been identified and the move-in process is underway. When the pre-CTI work is being handled by someone other than the CTI worker, the CTI worker should nevertheless meet the client at least once or twice before the move-in date. These meetings facilitate the development of an effective working relationship between worker and client and expedite the worker's assessment of clients' strengths and needs. In keeping with CTI's original emphasis on *timing* as a key factor in successful intervention, and given CTI-RRH's abbreviated timeline, pre-CTI in a RRH context is an opportunity to begin developing key community support connections early. These connections are then deepened, tested, and revaluated over the subsequent three phases.

Implementation Challenges

As noted earlier, CTI relies primarily on mobilizing, maximizing, and organizing existing services and supports, rather than creating housing, income, treatment, or other resources. Since communities differ significantly on the availability of such resources, CTI's effectiveness can also be expected to differ from place to place. However, the objective of the model is to magnify the impact of services and supports that are present.

The primary goal of CTI is to improve the client's capacity to remain housed during program participation and beyond by effectively connecting them with crucial community supports and helping them to attain greater economic stability. CTI is not designed to resolve poverty, and in many cases, clients' housing may remain precarious. Instead, CTI aims to best position the client for ongoing housing stability by maximizing available resources and supports. In order to achieve this, the intervention focuses exclusively on factors that directly influence housing stability: obtaining and coordinating financial benefits; accessing health care, child care, employment, and education services; improving management of financial resources; and connecting clients to effective social and community supports that can address other barriers to maintaining stable housing.

In order to achieve long-term housing stability, CTI workers create plans in partnership with their clients to increase economic resources. This may be through employment but could also be through access to benefits, room-sharing, or re-establishing relationships with family. The time-limited nature CTI can be both stressful and motivating for the client and worker, and the clearly defined end to CTI in this context can be difficult to accept. A unique aspect of CTI in general is that phases move along based on time, not on the resolution of goals. A regular review of cases in the context of supportive supervision is critical to ensure the case management stays on track and the worker feels supported as they move clients through the phases.

Summary

CTI is a time-limited, phased approach that was originally designed to support individuals and families transitioning from homelessness to independent living. In this chapter, evidence for CTI's effectiveness, its core principles, and its three phases were described. CTI's focus on identifying and maximizing existing resources to build long-term housing stability is an approach now being adapted for use with individuals and families during a wide variety of transitions. This chapter described one such application of CTI currently underway in the context of Rapid Re-Housing. The material presented is intended to encourage readers to think critically about how CTI achieves the goal of housing stability and the challenges CTI workers and clients experience in the field.

References

Herman, D. B., Conover, S., Gorroochurn, P., Hinterland, K., Hoepner, L., & Susser, E. S. (2011). Randomized trial of critical time intervention to prevent homelessness after hospital discharge. *Psychiatric Services, 62*(7), 713–719.

National Alliance to End Homelessness (2016). Resources. https://endhomelessness.org/resource/conference-presentations-from-the-2016-national-conference-on-ending-family/. Accessed 16 April 2018.

Samuels, J., Fowler, P. J., Ault-Brutus, A., Tang, D. I., & Marcal, K. (2015). Time-limited case management for homeless mothers with mental health problems: Effects on maternal mental health. *Journal of the Society for Social Work and Research, 6*(4), 515–539.

Shinn, M., Samuels, J., Fischer, S. N., Thompkins, A., & Fowler, P. J. (2015). Longitudinal impact of a family critical time intervention on children in high-risk families experiencing homelessness: A randomized trial. *American Journal of Community Psychology, 56*(3–4), 205–216.

Susser, E., Valencia, E., Conover, S., Felix, A., Tsai, W. Y., & Wyatt, R. J. (1997). Preventing recurrent homelessness among mentally ill men: A "critical time" intervention after discharge from a shelter. *American Journal of Public Health, 87*(2), 256–262.

Tomita, A., & Herman, D. B. (2012). The impact of critical time intervention in reducing psychiatric rehospitalization after hospital discharge. *Psychiatric Services, 63*(9), 935–937.

United States Interagency Council on Homelessness (2015). Rapid re-housing. https://www.usich.gov/solutions/housing/rapid-re-housing. Accessed 16 April 2018.

Valencia, E., Susser, E., Torres, J., Felix, A., & Conover, S. (1997). Critical time intervention for homeless mentally ill individuals in transition from shelter to community living. In W. R. Breakey & J. W. Thompson (Eds.), *Mentally ill and homeless: Special programs for special needs* (pp. 75–94). London: Routledge.

Chapter 12
Multisectoral Collaborations to Address Homelessness

Wonhyung Lee and Kristin M. Ferguson

Introduction

Homelessness is a multidimensional problem that requires intervention and support from multiple domains. By definition, homeless populations need affordable housing, but their needs often surpass housing; people also need access to health and mental health care, employment opportunities, social networks, and community-based supports. Moreover, the growing popularity of the Housing First approach, which requires coordinated support services that must be flexible and tailored to meet specific needs of individual clients, prompts increased cross-sector collaboration (Culhane and Byrne 2010).

Intervention efforts, especially for people experiencing chronic homelessness,[1] require collaboration from a wide range of sectors, with the government, law enforcement, local businesses, nonprofit service providers, and civil advocates

Electronic supplementary material: The online version of this chapter (https://doi.org/10.1007/978-3-030-03727-7_12) contains supplementary material, which is available to authorized users.

[1] Nearly 85,000 people (15% of the overall homeless population) experience chronic homelessness, more than 60% of whom are unsheltered (i.e., living outdoors or in places not meant for habitation; National Alliance to End Homelessness 2015). A person experiencing chronic homelessness is defined as "either (1) an unaccompanied homeless individual with a disabling condition who has been continuously homeless for a year or more, or (2) an unaccompanied individual with a disabling condition who has had at least four episodes of homelessness in the past 3 years" (US Department of Housing and Urban Development 2007 p.3).

W. Lee (✉)
University at Albany, State University of New York, Albany, NY, USA
e-mail: whlee@albany.edu

K. M. Ferguson
Arizona State University, Tempe, AZ, USA
e-mail: kristin.ferguson@asu.edu

H. Larkin et al. (eds.), *Homelessness Prevention and Intervention in Social Work*, https://doi.org/10.1007/978-3-030-03727-7_12

implementing various policies and programs. While these sectors may share the same goal of helping homeless people or reducing homelessness, challenges exist when these entities represent varying constituencies and competing interests. One of these challenges is demonstrated through the example of handling homeless people's belongings in the public space. Although the US Constitution forbids randomly seizing and destroying homeless people's belongings on city streets (Dolan 2012), how to approach homeless people and their belongings continues to be a sensitive topic for different sectors. In 2013, the City of Los Angeles asked the US Supreme Court to overturn a ruling on this issue, yet the final decision was made that homeless people's possessions could be taken only if they posed an immediate threat to public safety or health or if such possessions constituted criminal evidence. The order also requires the city to give owners a chance to reclaim their property before it is destroyed (Holland 2013). As shown in this example, the direction of homeless intervention practices is influenced by multiple agents (e.g., federal and local governments, property owners, business owners, private security guards, police officers, service providers, homeless advocates, and homeless populations), and thus the attempts to implement those practices require sensitive awareness of the multisectoral surroundings.

In this chapter, we discuss multisectoral collaboration in the context of attempts to address homelessness. First, we briefly explain multisectoral collaboration, and then we discuss examples by which multiple sectors collaborate to engage homeless populations and reduce homelessness. Our focus is on interagency collaborations and collaboration with the business sector. The content and findings presented regarding the business sector are from the chapter authors' fieldwork and research in Washington, D.C., and Los Angeles, CA. Finally, we suggest social work skills that are useful for collaboration.

Multisectoral Collaboration

The term *multisectoral collaboration* refers to situations in which more than one sector works together to achieve a common goal. In this sense, multisectoral collaborations can also be referred to as *cross-sector collaborations*, which are defined as "partnerships involving government, business, nonprofits and philanthropies, communities, and/or the public as a whole" (Bryson et al. 2006, p. 44). Similar concepts in public policy and nonprofit/business management, such as interorganizational or interagency collaborations (Sowa 2008), social partnerships (Waddock 1991), or cross-sector social partnerships (Clarke and Fuller 2010; Selsky and Parker 2005), share the essence of the values and principles of multisectoral collaboration. Despite differences in terminologies, these concepts share the common component of voluntary cooperation among two or more sectors to solve a problem or issue of mutual concern while sharing resources, commitments, costs, and responsibilities.

Multisectoral collaboration has become an important phenomenon and concept in public administration and nonprofit/business management, especially in the past two decades. During that time, the entities that provide services have diversified and fragmented—from the sole leadership of the government to the involvement of numerous private and nonprofit entities (Bryson 2011; Gazley 2008; Salamon 1995; Young 2006). The dramatic increase of non-governmental entities in service delivery, however, has given rise to an environment that is difficult for collaboration. For example, challenges reside in the following factors: separate organizations are involved in one project; organizations lack communication or transparency; organizations in various sectors compete for the same funding; parameters for collaboration goals and evaluations frequently change; and organizations may experience a clash of cultures. In this context, multiple sectors at various levels (i.e., local, state, and federal) prefer to exist and work separately, which is commonly described as organizations being "siloed" (Horvitz-Lennon et al. 2006; Kernaghan 2005).

Despite such barriers that often limit cross-sector collaborations, various sectors can be motivated or incentivized by policies or funders to work around a shared goal or a common focus. Conceptually, Lawson (2004) suggested that collaboration could yield multiple benefits, namely, "*effectiveness gains* (e.g., improved results and enhanced problem-solving competence); *efficiency gains* (e.g., eliminating redundancy); *resource gains* (e.g., more funding); *capacity gains* (e.g., weaknesses are covered and workforce retention improves); *legitimacy gains* (e.g., power and authority are enhanced, and jurisdictional claims are supported); and *social development benefits* (e.g., social movements are catalyzed)" (p. 225).

Collaboration can take various forms and includes a range of activities. Some organizations collaborate through informal networking and client referrals, whereas others collaborate through more formalized partnerships, such as co-locating services or implementing a project across a multisectoral coalition of organizations. Prior literature has classified various forms of collaboration based on a continuum of formalization, integration, and interdependence. On the lower end of this continuum, collaboration functions as information sharing, joint efforts, or service referrals, whereas, on the higher end of the continuum, collaboration can take place as a coalition, as a full partnership, and even as a merger (Guo and Acar 2005; Mandell and Steelman 2003). The collaboration types that we discuss in this chapter (i.e., interagency and for-profit-nonprofit) are mainly formalized collaborations with varying degrees of systemic integration. In terms of participating sectors, the first example is centered around the role of government, whereas the second example focuses on the role of businesses.

Interagency Collaboration

Several interagency collaborative attempts have been adopted to address homelessness. One structure that naturally stimulates interagency collaboration is the US Department of Housing and Urban Development's Continuum of Care (CoC) Program, which funds local planning bodies (consisting of nonprofits, state and local government entities, public housing agencies, and other key stakeholders) that coordinate homeless assistance. Introduced in 1994, CoCs coordinate multi-tier homeless assistance services for various subgroups of homeless clients (U.S. Interagency Council on the Homelessness 1994), and the level of coordination has expanded over time. More recently, the Homeless Emergency Assistance and Rapid Transition to Housing Act of 2009 (HEARTH Act) further consolidated three separate homeless assistance programs (i.e., Supportive Housing, Shelter Plus Care, and Section 8 Moderate Rehabilitation Single Room Occupancy (SRO)) into the CoC program (U.S. Department of Housing and Urban Development 2012). Throughout these developments, the government has emphasized the importance of interorganizational or interagency collaboration to provide comprehensive and long-term care for homeless populations (Wong et al. 2006).

Another structure that demonstrates interagency collaborative efforts is the US Interagency Council on Homelessness (USICH). Originally authorized in 1987 and reauthorized by the HEARTH Act of 2009, USICH leads the implementation of the federal strategic plan to prevent and end homelessness. Currently, USICH combines efforts from 19 federal member agencies along with every level of government and the private sector. They hold quarterly meetings among member agencies to "advance federal collaboration and support state and local activities" (USICH 2017a, p.1). USICH supports state and local partners to implement best practices by developing tools that can guide their practices and by publishing reports, case studies, and guidebooks for providers. USICH also builds a vision for preparing the comprehensive and coordinated response to homelessness. One example is illustrated in Fig. 12.1, which demonstrates how various sectors and agencies can work together to prevent and end

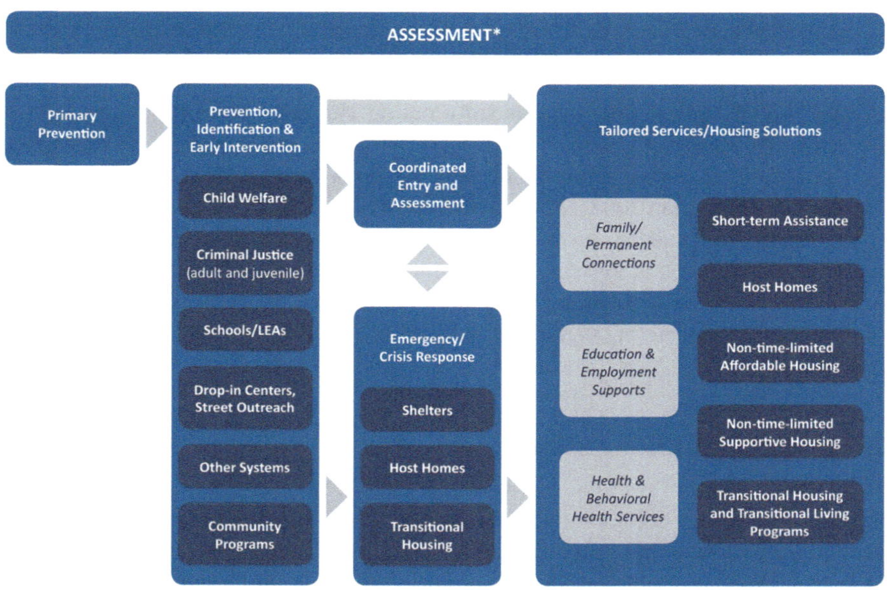

Fig. 12.1 A coordinated community response that will be necessary to prevent and end youth homelessness. (U.S. Interagency Council on Homelessness 2015)

youth homelessness. USICH actively encourages every state and local government to establish interagency councils to facilitate state-wide and local planning to build a coordinated and comprehensive community response to homelessness.

Structures such as CoCs and interagency councils provide foundations for government-involved collaborations. These interagency structures are designed to facilitate the implementation of federal strategies, to provide expert guidance to state and local leaders, and to communicate best practices across municipalities. For example, USICH's Mayors Challenge to End Veteran Homelessness drew more than 880 mayors, city and county officials, and governors from 50 communities across 26 states to join the call to action to achieve a common goal (USICH 2017b). Furthermore, interagency councils foster multisectoral collaboration not only among government agencies but also across sectors. USICH underscores that "it will take all of us—government, nonprofits, business, and philanthropy—to make sure every community has the capacity to achieve the goal" (USICH 2015, p. 1).

For-Profit-Nonprofit Collaboration

The business community is often viewed as a force that opposes, discriminates against, and even supports the criminalization of homeless populations in commercial areas. But recently, new approaches have emerged whereby local businesses collaborate with service providers to address chronic homelessness. To understand the role of the business sector in addressing chronic homelessness, we present two models of multisectoral collaboration in which the local business community has worked with service providers, clients, and advocates in a synergistic relationship: (1) a business improvement district (BID) and (2) a social enterprise (SE). We present qualitative insights gained from our field research in Washington, D.C., and Los Angeles, CA (see the box below), carrying voices from local business leaders and street outreach workers with the BID approach as well as nonprofit homeless advocates and homeless youth with the SE approach. Below we discuss each model in depth.

Homelessness in *Washington, D.C.*, has been a continuous issue. The downtown area, where shelters and food programs are concentrated, has historically attracted a number of homeless individuals (Simpson 2015). Even after some of these services were relocated, many parks and high-traffic tourist areas located downtown attract homeless individuals. According to the most recent point-in-time count results, there are 8,350 homeless persons in D.C. on any given night, including 318 unsheltered persons, 6,259 persons in

(continued)

emergency shelters, and 1,773 persons in transitional housing facilities (Community Partnership for the Prevention of Homelessness 2016). From 2015 to 2016, the number of persons experiencing homelessness increased by 14.4%, which is 45% higher than it was 8 years ago (Wogan 2015).

The 2016 *Los Angeles* Homeless Count estimated that 46,874 people in the Greater Los Angeles area experience homelessness, comprised of 34,701 unsheltered individuals and 12,173 sheltered individuals. These figures represent a 5.7% increase from 2015. The increase in homelessness rates in Los Angeles has been particularly notable among young adults (ages 18–24) and adults (ages 25–54), whose rates increased by 12% from 2015 to 2016 (Los Angeles Homeless Services Authority 2016). Social service agencies working with unaccompanied homeless youth in Los Angeles report that there are an estimated 12,000–15,000 youth who experience homelessness each year (Covenant House California 2007).

Business Improvement Districts

Business improvement districts (BIDs) are local organizations that aim to improve the social and physical environment of commercial areas (Briffault 1999; Houstoun 2003). BIDs are typically initiated by property owners or business owners who are willing to pay a fee to make the commercial area cleaner and safer. Once a BID is established, yearly fees become compulsory for all property owners within the delineated BID area. The money generated from these fees is spent on services, including street cleaning, security, and beautification of the area. BIDs have gained notable popularity since the 1990s as a response to accumulated urban problems as well as due to redevelopment booms across the country. More than 1,000 BIDs are active in the USA. As of 2017, there are 10 BIDs in Washington, D.C., and 42 in Los Angeles. The following introduces two areas through which BIDs have collaborated with the nonprofit sector to address homelessness.

Street Engagement and Pathways to Housing

Recently, the business community has joined the street outreach process in collaboration with local housing programs. A number of BIDs in Washington, D.C. and Los Angeles provide exemplary cases for this outreach effort. Several years ago, the Downtown DC BID started street outreach services, realizing that outreach leads to a more permanent solution for homeless individuals and business owners. Through a partnership with a local agency, Pathways to Housing DC, the Downtown DC BID began working with clinically based outreach workers to get to know the homeless populations and connect them to needed services. In addition, the Downtown DC

BID trains its own workforce to become familiar with the issue of homelessness and is equipped to offer human services. In fact, the Downtown DC BID has a separate unit called the Homeless Outreach Service Team (HOST), which is trained by Pathways to Housing DC, law enforcement, and other outreach social workers from the city to work closely with homeless individuals. These outreach efforts helped 51 homeless individuals move off the streets and into secure permanent supportive housing from 2012 to 2015 (Hartman 2015). On a daily basis, the outreach team builds relationships with homeless people and provides assessments, direct resources, interventions, and referrals. The outreach effort has been expanded to an adjacent BID—the Golden Triangle BID.

The Downtown BID in Los Angeles has a similar outreach approach. The mission of the outreach team is to contact, interview, and assist homeless individuals living on the west side of downtown. The outreach team encourages everyone to start on the path to permanent housing. One *Los Angeles Times* article defined this outreach as "a collaboration of the private and nonprofit sectors in one facet of the city's response to homelessness" (Smith 2017, p. 16). In this collaboration, the BID, which represents the private interests of property owners, collaborates with social service agencies, such as People Assisting the Homeless (PATH), a Los Angeles-based organization that provides services including street outreach, shelter, and housing construction. According to the same article, the team placed 36 people into permanent housing and enrolled 56 in PATH's housing services. Ninety percent of them are still housed, according to the BID's records (Smith 2017).

Policymaking and Advocacy

Multisectoral collaboration can be a driving force that carries policy agendas forward. As BIDs represent the interest of the business community, they can add leverage to certain policies or guidelines that have a stake in economic development or streetscape improvement. Because street homelessness is linked to the ambiance of the area, BIDs typically would be motivated to reduce homelessness in their areas. Instead of pushing an anti-homeless agenda, such as encouraging criminalization tactics, BIDs can be effective advocates for a Housing First approach. For example, the Downtown DC BID authored a position paper about actions they believe must be undertaken to end homelessness in the downtown area and in the city as a whole (Downtown Business Improvement District 2010). The Executive Director of the D.C. Business Improvement Districts Council, an association of the city's 10 business improvement districts, wrote an Op-Ed in *The Washington Post* to align the position of BIDs with the Housing First approach (Avery 2015). When BIDs added their voices to support the Housing First model, advocacy efforts for permanent supportive housing received a heightened level of attention from political leaders. Some of these advocacy methods included endorsing proposals or campaigns and publishing newsletters or other publications via various media. These examples demonstrate that BID leadership can promote a long-term solution for homelessness through its communication channels to BID members and more broadly to the business, nonprofit, and political communities.

At the same time, BIDs can advocate for homeless populations as a mediator. In Washington, D.C., BIDs serve an important role in educating the business community about who homeless people are and what their rights are from a humane and sustainable perspective. When members of the business community hold narrow views of homelessness and worry about a person asking for money in public spaces or sleeping in front of their storefront, BID staff can communicate to members that pushing someone off one corner of the district neither solves the problem of that person's situation nor achieves a collective goal as a community. One government official in Washington, D.C., echoed this sentiment about the role of BIDs:

> BIDs play an important role in educating their individual members. There are business owners who don't know a lot of details about homelessness. But what I find is the more people understand the issue and what we are doing about it, they become much more tolerant.

In addition, BIDs create a space for various law enforcement departments to communicate with one another and with BID service teams. In Washington, D.C. and Los Angeles, BIDs host periodic meetings where officers can share information about the neighborhood condition and update one another about how each unit is working on the same issue. These meetings have served an important role in stimulating coordination among various law enforcement units and BID service teams when it comes to responding to homeless persons in the public space with full consideration of discretion and emergency.

Social Enterprise

Social enterprises can refer to a nonprofit organization with a for-profit component, a socially responsible business, or a revenue-generating venture established to create positive social impact (Dees 1998; Krupa et al. 2003; Warner and Mandiberg 2006). The underlying principles of SEs include focusing on vulnerable populations, applying concepts from business entrepreneurship, creating innovative solutions to challenging social problems, and valuing social improvement over profit (Anderson 2014).

The Social Enterprise Intervention (SEI) is one type of social enterprise developed and evaluated by the second author of this chapter with homeless youth (ages 16–24) at one homeless youth organization in Los Angeles. There are four stages in the 20-month SEI model: (a) *vocational skill acquisition* is a 4-month course in which youth receive technical training concerning specific vocational skills; (b) *small-business skill acquisition* is a separate 4-month course that focuses on business-related skills needed to start a social enterprise, such as accounting, budgeting, marketing, and management; (c) *social enterprise formation and distribution* is the 12-month phase in which participating youth establish a goods-producing social enterprise in a supportive, empowering, and community-based setting; and (d) *clinical services* are the mental health component provided by the SEI clinician and/or case manager, which is woven throughout all stages over 20 months. In the SEI pilot study, the youth participants learned graphic design and Photoshop software skills that they used to embroider and silkscreen images onto apparel, which they then sold through the host organization and in local flea markets. The collaborative procedures for developing the SEI and methods for selecting the target products and data collection are described elsewhere in more detail (Ferguson 2007; Ferguson and Islam 2008).

The collaboration between the local business community and a homeless youth organization's staff and clients in a SE provides us with three areas of insights about the role of the local business community in addressing homelessness: employment, mentoring, and networking.

Employment

The local business community is well-positioned to connect difficult-to-employ youth to employment and initial work opportunities. Over the course of the SEI pilot study, various youth secured freelance positions with local businesses based on the skills they were learning in the vocational skill acquisition stage of the SEI (i.e., Photoshop, graphic design, embroidery, and silk-screening). Business leaders sought many of the youths' vocational skills for their own businesses, as one SEI youth noted: "I'm using what I learned in this class to help [a local business leader] make a website. I am making up letterings, different styles of letters, and images for his business, stuff like that." In some cases, youth were concurrently employed in the community, yet their skills were noticed by other business leaders and solicited for freelance work.

Mentoring

The business community can connect youth to business mentoring, skill-building opportunities, and resources to succeed in starting and running a business. SEI participants learned business skills through the small-business skill acquisition stage of the SEI, including marketing, accounting, management, and publicity. Many of these topics were taught using guest speakers from the local business community, who taught from their lived experiences. It was common that the youth developed mentee relationships with local business owners, in particular those owners who grew up in the local community, had experienced housing instability themselves, or were of a similar generation to the youth (i.e., those born in the 1980s and 1990s). One SEI youth's testimony mirrored the shared gratitude expressed by the youth for the mentorship by local business leaders: "If it wasn't for him [referring to a local business leader who mentored youth from the SEI Program] wanting to teach us, I never would know about these things, so I personally appreciate what he's done for me and I'm saying thank you because it's done a whole lot of other good stuff in my life right now."

Staff also noted the formative role of business leaders in mentoring youth in developing their own career goals and skills. Staff and volunteers agreed that business leaders were helpful in exposing the youth to new career paths by talking to the youth about a typical day in the life of the particular business leader and what professional and academic experiences contributed to the business leader's current position. This is illustrated by one host agency staff's comment:

> Also, the SEI Program gives the youth an opportunity to educate themselves about what other positions exist in the industry that they might not be aware of. Like [name of youth] who always imagined himself as the owner of his own business but now has learned about marketing and public relations from [name of business leader] and is now more interested in that area.

Networking

Local business leaders can expand the youths' existing employment network. Youth collectively considered their network or their "connections" or "people backing them up" to be more valuable to their success than any particular skill they possessed. One SEI youth said, "We are where we are now not because of *what* we know, but *who* we know."

In expanding their network, the youth met local business leaders through the SEI Program (i.e., as instructors, mentors, volunteers, or donors) and quickly incorporated these people in their network. In some cases, the youths' expanded networks resulted in new work orders for the social enterprise: "Well, I got a story where I have a friend who her old man is making a movie, and he wants some hoodies done for himself and his crew" (SEI youth). Similarly, another SEI participant, whose youthful perspective and creativity were coveted by a music producer who was catering to Millennials' tastes in a new release, noted: "I knew the producer. They wanted to do a logo for their company. Their logo was so old. It was like from the 1980s, and I knew he wanted a new one for that cover." In other cases, youth described situations in which they used their networks to help them better publicize their work in anticipation of attracting new customers: "I met this woman outside [on the local business strip] who will be filming here, and she bought a beanie for herself. So, then I asked her if I could just give her some other beanies, so she could give them to other people, just so she can network for me" (SEI youth).

Lessons for For-Profit-Nonprofit Collaboration

From these cases involving BIDs and an SE, we identify three lessons that could guide future multisectoral collaborations in addressing homelessness. First, in both cases, the business community served as a vital extension of social work in engaging and retaining clients in employment and in facilitating positive outcomes.

Business leaders largely succeeded in engaging homeless populations and working with them to achieve mutual goals (i.e., for business, reducing homeless populations on the streets; for homeless individuals, connecting with service or employment opportunities that increase their quality of life). In future multisectoral partnerships, it is important for each sector involved to identify its goals regarding consumer engagement, retention, and outcomes as well as to delineate ways in which each sector can complement and extend the roles of the other sector.

Second, these collaborative efforts yielded intervention outcomes at multiple levels, not merely related to employment but also behavioral and societal outcomes (Ferguson and Islam 2008). In the case of BIDs, communities and systems (e.g., law enforcement) were positively influenced through sensitizing business owners about the assets of homeless populations and enhancing collaboration with local homeless advocates and human service agencies. In the case of the SE, youth commonly noted improvements in their mental health, self-esteem, and behavior. Staff also reported enhanced relationships between their agency and the local business community, which resulted in monetary and in-kind donations. Future partnerships should thus consider adopting a holistic and client-centered evaluation approach through which outcomes can be tracked and communicated across multiple levels: client, nonprofit organization, for-profit business, and society (Rapp and Poertner 1992).

Third, both case studies imply that the collaborative approach contributed to transforming the perceptions and attitudes of the business community regarding homelessness in general and about individuals experiencing homelessness in particular. Through involvement in a BID or SEI, business stakeholders became more knowledgeable about homeless populations in their districts, more interested in helping them in a sustainable way, and more aware of the assets of homeless individuals and how they could be applied in business settings. Going forward, social work interventions addressing homelessness are encouraged to consider the expertise and resources of the business community and to engage the for-profit sector both as partners in providing services to and advocating for individuals experiencing homelessness and as sources of employment and mentoring for this population.

Social Work Skills for Multisectoral Collaboration

There are various skills that will be useful for social workers engaging in multisectoral collaborations. This skillset includes macro-level systems thinking and the generalist skills that bridge micro and macro social work practice. First, it is fundamental for anyone who plans to work on ending homelessness to become familiar with systems thinking. Systems thinking differs from conventional thinking in that it recognizes that homelessness is a complex problem that cannot be tackled by a policy designed to achieve only short-term success. Systems thinking consultants teach us that most quick fixes have unintended consequences that often make the situation worse in the long run (Stroh 2015). To make large system-level changes, practitioners must understand how an effort to solve one problem may link to a

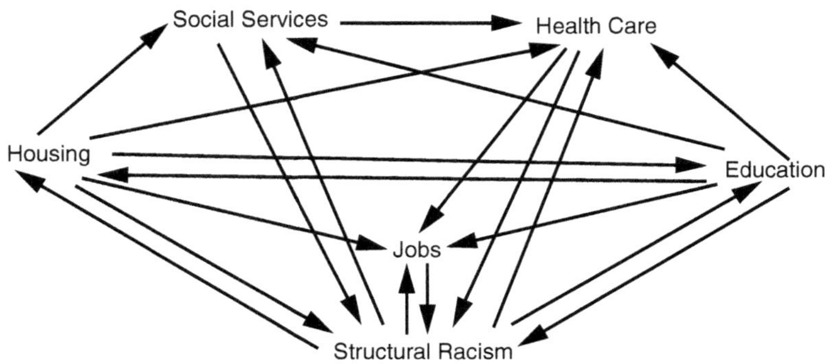

Fig. 12.2 Simple interdependence map related to homelessness. (Stroh 2015)

factor that perpetuates homelessness (see Fig. 12.2). Systems thinking can be used to help diverse stakeholders build a common agenda, pursue collective impact, and work together using continuous communication and a mutual learning environment.

In the process of understanding system-level relationships, it is important for practitioners to engage every stakeholder that shares a similar vision on ending homelessness. In the case example of a homeless coalition meeting (Stroh 2015, p. 80), for example, key stakeholders (i.e., an elected official, a business leader, a homeless shelter director, a director of Health Care for the Homeless, an affordable housing advocate, a funder, a concerned citizen, and a homeless person) came together to sort out their espoused purpose and hidden priorities. These stakeholders may have differing views and priorities, but through the process of identifying why they came together and how they can solve the problem, the group can establish a common ground to move forward.

The identification of initial roles and goals also needs to accompany the activities that facilitate the progression of collaboration by keeping partners engaged in and committed to the end goal. Claiborne and Lawson (2005) suggested eight "C Words" that support and strengthen collaboration: communicating, connecting, cooperating, consulting, coordinating, co-locating, community building, and contracting. In this model, each concept is a separate phase of collaboration, yet each interacts with other phases with increasing complexity as collaboration progresses. For example, in the beginning phases of forming a collaboration, actors need strong communication and interpersonal skills to engage partners, identify their strengths and assets, assign roles that enable them to apply these strengths, and build commitment to an issue or goal. During the collaboration, actors will begin more complex activities, such as service coordination or community building that require strong leadership and community engagement skills as well as efforts to sustain partners' commitment to the issue or goal. In the later phases of collaborations, actors can formalize their leadership by establishing a governance structure and new organizational structures, with a higher degree of shared liability and costs, as well as collective identity. In this phase, it is key that collaborators possess strong administrative and management skills.

	Service Agencies	*Faith-based Agencies*	*Advocacy Groups*	*Homeward Staff*	*Business*	*Local Government*
Diagnostic frames						
What is homelessness?/ Who are the homeless?						
• *Real homeless*			X		X	X
• *Diverse population*	X	X		X		
What is the primary cause of homelessness?						
• *Personal limitations*						
a) Over which the homeless have some control	X	X			X	
b) Over which the homeless have little/no control	X	X	X		X	X
• *Multiple factors*	X	X	X	X		
• *Structural conditions*		X	X	X		
Prognostic frames						
What should be done to address homelessness?						
• *Working together*	X	X	X	X	X	X
• *Effective system*	X			X	X	
• *Comprehensive holistic approach*	X	X				
• *On-demand services*	X		X		X	

Fig. 12.3 Summary of select frames most often used, by type of coalition participant. (Croteau and Hicks 2003)

Lastly, strong community organizing skills in framing issues and launching media campaigns are useful for social workers engaged in multisectoral collaborations to communicate and publicize their social issues, strategies, activities, and outcomes to policymakers, funders, and the broader society. Framing is the process by which we use words and ideas to shape the way we want others to see our issues and the need for our solutions. By selecting strategic language to communicate issues and solutions, we influence how policymakers, funders, and the broader society view—and respond to—our issues (Lakoff 2014). Social workers who address controversial or polarized social issues like homelessness would benefit from having communication and persuasion skills to frame their issues in language that elicits favorable political, economic, and philanthropic responses. Similarly, their ability to reframe unpopular issues using new language might help others see such issues in a more favorable manner. Figure 12.3 summarizes common homelessness frames used by various actors involved in multisectoral collaborations.

In addition to framing skills, social workers involved in multisectoral collaborations benefit from skills related to designing and implementing successful media campaigns. Media campaigns refer to the use of mass media (social and traditional media) to disseminate a message that captures the attention of an intended audience, builds their interest in the message, and stimulates their intention to act in a way that aligns with the group's goals. Media campaigns can be used to educate the public about social and policy issues, change public perceptions about issues, and motivate people to take action in a desired direction (Woods-Waller 2008). In the case of addressing homelessness, social media campaigns such as Miracle Messages in San Francisco attempt to connect people experiencing homelessness with friends and family through disseminating their messages via social media and crowdfunding to finance their relocation expenses (O'Connor 2015). In developing and implementing successful media campaigns, social workers need to be knowledgeable of local, regional, and national media sources and comfortable contacting and working with media figures. Additionally, social workers who launch successful media campaigns possess additional skills in agenda setting, communications, member recruitment, advocacy, and technology use (e.g., social media platforms).

Conclusion

In this chapter, we introduced multisectoral collaborations, or partnerships among more than one sector (i.e., government, private for-profit, private nonprofit), and described their characteristics. We then presented two overall multisectoral collaborative approaches (i.e., interagency collaborations and For-profit-nonprofit collaborations) designed to address homelessness. We used the Continuum of Care and US Interagency Council on Homelessness models to illustrate interagency collaborations as well as business improvement district and social enterprise models as examples of for-profit-nonprofit collaborations. We concluded the chapter by providing an overview of the macro and generalist skills that are useful for social workers engaged in multisectoral collaborations.

References

Anderson, S. G. (2014). *New strategies for social innovation: Market-based approaches for assisting the poor*. New York: Columbia University Press.

Avery, N. (2015, May 1). A new energy on combating homelessness. https://www.washingtonpost.com/opinions/a-new-energy-on-combating-homelessness/2015/05/01/9882119a-edf1-11e4-8abc-d6aa3bad79dd_story.html?utm_term=.4a849148b8bf. Accessed 15 June 2018.

Briffault, R. (1999). A government for our time? Business improvement districts and urban governance. *Columbia Law Review, 99*, 365.

Bryson, J. M. (2011). *Strategic planning for public and nonprofit organizations: A guide to strengthening and sustaining organizational achievement* (Vol. 1). San Francisco: John Wiley & Sons.

Bryson, J. M., Crosby, B. C., & Stone, M. M. (2006). The design and implementation of cross-sector collaborations: Propositions from the literature. *Public Administration Review, 66*, 44–55.

Claiborne, N., & Lawson, H. A. (2005). An intervention framework for collaboration. *Families in Society, 86*(1), 93–103.

Clarke, A., & Fuller, M. (2010). Collaborative strategic management: Strategy formulation and implementation by multi-organizational cross-sector social partnerships. *Journal of Business Ethics, 94*, 85–101.

Community Partnership for the Prevention of Homelessness (2016). Facts & figures. http://www.community-partnership.org/facts-and-figures. Accessed 5 Sept 2016.

Covenant House California (2007). Statistics. http://www.covenanthouseca.org. Accessed 30 June 2018.

Croteau, D., & Hicks, L. (2003). Coalition framing and the challenge of a consonant frame pyramid: The case of a collaborative response to homelessness. *Social Problems, 50*(2), 251–272.

Culhane, D. P., & Byrne, T. (2010). Ending chronic homelessness: Cost-effective opportunities for interagency collaboration. University of Pennsylvania. http://repository.upenn.edu/spp_papers/143. Accessed 15 June 2018.

Dees, J. G. (1998). Enterprising nonprofits. *Harvard Business Review, 76*, 54–69.

Dolan, M. (2012, September 5). Court rules that L.A. can't destroy homeless people's property. Los Angeles Times. http://articles.latimes.com/2012/sep/05/local/la-me-0906-homeless-lapd-20120906. Accessed 15 June 2018.

Downtown Business Improvement District (2010). Ending chronic homelessness in DC: A unified strategy. https://www.downtowndc.org/wp-content/uploads/2017/06/leadershiphomelessness2.pdf. Accessed 15 June 2018.

Ferguson, K. M. (2007). Implementing a social enterprise intervention with homeless, street-living youths in Los Angeles. *Social Work, 52*(2), 103–112.

Ferguson, K. M., & Islam, N. (2008). Conceptualizing outcomes with street-living young adults: Grounded theory approach to evaluating the social enterprise intervention. *Qualitative Social Work, 7*(2), 217–237.

Gazley, B. (2008). Beyond the contract: The scope and nature of informal government–nonprofit partnerships. *Public Administration Review, 68*(1), 141–154.

Guo, C., & Acar, M. (2005). Understanding collaboration among nonprofit organizations: Combining resource dependency, institutional, and network perspectives. *Nonprofit and Voluntary Sector Quarterly, 34*(3), 340–361.

Hartman, R. R. (2015). 51 homeless individuals secured housing through BID and Pathways to Housing DC. Downton DC BID. http://www.downtowndc.org/news/51-homeless-individuals-secured-housing-through-bid-and-pathways-housing-dc. Accessed 7 July 2017.

Holland, G. (2013, June 24). Court refuses to allow L.A. to cart off homeless' belongings. Los Angeles Times. http://www.latimes.com/local/lanow/la-me-ln-homeless-belongings-20130624-story.html. Accessed 15 June 2018.

Horvitz-Lennon, M., Kilbourne, A. M., & Pincus, H. A. (2006). From silos to bridges: Meeting the general health care needs of adults with severe mental illnesses. *Health Affairs, 25*(3), 659–669.

Houstoun, L. O. (2003). *BIDs: Business improvement districts* (2nd ed.). Washington, D.C.: Urban Land Institute.

Kernaghan, K. (2005). Moving towards the virtual state: Integrating services and service channels for citizen-centered delivery. *International Review of Administrative Sciences, 71*(1), 119–131.

Krupa, T., Lagarde, M., & Carmichael, K. (2003). Transforming sheltered workshops into affirmative businesses: An outcome evaluation. *Psychiatric Rehabilitation Journal, 26*(4), 359.

Lakoff, G. (2014). *The all new don't think of an elephant!: Know your values and frame the debate*. White River Junction: Chelsea Green Publishing.

Lawson, H. A. (2004). The logic of collaboration in education and the human services. *Journal of Interprofessional Care, 18*(3), 225–237.

Los Angeles Homeless Services Authority. (2016). *2016 homeless count results*. Los Angeles: Author.

Mandell, M., & Steelman, T. (2003). Understanding what can be accomplished through interorganizational innovations: The importance of typologies, context and management strategies. *Public Management Review, 5*(2), 197–224.

National Alliance to End Homelessness. (2015). *The state of homelessness of America 2015: An examination of trends in homelessness, homelessness assistance, and at-risk populations at the national and state levels*. Washington, D.C.: Author.

O'Connor, L. (2015, January 29). Social media campaign helps connect homeless people with loved ones. Huffington Post. https://www.huffingtonpost.com/2015/01/29/san-francisco-homeless-videos_n_6575074.html. Accessed 15 June 2018.

Rapp, C. A., & Poertner, J. (1992). *Social administration: A client-centered approach*. New York: Allyn and Bacon.

Salamon, L. M. (1995). *Partners in public service: Government-nonprofit relations in the modern welfare state*. Baltimore: Johns Hopkins University Press.

Selsky, J. W., & Parker, B. (2005). Cross-sector partnerships to address social issues: Challenges to theory and practice. *Journal of Management, 31*(6), 849–873.

Simpson, J. (2015). Police and homeless outreach worker partnerships: Policing of homeless individuals with mental illness in Washington, D.C. *Human Organization, 74*(2), 125–134.

Smith, D. (2017). Downtown L.A. businesses try outreach to find permanent housing for the homeless. The Los Angeles Times. http://www.latimes.com/local/lanow/la-me-ln-bid-homeless-outreach-20161221-story.html. Accessed 15 June 2018.

Sowa, J. E. (2008). Implementing interagency collaborations exploring variation in collaborative ventures in human service organizations. *Administration & Society, 40*(3), 298–323.

Stroh, D. P. (2015). *Systems thinking for social change: A practical guide to solving complex problems, avoiding unintended consequences, and achieving lasting results*. White River Junction: Chelsea Green Publishing.

U.S. Department of Housing and Urban Development. (2007). *Defining chronic homelessness: A technical guide for HUD programs*. Washington, D.C.: Author.

U.S. Department of Housing and Urban Development (2012). Introductory guide to the continuum of care (CoC): Understanding the CoC Program and the requirements of the CoC Program Interim Rule. https://www.hudexchange.info/resources/documents/CoCProgramIntroductoryGuide.pdf. Accessed 10 July 2017.

U.S. Interagency Council on Homelessness (2015). Preventing and ending youth homelessness: A coordinated community response. https://www.usich.gov/resources/uploads/asset_library/Youth_Homelessness_Coordinated_Response.pdf. Accessed 10 July 2017.

U.S. Interagency Council on Homelessness (2017a). USICH fact sheet. https://www.usich.gov/resources/uploads/asset_library/USICH_Fact_Sheet_2017.pdf. Accessed 10 July 2017.

U.S. Interagency Council on Homelessness (2017b). Mayors challenge to end veteran homelessness. https://www.usich.gov/solutions/collaborative-leadership/mayors-challenge. Accessed 10 July 2017.

U.S. Interagency Council on the Homelessness. (1994). *Priority: Home! The federal plan to break the cycle of homelessness*. Washington, D.C: Author.

Waddock, S. A. (1991). A typology of social partnership organizations. *Administration & Society, 22*(4), 480–515.

Warner, R., & Mandiberg, J. (2006). An update on affirmative businesses or social firms for people with mental illness. *Psychiatric Services, 57*(10), 1488–1492.

Wogan, J. B. (2015). Why homelessness is rising in D.C. but declining elsewhere. Governing the States and Localities. http://www.governing.com/topics/health-human-services/gov-dc-turnaround-homelessness-problem-human-services-director.html. Accessed 15 June 2018.

Wong, Y.-L. I., Park, J. M., & Nemon, H. (2006). Homeless service delivery in the context of continuum of care. *Administration in Social Work, 30*(1), 67–94.

Woods-Waller, G. (2008). Media campaigns. In T. Mizrahi & L. E. Davis (Eds.), *Encyclopedia of social work* (20th ed., pp. 195–198). New York: NASW and Oxford University Press.

Young, D. R. (2006). Complementary, supplementary, or adversarial? Nonprofit-government relations. In E. T. Boris & C. E. Steuerle (Eds.), *Nonprofits and government: Collaboration and conflict* (3rd ed., pp. 37–80). Washington, D.C.: The Urban Institute Press.

Chapter 13
Trauma-Informed Care in Homelessness Service Settings: Challenges and Opportunities

Cassandra Bransford and Michael Cole

> The ache for home lives in all of us, the safe place where we can go as we are and not be questioned. (Angelou 1991, p. 196)

Home is generally considered to be a place of refuge, warmth, and safety, where one can find shelter, relax, and de-stress from everyday life. Sadly, this basic and fundamental human need is unmet for increasing numbers of homeless people. Indeed, according to the US Department of Housing and Urban Development (HUD), 553,742 persons were homeless on a given night in 2017, an increase of approximately 1% from 2016. One third of those were living in unsheltered settings. In the USA alone, homelessness affects approximately 10 million people annually (National Law Center on Poverty and Homelessness 2015).

The human toil and suffering resulting from homelessness is devastating. Not only are persons deprived of their basic need for a place of their own, but they are also at an increased risk for assault, injury and death (Jetelina et al. 2017; Morrison 2009), infectious and other diseases (Rimawi et al. 2014), mental illness (Oppenheimer et al. 2016), substance abuse (Johnson and Chamberlain 2008), incarceration (Gowan 2002), and sex trafficking (Murphy 2017). While homelessness puts people at risk for trauma, prior traumatic experiences, including adverse childhood experiences, predispose individuals to homelessness (Roos et al. 2013). Indeed, people who have had early and/or untreated past experiences of trauma are at the greatest risk for becoming homeless (SAMSHA 2016). Given the high rates of trauma experienced by individuals and families affected by homelessness, it is imperative that organizational settings providing services to them become trauma informed. This chapter will provide an overview of trauma, its reciprocal

---

Electronic supplementary material: The online version of this chapter (https://doi.org/10.1007/978-3-030-03727-7_13) contains supplementary material, which is available to authorized users.

C. Bransford (✉) · M. Cole
Binghamton University, Binghamton, NY, USA
e-mail: cbrans@binghamton.edu; mcole5@binghamton.edu

H. Larkin et al. (eds.), *Homelessness Prevention and Intervention in Social Work*, https://doi.org/10.1007/978-3-030-03727-7_13

relationship with homelessness, and the need for and use of trauma-informed care (TIC) in prevention and intervention settings.

The Substance Abuse and Mental Health Services Administration (SAMHSA) defines trauma as "resulting from an event, series of events, or set of circumstances that is [are] experienced by an individual as physically or emotionally harmful or life threatening and that has [have] lasting adverse effects on the individual's functioning and mental, physical, social, emotional, or spiritual well-being" (SAMHSA 2017, para. 3). Effects of trauma can include feelings of isolation, powerlessness, changes in worldview, devastating fear, and feelings of shame and guilt, which can be especially crippling for those also traumatized by the experience of homelessness (Chrystal et al. 2015; Deck and Platt 2015).

Homelessness, as defined within the US Department of Housing and Urban Development's implementation of the HEARTH Act, consists of the following four categories:

1. Individuals and families who lack a fixed, regular, and adequate nighttime residence and include a subset for an individual who resided in an emergency shelter or a place not meant for human habitation and who is exiting an institution where he or she temporarily resided
2. Individuals and families who will imminently lose their primary nighttime residence
3. Unaccompanied youth and families with children and youth who are defined as homeless under other federal statutes who do not otherwise qualify as homeless under this definition
4. Individuals and families who are fleeing, or are attempting to flee, domestic violence, dating violence, sexual assault, stalking, or other dangerous or life-threatening conditions that relate to violence against the individual or a family member (Federal Register 2011)

Homelessness and Trauma

Decades of research have shown that, much like poverty (East and Roll 2015) and substance abuse (Flanagan et al. 2015), trauma and homelessness have a close, often cyclical relationship (Deck and Platt 2015). Experiencing homelessness can be traumatic in and of itself; the social disaffiliation and learned helplessness that accompany it can produce symptoms similar to those described by physical and sexual abuse survivors (Goodman et al. 1991).

Prior experiences with trauma can increase the risk for experiencing homelessness. Those facing housing instability consistently report higher rates of lifetime trauma (Sundin and Baguley 2015) and are subject to higher rates of premature death (Lakeman 2011), as compared to the general population. Lifetime exposure to trauma has also been found to have powerful predictive effects on numbers of days homeless, job training outcomes, unemployment, and first episode of homelessness (Alexander 2011; Mar et al. 2014; Tsai et al. 2012). Additionally, the timing of homelessness shapes future lifetime experiences of trauma, with those facing homelessness before age 50 reporting greater life adversity overall (Brown et al. 2016). Lifetime trauma exposure has also been linked to higher rates of depression in homeless mothers (Bassuk and Beardslee 2014).

Emerging studies have shown that a variety of traumatic experiences, particularly childhood maltreatment, have effects that span time. For example, parents with higher rates of adverse childhood experiences (ACEs) were found more likely to maltreat their children in a sample of families in emergency shelters, suggesting a continuity of intergenerational trauma that predisposes families to further problems and pain (Narayan et al. 2017).

Types of trauma and chronicity of traumatic stress may also impact populations differently. For example, experiences of discrimination, poly-victimization, and violent victimization, as well as repeated systemic failures, have been found to put LBGT homeless youth at increased risk for juvenile and criminal justice involvement and revictimization (Snyder et al. 2016). For older adults, the chronicity of traumatic stress can lead them to physically age faster than their chronological age, suggesting a need for a different approach as baby boomers continue to age over time. Common factors related to homelessness in elders include relationship breakdown, financial problems, and subsequent eviction. Other stressors include lack of affordable housing, service barriers, and failing health (Woolrych et al. 2015).

Veterans, particularly female veterans, also face unique traumas before and during their time in the military. One study found homeless female veterans faced a median average of 31 previous traumas, and military sexual trauma was significantly and independently associated with post-deployment homelessness (Brignone et al. 2016). Assessing for these experiences is vital in contextualizing these unique events within the framework of what we currently understand about trauma and in fully conceptualizing the role of trauma in each client's life (Hamilton et al. 2013; Tsai et al. 2012).

The trauma experienced by homeless people impacts their well-being. Young children experiencing homelessness face greater exposure to traumatic events within shelters, overwhelming their stress response systems (Herbers et al. 2014). Childhood traumas have also been linked to mental health problems in homeless adults, with 87% reporting one adverse childhood event and more than half reporting four or more, replicating findings from past studies (Larkin and Park 2012). Similar results have been found in samples of homeless youth (Jordan 2012). The combination of homelessness and trauma creates a unique vulnerability to psychopathology and necessitates a change in organizational and professional perspectives to recognize persons' needs (Davies and Allen 2017).

Trauma-Informed Care

Working in settings that serve people experiencing homelessness can be enormously stressful. Despite the often-well-meaning intentions of service providers, re-traumatization can and often does occur (Jennings 2008). Trauma-informed care (TIC) models are unique in that they seek to support the needs of both clients and service providers in organizational settings. Over the last 30 years, TIC has gained meaningful ground in its efforts to reform care contexts. These contexts include child welfare, substance abuse, mental health, school systems, and criminal justice institutions (Conners-Burrow et al. 2013; Kramer et al. 2015; Langley et al. 2013).

Trauma-informed care (TIC) has been defined as follows: Trauma-informed care is a strengths-based framework that is grounded in an understanding of and responsiveness to the impact of trauma that emphasizes physical, psychological, and emotional safety for both providers and survivors and that creates opportunities for survivors to rebuild a sense of control and empowerment (Hopper et al. 2010, p. 82).

TIC seeks to transform the overall organizational care system and culture to minimize re-traumatization of service recipients and reduce vicarious or secondary trauma of service providers. While important in all care settings, TIC is particularly relevant to individuals experiencing homelessness (Guarino et al. 2014). A primary goal of TIC is that it seeks specifically to create safe, healthy, and caring environmental contexts for those who may have experienced toxic early home environments and interpersonal trauma. Moreover, for those who have experienced the traumatic effects of homelessness, effectively implemented TIC settings can provide a healing and remediating milieu (Hodgdon et al. 2013; Hopper et al. 2010).

Evolution of Trauma-Informed Care

A body of formal knowledge about trauma only began to develop in the USA in the latter half of the twentieth century. This is likely due to the enormous difficulty society has had, and continues to have, in acknowledging the existence of child sexual abuse and other violent atrocities perpetrated by people against one another. The lack of acknowledgment of trauma has not only impeded the development and adaptation of TIC programs and policies in organizational settings but has also delayed a more universal acknowledgment about the existence of trauma in the lives of service recipients and providers.

Nonetheless, the study of trauma has grown over the last several decades. Thanks to the work of feminist activists and scholars supporting survivors of rape, domestic violence, and childhood sexual abuse (Webster and Dunn 2005), and medical professionals and social scientists treating and studying veterans of the Vietnam War (Laufer et al. 1984), researchers began to seriously consider how best to support populations with severe trauma histories. A brief discussion of the evolution of trauma theory will highlight society's historical resistance to fully acknowledging the existence of trauma.

Historical Epochs

Herman (1992) identified three fundamental historical epochs, or significant time periods, in the development of trauma theory over the past century: (1) the study of hysteria and the development and later abandonment of Freud's seduction theory, (2) the study of war neurosis from World War I through the Vietnam War era, and (3) the women's movement. Within these epochs, an initial recognition of trauma was later followed by a collective public denial and general disbelief that atrocities, such as sexual abuse, war trauma, or domestic violence, could actually exist. Characterizing this denial as *social amnesia*, Herman compared it to the repressive amnesia often experienced by trauma survivors. Herman explained, "to study psychological trauma is to come face to face with human vulnerability in the natural world and with the capacity for evil in human nature" (p. 7). Herman (1992) thus described the tendency of humans to disbelieve the unimaginable: "In the absence of strong political movements for human rights, the active process of bearing witness inevitably gives way to the active process of forgetting. Repression, dissociation, and denial are phenomena of social as well as individual consciousness" (p. 9).

First Epoch: Late Nineteenth Century – The Study of Hysteria and Development of Seduction Theory

Freud's initial development and later abandonment of seduction theory illustrates the enormous pressure wielded by society to deny the existence of sexual trauma. Freud developed seduction theory based upon case notes amassed from his work with female patients who exhibited symptoms of hysteria. These symptoms typically involved the loss of specific bodily functions, such as speech or the ability to move limbs, despite the absence of any medical basis for these impairments. Freud subsequently found that the women exhibiting these symptoms had been subjected to sexual abuse, assault, and incest (Herman 1992). Following the publication of his groundbreaking paper, *The Aetiology of Hysteria* (1896), which documented his findings, Freud increasingly became isolated and scorned. The uproar his theory generated among the upper echelon of late nineteenth-century Viennese society, who could not bear to acknowledge the prevalence of sexual abuse perpetrated by seemingly respectable persons from within their own ranks, caused Freud to abandon this theory (Masson 1984). He subsequently developed his theory of infantile sexuality, which relegated the origin of hysterical symptoms to the unsatisfied sexual desires and fantasies of his female patients, rather than the real-world perpetrators of sexual violence and abuse.

Second Epoch: Post World War I to the Vietnam War

The protracted ravages of World War I left many combatants suffering symptoms not unlike those of nineteenth-century women previously diagnosed with hysteria. Many soldiers had witnessed the death of their comrades and were subjected to situations in which they were rendered helpless, captive to the horrors of war. Their symptoms included unrelenting weeping, catatonia, muteness, amnesia, and emotional cutoffs (Herman 1992). While these symptoms were initially viewed as resulting from exposure to exploding shells, or shell shock, later, military psychiatrists attributed these symptoms to the psychological trauma of war. Gradually, however, the symptoms exhibited by war veterans increasingly became viewed by society as representing signs of moral inferiority or cowardice rather than resulting from trauma. The treatments developed to cure them included shaming, ridicule, and aversion therapies, such as applying electrical currents to the throats of soldiers. Many soldiers were court-martialed for their supposed cowardice. And, again, the reality of trauma was largely denied, its victims viewed as deficient and blamed for their own suffering (Herman 1992).

During World War II, the use of brief treatments was initiated with soldiers exhibiting trauma symptoms. These brief treatments included hypnosis and the use of sodium amytal to facilitate rapid catharsis of intense war-related emotions. Prominent psychiatrists of the day argued that catharsis alone was insufficient to address the effects of war trauma and that integration of traumatic memories into consciousness was required. Additionally, an emphasis on the importance of human connections in facilitating recovery from trauma was stressed. The influential text *The Traumatic Neuroses of War* (Kardiner 1941) provided cogent psychological explanations for war and other trauma-related symptoms, as did its revised edition *War Stress and Neurotic Illness* (Kardiner and Spiegel 1947), but, nonetheless, a sustained public interest in trauma explanations soon waned. Scant attention was paid to returning veterans who continued to suffer from the lasting effects of war-related trauma, many of whom were forced to reside in the overcrowded backward of psychiatric hospitals. Again, society's appetite for acknowledging the realities of trauma receded (Herman 1992).

A serious and concerted effort to acknowledge war trauma did not occur again until the Vietnam War era, when anti-war activists spoke out publicly about the horrors of war and organized rap groups, which provided opportunities for veterans to acknowledge the traumas they underwent. The proliferation of rap groups in the 1970s yielded sufficient pressure on the Veteran's Administration to develop outreach centers across the country to provide peer-run services to veterans (Herman 1992).

Third Epoch: The Women's Movement

In the 1970s, second-wave feminists began speaking out about violence against women, and safe spaces were identified where women could begin to openly address their experiences of violence in the home. Just as peer-led rap groups validated experiences of war trauma for veterans, consciousness raising groups provided women with opportunities to speak about rape and other forms of violence that were taking place behind the so-called sanctity of closed doors (Herman 1992). Spearheaded by the National Organization for Women, rape reform legislation was initiated in the 1970s, leading to the development of rape crisis centers across the country. Rape came to be seen as an act of power and violence rather than a sexual act. The symptoms related to rape were found to be similar to those related to war trauma and included startle response, insomnia, and dissociation. These reforms were closely followed by legislation on domestic violence and child sexual abuse. Walker (1979) coined the term "battered woman syndrome" to describe the constellation of trauma symptoms experienced by victims of domestic violence.

Trauma in the 1980s and Beyond

The aforementioned efforts resulted eventually in the 1980 inclusion of post-traumatic stress disorder (PTSD) into the third edition of the *Diagnostic and Statistical Manual of Mental Disorders* (*DSM-III*; APA 1980). Moreover, in 1985, the International Society for Traumatic Stress Studies came together to seek greater understanding about trauma and how to treat it. This led directly to the creation of the National Center for Post-Traumatic Stress Disorder. The official recognition of the role of trauma in many women's issues by the Substance Abuse and Mental Health Administration in the 1990s kicked off a boom in trauma-oriented research (Wilson et al. 2013).

Two large-scale studies conducted during this time helped practitioners to better understand both the widespread role of trauma in the early experiences of children and its relationship to mental health, substance abuse, suicidality, and health risks (Felitti et al. 1998) and also the importance of developing trauma-informed organizational models overtly designed to avoid retraumatizing female survivors (McHugo et al. 2005; SAMSHA 2007). This proliferating body of work guided social workers and other health and human service professionals to develop empirically based treatments for PTSD and to conceptualize how contexts of care can be informed by the experiences of clients.

Along with the studies referenced above, this new openness to the realities of trauma led to a wave of research in the 1990s and early 2000s. The work of Terr (1991), Herman (1992), van der Kolk (1994), van der Kolk et al. (1996), and others began to forge an understanding of the psychobiology of trauma. This understanding highlighted the relationship of traumatic stress to neurobiology (Perry 2006; Siegel 2001) and produced evidence that an abundance of traumatic stress, particularly in the early developmental years, affected multiple domains of functioning. The functional domains affected by traumatic stress included "disturbances in perception, information processing, affect regulation, impulse control, and personality development" (van der Kolk et al. 2005, p. 366). This constellation of functional difficulties resulting from childhood trauma during pivotal development periods has come to be known as complex trauma.

The National Child Traumatic Stress Network (n.d.) describes complex trauma as follows: The term complex trauma describes both children's exposure to multiple traumatic events, often of an invasive, interpersonal nature, and the wide ranging, long-term impacts of this exposure. These events are severe and pervasive, such as abuse or profound neglect. They usually begin early in life and can disrupt many aspects of the child's development and the very formation of a self. Since they often occur in the context of the child's relationship with a caregiver, they interfere with the child's ability to form a secure attachment bond. Many aspects of a child's health and physical and mental development rely on this primary source of safety and stability (para. 1–2).

A greater understanding of the antecedents and effects of traumatic stress, or complex trauma, has led to the development of TIC models. By incorporating research on disrupted attachment, childhood adversity, the effects of trauma on the brain, biological adaptation, relationships, self-esteem, and meaning making, the TIC movement seeks ultimately to create transformational systemic change in the provision of services to people impacted by trauma. The work of Sandra Bloom, and colleagues, who developed the Sanctuary Model, epitomizes this movement toward TIC (Bloom 2005, 2013; Bloom and Farragher 2013).

Understanding Trauma-Informed Care

Trauma-Informed Culture

Incorporating TIC in human service and mental health settings is forging a significant paradigmatic cultural shift in the way that symptoms and functional impairments are conceptualized. Instead of asking a client, "What is wrong with you?" the question instead becomes, "What has happened to you?" This important shift reconceptualizes symptoms as representing gallant efforts at adapting to severely adverse circumstances rather than reflective of internal deficiencies. Moreover, this reconceptualization signifies that persons can entirely overcome and heal from past trauma rather than simply learn to live with diminished expectations about one's future potential for a satisfying life.

Profound and fundamental to TIC is the active application of knowledge about trauma and how it impacts the lives of all individuals in care settings, including clients and staff at all levels of operations (Hopper et al. 2010; Guarino and Bassuk 2010). TIC providers approach their work with the assumptions that trauma is pervasive, affects clients broadly, shapes lives deeply, and perpetuates across generations (Fallot and Harris 2009). This is known as *trauma awareness*, and it is necessary at all levels of service work. This awareness ranges from designing intake assessments that integrate knowledge of trauma to a focus on how all staff relate to clients within the organization. Trauma awareness can be facilitated by using trauma-informed training procedures and supervision with all personnel to instill institutional knowledge about the role of trauma in all aspects of organizational life.

Key Assumptions

Important to understanding TIC is grasping what SAMHSA (2014a) describes as the three Es and four Rs of trauma. Thus, trauma is understood to consist of three linear components: (a) *events*, (b) *experience*, and (c) *effects*. Traumatic *events* can include actual threats of harm or life-threatening neglect and can occur once or repeatedly. Whether individuals consider an event to be traumatic is shaped by their *experiences* around it, including how they label and assign meaning to the event, whether they are subjectively disturbed by what happened, and whether there was anyone there to help them process and integrate the event. Together, these factors determine if the incident was traumatic (SAMSHA 2014a). Lastly, trauma is defined by its short- and long-term *effects*. It is assumed that it may take time for individuals to process and respond to what they have experienced, and that is normal. Effects can include an impaired ability to cope with normal stressors, difficulty in forming relationships, and changes in the person's neurobiological makeup (Cook et al. 2017).

With regard to the four Rs, staff within a TIC environment are expected to operate with an active *realization* about the ubiquity of trauma and an understanding of its effects on individuals, groups, families, and communities. Behavior, maladaptive or otherwise, is understood as shaped within the context of overcoming adversity. Providers acknowledge that trauma plays an important role in mental health and substance use issues and must be addressed systematically in human service and other institutional systems in order for these issues to be overcome. Workers within TIC organizations are thus trained to *recognize* the signs of trauma and *respond* by applying principles of TIC in all areas of systemic functioning with both staff and clients. Lastly, trauma-informed practitioners seek to resist *re-traumatization* of all individuals within the institutional context. Often organizations trying to implement TIC forget to be mindful of the trauma that those within the helping professions also experience, including the vicarious trauma experienced when listening to clients recount their experiences. This oversight can undermine the effectiveness of TIC programming. When properly implemented, TIC equips staff with tools to recognize traumatic organizational practices and to advocate for change whenever appropriate (SAMSHA 2014a).

Core Principles

According to SAMSHA, there are six core principles to TIC. *Safety* is first and fundamental, accomplished through the creation of environments that ensure both physical and emotional safety of all clients (Hopper et al. 2010). Examples of instilling safety include being mindful of how intake spaces are designed, providing locks for client dormitories, and setting clear and consistent boundaries upon admission. These changes are intended to help clients feel safe enough to be honest about what they have experienced, facilitating the relationship between clinicians and clients, as well as between clients and the agency itself (Beyer et al. 2010).

Trustworthiness and transparency are also crucial. This includes honoring confidentiality and being transparent regarding agency regulations and rules. When rules are broken, and action is taken, procedures should be communicated and put into effect in a clear and culturally competent manner. Homeless clients with trauma histories may come from families without clear boundaries, where rules constantly change. When clients know what to expect from care systems, their sense of safety is improved, as well as their chances at better outcomes (SAMSHA 2014a).

Empowerment, voice, and choice comprise another core principle, placing value on the right of consumers to make their own decisions regarding care and for their voices to be heard. Because control is often lost amidst trauma and real choices are limited, opportunities for consumers to make meaningful choices in predictable environments can result in low self-esteem and a lack of confidence in their ability to improve their lives. Using a strengths-based approach, providers identify what clients can already do and tap into their inner strengths. Clients are supported in building coping skills to help overcome life's challenges. Many clients find this approach to be affirming and hope inducing, validating their life experiences while still moving them toward the growth they need to thrive (SAMSHA 2014a).

The last three principles are *peer support*, *collaboration*, and *cultural, historical, and gender issues*. Creating opportunities for clients to support one another is crucial, as it can allow trauma survivors to develop sustainable communities and prevent relapse. Group models, such as the Trauma Recovery and Empowerment Model (TREM), exemplify the value of creating structured environments where clients can make sense of what has happened to them and heal together (Fallot and Harris 2002, SAMSHA 2014a). The principle of *collaboration* touches upon the need to involve all clients in the planning and implementation of care plans. By sharing the decision-making power, clients are given the skills to begin to pursue their own long-term growth. While the process of eliciting buy-in is lengthy and resource intensive at times, ultimately, when providers and clients work together, it can lead to better outcomes (Signorelli et al. 2017).

The final principle, *cultural, historical, and gender issues*, refers to applying a sociocultural lens to conceptualizing trauma. Thus, trauma is defined not only by individual experiences but also by shared understandings of the meaning of trauma by members of different cultural groups and the development of historical narratives. Gender identity is also important, as some groups are more likely to experience a specific type of trauma (Hetzel-Riggin and Roby 2013). Cultural background and ethnicity can also shape beliefs around appropriate help-seeking behaviors and serve as sources of strength (Tummala-Narra et al. 2014; Al-Krenawi and Kimberly 2014). TIC providers and agencies can support clients' recovery by incorporating culturally responsive practices at every level of practice. By incorporating these principles, providers and researchers can better ensure that trauma interventions are evidence-based and culturally competent (SAMSHA 2014a).

Implementing Trauma-Informed Care in Homelessness Service Settings and Beyond

Impact of Trauma Work on Providers

While there is always a risk of psychological harm in providing services to clients, this danger may be exacerbated when working with clients in the homelessness service sector. However, the vulnerabilities of the organizational workforce are often overlooked. In fact, a greater trauma history among personnel is associated with worsened vicarious trauma symptoms (Knight 2010; Agllias 2012; Gilin and Kauffman 2015).

Additionally, social service providers are particularly susceptible to experiencing secondary traumatic stress, with a lifetime PTSD rate nearly three times that of the general population (Bride et al. 2009). Hearing clients recount painful histories can provide potentially meaningful valence to the work but may contribute to the stress that leads to burnout and high turnover (Hernandez et al. 2010; Middleton and Potter 2015). Leaving issues related to vicarious trauma and secondary stress unaddressed can make providers' adjustment to trauma-informed work greatly challenging, particularly in homelessness service settings (Newell and MacNeil 2010; Olivet et al. 2010).

There are multiple constructs used to describe the impact of trauma work on therapists and other frontline workers (Nimmo and Huggard 2013; Ray et al. 2013). These constructs include *vicarious trauma, secondary traumatic stress, compassion fatigue, compassion satisfaction,* and *vicarious resilience*.

Vicarious trauma has been defined as the negative transformational processes that occur within providers resulting from empathizing and engaging with clients. These negative processes include loss of meaning and hope (Pearlman and Caringi 2009). *Secondary traumatic stress* refers to the stress response symptoms experienced by workers who are witnessing or hearing about the traumatic experiences of their clients (Huggard 2003). *Compassion fatigue* is the reduced ability to be effective with clients, as a result of hearing about or witnessing their distress, coupled with organizational contexts that are not supportive (Figley 1995). *Compassion satisfaction* refers to the positive effects of working with people affected by trauma. These positive effects include gratification and a personal sense of reward (Stamm 2005, 2009).

If adequately supported by organizational policies and supports, providers can build resilience to the negative effects of working with clients experiencing trauma. TIC organizational strategies, such as cognitive empathy, training and support (Yu et al. 2016), lower caseloads, regular supervision, and the introduction of mindfulness-based interventions, such as meditation stress reduction training (Kabat-Zinn 2003), have been found to be effective in reducing compassion fatigue (Turgoose and Maddox 2017) and work stress (dos Santos et al. 2016) and increasing self-compassion and satisfaction (Duarte and Pinto-Gouveia 2016) among nurses and other frontline workers. This may support the development of *vicarious resilience*, the process by which healthcare professionals can be inspired and transformed by their clients' endurance and resilience in the face of grave adversity (Hernández et al. 2010). Many experienced providers attest to being moved by the work they do, sometimes even inspired by it (Ferris 2016). While trauma is often viewed as negative and painful in therapeutic contexts, working through it in the right setting can be empowering for all those involved in this work.

The ways that individuals respond to bearing witness to traumatic life experiences of clients vary greatly. How agencies train and address worker stress can make or break efforts to implement TIC. Encouraging providers only to practice the social work panacea of self-care has been found to be insufficient in reducing PTSD symptoms, vicarious trauma, and burnout (Adams and Riggs 2008).

Lack of regular organizational debriefings has been reported as an issue confounding management of the emotional impacts of trauma work and has been correlated with slow rates of client improvement, increased work pressure, and boundary issues between workers and clients (Olivet et al. 2010; Bermingham 2014). While implementing trauma-informed principles for clients is the goal, ensuring that a framework is in place for staff is equally important in promoting organizational sustainability.

Culture Clash

Another obstacle to successful implementation of TIC is a failure to consider the cultural needs of large, multifaceted organizations. While social work values organizational change in terms of social justice and antiracism work, organizational discourse and climate development are also important components in the creation of effective TIC settings (Mattar 2010; Wolf et al. 2014; Bateman et al. 2013). Organizational discourse has been defined as "the languages and symbolic media we employ to describe, represent, interpret, and theorize what we take to be the facticity of organizational life" (Grant et al. 1998, p. 1). How clinicians understand the work they do and how an agency fits within a broader cultural context is key to making long-term changes in how services to homeless clients are provided. For example, embedded professional cultural practices and beliefs were obstacles in efforts to successfully apply TIC in mental health settings in Australia. Recalcitrant organizational policies and cultural practices, such as a "diagnose and treat" approach, staff disbelief in clients' self-reported abuse, a societal inclination toward victim blaming, and the use of coercive, paternalistic interventions, impeded organizational change (Bateman et al. 2013).

A single training session on TIC is insufficient. Broader infrastructure changes are necessary to support cultural transformation. Capacity building to create a trauma-informed workforce is crucial, and not doing so can contribute to burnout and an ineffective use of human services expenditures (Guarino et al. 2014). Moreover, failing to consider the unique cultural needs of some client populations can limit a successful implementation of TIC in settings serving people experiencing homelessness. Not enough social science research from the past century has been conducted with diverse populations, and trauma theory is no exception. Limited dialogue between evidence-based practitioners and proponents of culturally competent practice in the field of trauma-informed services can impede the development of a more inclusive trauma-informed culture that meets the needs of those disproportionately impacted by trauma (SAMSHA 2014a; Ardino 2014). Also, the fact that many training models are based on worker objectivity is also a barrier, as such theoretical approaches clash deeply with some cultural groups. Also of concern are narrow notions of what constitutes culture or the definition of "other" within US research and the hegemony, or continuing dominance, of Western expertise (Mattar 2010).

Cultural competency can also include awareness of cultures specific to certain subgroups of homeless populations, such as street youth. Recent work incorporating the unique perspectives of homeless youth with complex trauma histories has proved hopeful (Bender et al. 2015; McManus and Thompson 2008; Narendorf et al. 2016). Homeless youth have also shared that unsafe or disruptive settings, rigid rules, disrespectful staff, and a lack of targeted programming hinder services designed with them in mind (Heinze et al. 2010). Developing more effective trauma-based interventions will require further research about how trauma is experienced across different groups and careful tweaking to address those differences in a culturally competent manner.

Logistical Issues

Multiple issues impede successful implementation of TIC in organizations, including the absence of clear guidelines. This can contribute to haphazard implementation of the principles of TIC, including a failure to include the whole staff (Wolf et al. 2014). The success of a TIC program depends ultimately on strong administrators who uphold and model the principles of TIC. Thus, a strong agency administration is key to organizational transformation.

Access to TIC also poses a challenge, particularly in rural regions, where efforts to implement online trainings are tested by problematic clinician attitudes, high costs, and lack of ongoing support (Fritz et al. 2013). Moreover, at the present time, SAMHSA's (2014b) "Trauma-Informed Care in Behavioral Health Services" is perhaps the only freely available guidebook describing how to apply TIC.

Issues have also been reported in efforts to train frontline workers to incorporate trauma- informed principles into their practice. These issues include resistance to new modalities, excessive caseloads, personal stress, hostile or toxic work environments, physical fatigue, stress about policy requirements, and low prioritization of completing trainings due to ongoing crisis management (Kramer et al. 2015). Initiative fatigue is also an issue in efforts to implement change, as staffs are reluctant to add "one more thing: to the often-changing training roster (Hanson et al. 2016). Other barriers include a lack of communication, money constraints, and resistance to changes in standards within agency practice (Conners-Burrow et al. 2013). Implementing TIC with staff working directly with clients will not just require a clearer framework but also the creation of work environments that support reflection, exploration, and growth in practitioners.

Strategies and Solutions

Making TIC More Responsive to Client Needs

Policies and the ways in which care is structured for clients can improve services to homeless clients within trauma-informed frameworks. Sometimes the issue is as simple as the context within which trauma treatment is provided. One study found location to be a salient variable, with school-based treatments significantly more effective than clinic-based interventions for young children (Langley et al. 2013). Along the same lines, access can also be addressed by bringing services directly to client populations. For example, increasing access to TIC in rural communities may require establishing satellite offices in those communities. Similarly, providing targeted services within correctional facilities and working with reentry programs to provide TIC to current or formerly incarcerated trauma survivors may improve access.

Moreover, it has been suggested that shelter policies, such as zero tolerance for pets or substance use, could be reconsidered as part of implementing TIC in order to increase access to needed services, especially considering the high rates of pet ownership and substance use among people experiencing homelessness (Rhoades et al. 2015). In a sample of homeless Canadian adults, 92.8% of participants met criteria for a mental health disorder and 82.6% for substance dependence (Krausz et al. 2013). Unwillingness to challenge long-standing policies can easily undo positive interventions by excluding people from the help they need to overcome challenges and thrive.

Client-Centered Care for Specialized Populations

Structural design and service rules need to be more accommodating and better attuned to the unique qualities and needs of specific subpopulations. For example, in working with youth, institutional estrangement has been reduced through youth-centered programming that incorporates trauma-informed principles to address cultural differences. These principles include promoting a sense of belonging and efficacy through care structured around encouraging and preserving relationships (Heinze et al. 2010; Riebschleger et al. 2015) and inclusion of more age-appropriate strength-building resources (Eccles and Gootman 2002).

Youth have identified a desire for structured housing options, trauma-focused interventions, and victimization prevention training (Bender et al. 2015). Some tentative success has been found with self-guided models, particularly in areas where there are not enough staff to provide specialty services (Held and Owens 2015). Attitudes about street youth should be challenged through outreach to encourage use of existing services (Ha et al. 2015). In working with LGBTQ youth, care must be taken to incorporate inclusive, nondiscriminatory policies, for example, providing accommodations that are not based upon sex assignment at birth, avoiding unnecessarily isolating youth from other residents, and displaying supportive signs and symbols, such as pink triangles and safe zone stickers (Cochrane et al. 2002).

Community-based participatory action research (PAR) methods can provide strategies that can be used with marginalized homeless populations to both empower them in their path toward recovery and help workers ensure that homeless services are appropriate. PAR strategies privilege the perspectives of service recipients in all aspects of designing, implementing, and evaluating services. Moving toward more client-centered, long-term services holds promise. Both providers and service recipients value consistency in care without rigid adherence to policies and practices that do not work (Archard and Murphy 2015). TIC coupled with culturally competent services appears to be a promising path forward.

Trauma-Informed Education

Within the broader field, we need to begin injecting principles of trauma awareness into the curriculum of bachelor and master's programs of social work to better prepare students to bring trauma knowledge and skills into the field and to equip them to deal with secondary stress. Creating trauma-informed learning spaces for students is paramount, as is the careful selection of content, context, and teaching methods used to convey sensitive material with students who may have trauma histories themselves (Cunningham 2004). Effective self-care could be an active part of coursework, and techniques around how to manage secondary stress could be implemented throughout program content (Hernández et al. 2010; Gilin and Kauffman 2015). Students could be better screened for compassion fatigue by program faculty, and field instructors could actively engage students in developing self-care plans, perhaps even integrating stress management content into their learning contract (Harr and Moore 2011).

There is also a need to identify classroom pedagogies that better assist students to recognize and address trauma symptoms in their clients (Fritz et al. 2013) and to develop advocacy skills for system change within homelessness services, including the institution of TIC principles (Conner-Burrow et al. 2013). The cultural change needed in our organizations and community will require multiple linked efforts that support both the theoretical tenets of TIC and the staff working at all organizational levels to implement it.

Communities of Care

In addition to creating new services, we can choose to set an example by weaving finer mesh in our social safety net, linking existing services together, and ensuring that even non-TIC agency personnel are trained to direct homeless clients toward environments where they can get needed support. Some have described this as the "no wrong door approach" to care, and this is accomplished through coordination across multiple care systems (Bateman et al. 2013). This work includes developing buy-in from staff within organizations and in the community itself around the value of utilizing a trauma-informed approach with homeless individuals in our communities (Langley et al. 2013). One model showing promise in reducing provider strain and leading to better outcomes in implementing TIC in homelessness programs has been the use of communities of practice. This model involves building a network of different professionals to share knowledge and experience, leading to opportunities for interprofessional collaboration (Cornes et al. 2014). Ongoing engagement and follow-up with constituents are important, as is follow-up with clients during and after their contact with services. As providers, it is important to stay aware of trends in trauma recovery and relapse and to develop contingency plans when appropriate (Helfrich et al. 2011).

Politically oriented frameworks like the Strengths, Prevention, Empowerment, and Community (SPEC) model have also been useful in extending the TIC model further and tackling societal and structural limitations, such as lack of income supports (Mckenzie-Mohr et al. 2012). Some suggest that truly implementing a trauma-informed framework will mean transforming not only our social agencies but also the political fabric of our society.

Concluding Thoughts

Bolder Science

There is a need for bolder research within agencies advancing innovation to better understand how organizations can support staff and clients through a trauma-informed lens. Among homeless veterans, for example, there is a serious deficit in trauma-informed case management services, despite high levels of PTSD and related trauma symptoms among this population (Dinnen et al. 2014). Even in subpopulations, such as children, where some interventions have shown promise, we still need to develop a better understanding of shortcomings in the current models (Bassuk et al. 2014).

New barriers are emerging within care systems as the political contexts within which services are provided are changing (Deck and Platt 2015). Future research may benefit from including more perspectives from frontline staff working to implement TIC and seeking to transform organizational culture and leadership (Middleton et al. 2015). Developing a more extensive literature around applying TIC within homelessness programs will ultimately strengthen efforts to advocate for this framework, both with long-standing health service professionals and with the broader communities they serve.

Hopeful Paths Forward

While the challenges of implementing TIC in the homelessness sector are significant, the struggles of both researchers and social workers have provided a wealth of literature to guide future efforts. Much of this research carries with it a common message. There is a desire across multiple subpopulations of people experiencing homelessness for interventions that provide a sense of control, that empower clients to reclaim their lives, and that truly honor their experiences (Lewinson et al. 2014; Schmidt et al. 2015). Beyond changing policies and implementation guidelines, there is an urgent institutional need in the field of homelessness services to challenge trends within Western culture that pathologize people who are impoverished, victimized, and homeless. Truly bringing TIC into homelessness service agencies will mean also addressing long-standing organizational issues, like high turnover and the chronic overworking of staff. Telling current and future social workers to simply take care of themselves is not a sufficient way to address toxic work environments. In fact, TIC recognizes that the intentional development of a restorative organizational context, one that is characterized by mutual respect, empathy, encouragement, and caring for all staff and clients, is a fundamental imperative for healing and recovery from trauma. We cannot expect homeless service agencies to ever be truly trauma informed if they are not continuously striving to achieve these goals. Similarly, trauma-informed schools of social work can work toward providing restorative experiences that support the students in the classroom and also set an example for the agencies within which students are placed.

References

Adams, S. A., & Riggs, S. A. (2008). An exploratory study of vicarious trauma among therapist trainees. *Training and Education in Professional Psychology, 2*(1), 26.

Agllias, K. (2012). Keeping safe: Teaching undergraduate social work students about interpersonal violence. *Journal of Social Work Practice, 26*(2), 259–274.

Alexander, P. P. (2011). Childhood maltreatment, intimate partner violence, work interference, and women's employment. *Journal of Family Violence, 26*(4), 255–261.

Al-Krenawi, A., & Kimberley, D. (2014). Palestinian youth and their families: Paradoxes of resilience in the cultural and sociopolitical context of conflict, stress, and trauma in the Middle East. *International Journal of Child Health and Human Development, 7*(2), 101.

American Psychiatric Association. (1980). *Diagnostic and statistical manual of mental disorders* (3rd ed.). Washington, DC: American Psychiatric Association.

Angelou, M. (1991). *All God's children need traveling shoes*. New York: Vintage.

Archard, P. J., & Murphy, D. (2015). A practice research study concerning homeless service user involvement with a programme of social support work delivered in a specialized psychological trauma service. *Journal of Psychiatric and Mental Health Nursing, 22*(6), 360–370.

Ardino, V. (2014). Trauma-informed care: Is cultural competence a viable solution for efficient policy strategies? *Clinical Neuropsychiatry, 11*(1), 45–51.

Bassuk, E. L., & Beardslee, W. R. (2014). Depression in homeless mothers: Addressing an unrecognized public health issue. *American Journal of Orthopsychiatry, 84*(1), 73–81.

Bassuk, E. L., DeCandia, C. J., Beach, C. A., & Berman, F. (2014). America's youngest outcasts: A report card on child homelessness. The American Institutes for Research. http://www.air.org/sites/default/files/downloads/report/Americas-Youngest-Outcasts-Child-Homelessness-Nov2014.pdf. Accessed 22 June 2018.

Bateman, J., Henderson, C., & Kezelman, C. (2013). Trauma-informed care and practice: Towards a cultural shift in policy reform across mental health and human services in Australia, a national strategic direction. Mental Health Coordinating Council. http://www.mhcc.org.au/media/44467/nticp_strategic_direction_journal_article__vf4_-_jan_2014_.pdf. Accessed 22 June 2018.

Bender, K., Thompson, S., Ferguson, K., Yoder, J., & DePrince, A. (2015). Risk detection and self-protection among homeless youth. *Journal of Research on Adolescence, 25*, 352–365.

Bermingham, A. (2014). Youth homelessness: An investigation into the emotional effects on social care workers. Dublin Business School. http://esource.dbs.ie/bitstream/handle/10788/2287/ba_bermingham_a_2014.pdf?sequence=1. Accessed 22 June 2018.

Beyer, L., Murphy, H., & McWilliam, S. (2010). An introduction to trauma informed care: Creating physically and emotionally safe environments for client, families and staff. IWK Health Center. http://yourexperiencesmatter.com/wp-content/uploads/2016/02/An_Introduction_to_Trauma_Informed_Care3.pdf. Accessed 22 June 2018.

Bloom, S. L. (2005). The Sanctuary Model of organizational change for children's residential treatment. therapeutic community. *The International Journal for Therapeutic and Supportive Organizations, 26*(1), 65–81.

Bloom, S. L. (2013). *Creating sanctuary: Toward the evolution of sane societies* (2nd ed.). New York: Routledge.

Bloom, S. L., & Farragher, B. (2013). *Restoring sanctuary: A new operating system for trauma-informed organizations*. New York: Oxford University Press.

Bride, B. E., Hatcher, S. S., & Humble, M. N. (2009). Trauma training, trauma practices, and secondary traumatic stress among substance abuse counselors. *Traumatology, 15*(2), 96.

Brignone, E., Gundlapalli, A. V., Blais, R. K., Carter, M. E., Suo, Y., Samore, M. H., et al. (2016). Differential risk for homelessness among US male and female veterans with a positive screen for military sexual trauma. *JAMA Psychiatry, 73*(6), 582–589.

Brown, R. T., Goodman, L., Guzman, D., Tieu, L., Ponath, C., & Kushel, M. B. (2016). Pathways to homelessness among older homeless adults: Results from the HOPE HOME study. *PLoS One, 11*(5), e0155065.

Chrystal, J. G., Glover, D. L., Young, A. S., Whelan, F., Austin, E. L., Johnson, N. K., et al. (2015). Experience of primary care among homeless individuals with mental health conditions. *PLoS One, 10*(2), e0117395.

Cochrane, B. N., Stewart, A. J., Ginzler, J. A., & Cauce, A. M. (2002). Challenges faced by homeless sexual minorities: Comparison of gay, lesbian, bisexual, and transgender homeless adolescents with their heterosexual counterparts. *American Journal of Public Health, 92*(5), 773–777.

Conners-Burrow, N. A., Kramer, T. L., Sigel, B. A., Helpenstill, K., Sievers, C., & McKelvey, L. (2013). Trauma-informed care training in a child welfare system: Moving it to the front line. *Children and Youth Services Review, 35*(11), 1830–1835.

Cook, A., Spinazzola, J., Ford, J., Lanktree, C., Blaustein, M., Cloitre, M., et al. (2017). Complex trauma in children and adolescents. *Psychiatric Annals, 35*(5), 390–398.

Cornes, M., Manthorpe, J., Hennessy, C., Anderson, S., Clark, M., & Scanlon, C. (2014). Not just a talking shop: Practitioner perspectives on how communities of practice work to improve outcomes for people experiencing multiple exclusion homelessness. *Journal of Interprofessional Care, 28*(6), 541–546.

Cunningham, M. (2004). Teaching social workers about trauma: Reducing the risks of vicarious traumatization in the classroom. *Journal of Social Work Education, 40*(2), 305–317.

Davies, B. R., & Allen, N. B. (2017). Trauma and homelessness in youth: Psychopathology and intervention. *Clinical Psychology Review, 54*, 17–28.

Deck, S. M., & Platt, P. A. (2015). Homelessness is traumatic: Abuse, victimization, and trauma histories of homeless men. *Journal of Aggression, Maltreatment & Trauma, 24*, 1022–1043.

Dinnen, S., Kane, V., & Cook, J. M. (2014). Trauma-informed care: A paradigm shift needed for services with homeless veterans. *Professional Case Management, 19*(4), 161–170.

dos Santos, T. M., Kozasa, E. H., Carmagnani, I. S., Tanaka, L. H., Lacerda, S. S., Nogueira-Martin, L. A., East, J. F., & Roll, S. J. (2016). Positive effects of a stress reduction program based on mindfulness meditation in Brazilian nursing professionals: Qualitative and quantitative evaluation. *Explore, 12*(2), 90–99.

Duarte, J., & Pinto-Gouveia, J. (2016). Effectiveness of a mindfulness-based intervention on oncology nurses' burnout and compassion fatigue symptoms: A non-randomized study. *International Journal of Nursing Studies, 64*, 98–107.

East, J. F., & Roll, S. J. (2015). Women, poverty, and trauma: An empowerment practice approach. *Social Work, 60*(4), 279–286.

Eccles, J., & Gootman, J. A. (Eds.). (2002). *Community programs to promote youth development*. Washington, DC: National Academy Press.

Fallot, R. D., & Harris, M. (2002). The trauma recovery and empowerment model (TREM): Conceptual and practical issues in a group intervention for women. *Community Mental Health Journal, 38*(6), 475–485.

Fallot, R. D., & Harris, M. (2009). Community connections. Creating cultures of trauma-informed care: A self assessment with planning protocol. Community Connections. https://www.healthcare.uiowa.edu/icmh/documents/CCTICSelf-AssessmentandPlanningProtocol0709.pdf. Accessed 22 June 2018.

Federal Register. (2011). Rules and regulations. https://www.hudexchange.info/resources/documents/HEARTH_HomelessDefinition_FinalRule.pdf. Accessed 22 June 2018.

Felitti, V. J., Anda, R. F., Nordenberg, D., Williamson, D. F., Spitz, A. M., Edwards, V., Koss, M. P., & Marks, J. (1998). Relationship of childhood abuse and household dysfunction to many of the leading causes of death in adults: The adverse childhood experiences (ACE) study. *American Journal of Preventive Medicine, 14*(4), 245–258.

Ferris, L. J. (2016). The Florence Nightingale effect: Organizational identification explains the peculiar link between others' suffering and workplace functioning in the homelessness sector. *Frontiers in Psychology, 28*, 7–16.

Figley, C. R. (1995). *Compassion fatigue: Coping with secondary traumatic stress disorder in those who treat the traumatized*. New York: Hrunner/Mazel.

Flanagan, J., Sullivan, T., & Connell, C. (2015). Profiles of intimate partner violence victimization, substance misuse, and depression among female caregivers involved with child protective services. *Journal of Family Violence, 30*(8), 999–1005.

Fritz, R. M., Tempel, A. B., Sigel, B. A., Conners-Burrow, N. A., Worley, K. B., & Kramer, T. L. (2013). Improving the dissemination of evidence-based treatments: Facilitators and barriers to participating in case consultation. *Professional Psychology: Research and Practice, 44*(4), 225–230.

Gilin, B., & Kauffman, S. (2015). Strategies for teaching about trauma to graduate social work students. *Journal of Teaching in Social Work, 35*(4), 378–396.

Goodman, L. A., Saxe, L., & Harvey, M. (1991). Homelessness as psychological trauma: Broadening perspectives. *American Psychologist, 46*(11), 1219.

Gowan, T. (2002). The nexus: Homelessness and incarceration in two American cities. *Ethnography, 3*(4), 500–534.

Grant, D., Keeney, T., & Oswick, C. (1998). Defining organizational discourse: Of diversity, dichotomy and multidisciplinarity. In D. Grant, T. Keeney, & Oswick (Eds.), *Discourse and organization* (pp. 1–13). London: Sage.

Guarino, K., & Bassuk, E. (2010). Working with families experiencing homelessness: Understanding trauma and its impact. *Zero to Three (J), 30*(3), 11–20.

Guarino, K. M., Clervil, R., & Beach, C. A. (2014). Trauma-informed care for veterans experiencing homelessness: Building workforce capacity. The American Institute of Research. http://www.air.org/sites/default/files/Trauma-informed%20care%20for%20homeless%20veterans%20Building%20Workforce%20Capacity%20Nov%202014.pdf. Accessed 22 June 2018.

Ha, Y., Narendorf, S. C., Santa Maria, D., & Bezette-Flores, N. (2015). Barriers and facilitators to shelter utilization among homeless young adults. *Evaluation and Program Planning, 53*, 25–33.

Hamilton, A. B., Washington, D. L., & Zuchowski, J. L. (2013). Gendered social roots of homelessness among women veterans. *Annals of Anthropological Practice, 37*, 92–107.

Hanson, R. F., Lang, J. M., Campbell, K., Shanley, P., Crusto, C. A., & Connell, C. M. (2016). Building capacity for trauma-informed care in the child welfare system. *Child Maltreatment, 21*(2), 113–124.

Harr, C., & Moore, B. (2011). Compassion fatigue among social work students in field placements. *Journal of Teaching Social Work, 31*, 350–363.

Heinze, H. J., Jozefowicz, D. M. H., & Toro, P. A. (2010). Taking the youth perspective: Assessment of program characteristics that promote positive development in homeless and at-risk youth. *Children and Youth Services Review, 32*(10), 1365–1372.

Held, P., & Owens, G. P. (2015). Effects of self-compassion workbook training on trauma-related guilt in a sample of homeless veterans: A pilot study. *Journal of Clinical Psychology, 71*(6), 513–526.

Helfrich, C. A., Peters, C. Y., & Chan, D. V. (2011). Trauma symptoms of individuals with mental illness at risk for homelessness: Participating in a life skills intervention. *Occupational Therapy International, 18*(3), 115–123.

Herbers, J. E., Cutuli, J. J., Monn, A. R., Narayan, A. J., & Masten, A. S. (2014). Trauma, adversity, and parent-child relationships among young children experiencing homelessness. *Journal of Abnormal Child Psychology, 42*(7), 1167.

Herman, J. (1992). *Trauma and recovery: The aftermath of violence—from domestic abuse to political terror*. New York: Basic Books.

Hernández, P., Engstrom, D., & Gangsei, D. (2010). Exploring the impact of trauma on therapists: Vicarious resilience and related concepts in training. *Journal of Systemic Therapies, 29*(1), 67.

Hetzel-Riggin, M. D., & Roby, R. P. (2013). Trauma type and gender effects on PTSD, general distress, and peritraumatic dissociation. *Journal of Loss and Trauma, 18*(1), 41–53.

Hodgdon, H., Kinniburgh, K., Gabowitz, D., Blaustein, M., & Spinazzola, J. (2013). Development and implementation of trauma-informed programming in youth residential treatment centers using the ARC framework. *Journal of Family Violence, 28*, 679–692.

Hopper, E. K., Bassuk, E. L., & Olivet, J. (2010). Shelter from the storm: Trauma-informed care in homeless service settings. *The Open Health Services and Policy Journal, 3*, 80–100.

Huggard, P. (2003). Secondary traumatic stress; Doctors at risk. *New Ethicals Journal, 6*, 9–14.

Jennings, A. (2008). Models for developing trauma-informed behavioral health systems and trauma-specific services. NTAC and NASMHPD. http://www.annafoundation.org/MDT.pdf. Accessed 22 June 2018.

Jetelina, K. K., Gonzalez, J. R., Brown, C. R., Foreman, M. L., & Field, C. (2017). Acute alcohol use, history of homelessness, and intent of injury among a sample of adult emergency department patients. *Violence and Victims, 32*(4), 658–670.

Johnson, G., & Chamberlain, C. (2008). Homelessness and substance abuse: Which comes first? *Australian Social Work, 61*(4), 342–356.

Jordan, L. (2012). Spaces of trauma: Young people, homelessness and trauma. *Youth Studies Australia, 2*(4), 1–17.

Kabat-Zinn, J. (2003). Mindfulness-Based interventions in context: Past, present, and future. *Clinical Psychology Science and Practice, 10*(2), 144–156.

Kardiner, A. (1941). *The traumatic neuroses of war*. New York: Hoeber.

Kardiner, A., & Spiegel, H. (1947). *War, stress, and neurotic illness*. New York: Hoeber.

Knight, C. (2010). Indirect trauma in the field practicum: Secondary traumatic stress, vicarious trauma, and compassion fatigue among social work students and their field instructors. *Journal of Baccalaureate Social Work, 15*(1), 31–52.

Kramer, T. L., Sigel, B. A., Conners-Burrow, N., Worley, K. B., Church, J. K., & Helpenstill, K. (2015). It takes a state: Best practices for children exposed to trauma. *Best Practices in Mental Health: An International Journal, 11*(1), 14–24.

Krausz, R. M., Clarkson, A. F., Strehlau, V., Torchalla, I., Li, K., & Schuetz, C. G. (2013). Mental disorder, service use, and barriers to care among 500 homeless people in 3 different urban settings. *Social Psychiatry and Psychiatric Epidemiology, 48*(8), 1235–1243.

Lakeman, R. (2011). How homeless sector workers deal with the death of service users: A grounded theory study. *Death Studies, 35*(10), 925–948.

Langley, A., Santiago, C., Rodríguez, A., & Zelaya, J. (2013). Improving implementation of mental health services for trauma in multicultural elementary schools: Stakeholder perspectives on parent and educator engagement. *Journal of Behavioral Health Services & Research, 40*(3), 247–262.

Larkin, H., & Park, J. (2012). Adverse childhood experiences (ACEs), service use, and service helpfulness among people experiencing homelessness. *Families in Society: The Journal of Contemporary Social Services, 93*(2), 85–93.

Laufer, R. S., Gallops, M. S., & Frey-Wouters, E. (1984). War stress and trauma: The Vietnam veteran experience. *Journal of Health and Social Behavior, 25*(1), 65–85.

Lewinson, T., Thomas, M. L., & White, S. (2014). Traumatic transitions: Homeless women's narratives of abuse, loss, and fear. *Affilia, 29*(2), 192–205.

Mar, M. Y., Linden, I. A., Torchalla, I., Li, K., & Krausz, M. (2014). Are childhood abuse and neglect related to age of first homelessness episode among currently homeless adults? *Violence and Victims, 29*(6), 999–1013.

Masson, J. M. (1984). *The assault on truth, Freud's suppression of the seduction theory*. New York: Farrar, Straus, and Giroux.

Mattar, S. (2010). Cultural considerations in trauma psychology education, research, and training. *Traumatology, 16*(4), 48–52.

McHugo, G. J., Caspi, Y., Kammerer, N., & Mazelis, R. (2005). The assessment of trauma history in women with co-occurring substance abuse and mental disorders and a history of interpersonal violence. *The Journal of Behavioral Health Services & Research, 32*(2), 113–127.

McKenzie-Mohr, S. S., Coates, J., & McLeod, H. (2012). Responding to the needs of youth who are homeless: Calling for politicized trauma-informed intervention. *Children & Youth Services Review, 34*(1), 136–143.

McManus, H. H., & Thompson, S. J. (2008). Trauma Among unaccompanied homeless youth: The integration of street culture into a model of intervention. *Journal of Aggression, Maltreatment & Trauma, 16*(1), 92–109.

Middleton, J. S., & Potter, C. C. (2015). Relationship between vicarious traumatization and turnover among child welfare professionals. *Journal of Public Child Welfare, 9*(2), 195–216.

Middleton, J. S., Harvey, S., & Esaki, N. (2015). Transformational leadership and organizational change: How do leaders approach trauma-informed organizational change…twice? *Families in Society: The Journal of Contemporary Social Services, 96*(2), 155–163.

Morrison, D. S. (2009). Homelessness as an independent risk factor for mortality: results from a retrospective cohort study. *International Journal of Epidemiology, 38*(3), 877–883.

Murphy, L. T. (2017). Modern slavery research project, labor and sex trafficking among homeless youth.: A ten city study full report. Loyola University, New Orleans. https://oag.ca.gov/sites/all/files/agweb/pdfs/ht/murphy-labor-sex-trafficking-homeless-youth.pdf. Accessed 22 June 2018.

Narayan, A. J., Kalstabakken, A. W., Labella, M. H., Nerenberg, L. S., Monn, A. R., & Masten, A. S. (2017). Intergenerational continuity of adverse childhood experiences in homeless families: Unpacking exposure to maltreatment versus family dysfunction. *American Journal of Orthopsychiatry, 87*(1), 3–14.

Narendorf, S. C., Santa Maria, D., Ha, Y., Cooper, J., & Schieszler, C. (2016). Counting and surveying homeless youth: Recommendations from YouthCount 2.0! A community-academic partnership. *Journal of Community Health, 41*(6), 1234–1241.

National Child Traumatic Stress Network. (n.d.). Complex trauma. http://www.nctsn.org/trauma-types/complex-trauma. Accessed 22 June 2018.

National Law Center on Homelessness and Poverty (2015). Overview of homelessness: Data and causes. https://www.nlchp.org/documents/Homeless_Stats_Fact_Sheet. Accessed 22 June 2018.

Newell, J. M., & MacNeil, G. A. (2010). Professional burnout, vicarious trauma, secondary traumatic stress, and compassion fatigue. *Best Practices in Mental Health, 6*(2), 57–68.

Nimmo, A., & Huggard, H. (2013). A systematic review of the measurement of compassion fatigue, vicarious trauma, and secondary traumatic stress in physicians. *Australasian Journal of Disaster and Trauma Studies, 17*(1), 37–44.

Olivet, J., McGraw, S., Grandin, M., & Bassuk, E. (2010). Staffing challenges and strategies for organizations serving individuals who have experienced chronic homelessness. *The Journal of Behavioral Health Services & Research, 37*(2), 226–238.

Oppenheimer, S. C., Nurius, P. S., & Green, S. (2016). Homelessness history impacts on health outcomes and economic and risk behavior intermediaries: New insights from population data. *Families in Society, 97*(3), 230–242.

Pearlman, L. A., & Caringi, J. (2009). Living and working self-reflectively to address vicarious trauma). In C. A. Courtois & J. D. Ford (Eds.), *Treating complex traumatic stress disorders: An evidence-based guide* (pp. 202–224). New York: Guilford Press.

Perry, B. (2006). Applying principles of neurodevelopment to clinical work with maltreated and traumatized children: The neurosequential model of therapeutics. In N. B. Webb (Ed.), *Working with traumatized youth in child welfare* (pp. 27–52). New York: Guilford Press.

Ray, S. L., Wong, C., White, D., & Heaslip, K. (2013). Compassion satisfaction, compassion fatigue, work life conditions, and burnout among frontline mental health care professionals. *Traumatology, 19*(4), 255–267.

Rhoades, H., Winetrobe, H., & Rice, E. (2015). Pet ownership among homeless youth: Associations with mental health, service utilization and housing status. *Child Psychiatry & Human Development, 46*(2), 237–244.

Riebschleger, J., Day, A., & Damashek, A. (2015). Foster care youth share stories of trauma before, during, and after placement: Youth voices for building trauma-informed systems of care. *Journal of Aggression, Maltreatment & Trauma, 24*, 339–360.

Rimawi, B. H., Mirdamadi, M., & John, J. F. (2014). Infections and homelessness: Risks of increased infectious diseases in displaced women. *World Medical & Health Policy, 6*(2), 118–132.

Roos, L. E., Mota, N., Afifi, T. O., Katz, L. Y., Distasio, J., & Sareen, J. (2013). Relationship between adverse childhood experiences and homelessness and the impact of axis I and II disorders. *American Journal of Public Health, 103*(Suppl 2), S275–S281.

SAMHSA. (2007). Lessons learned from the women, co-occurring disorders, and violence study: Exploring how to best serve women survivors of violence and trauma. https://www.ncjrs.gov/App/publications/abstract.aspx?ID=241360.

SAMHSA. (2014a). SAMHSA's concept of trauma and guidance for a trauma informed approach. https://store.samhsa.gov/shin/content/SMA14-4884/SMA14-4884.pdf. Accessed 22 June 2018.

SAMHSA. (2014b). A treatment improvement protocol: Trauma-informed care in behavioral health services. https://store.samhsa.gov/shin/content/SMA14-4816/SMA14-4816.pdf. Accessed 22 June 2018.

SAMSHA (2016). SHIFT study highlights trauma's impact on homelessness. Retrieved from: https://www.samhsa.gov/homelessness-programs-resources/hpr-resources/traumas-impact-homelessness

SAMSHA. (2017). Trauma and violence. https://www.samhsa.gov/trauma-violence. Accessed 22 June 2018.

Schmidt, R., Hrenchuk, C., Bopp, J., & Poole, N. (2015). Trajectories of women's homelessness in Canada's 3 northern territories. *International Journal of Circumpolar Health, 74*, 1–9.

Siegel, D. (2001). Toward an interpersonal neurobiology of the developing mind: Attachment relationships, 'mindsight' and neural integration. *Infant Mental Health Journal, 22*(1–2), 67–94.

Signorelli, R. G., Gluckman, N. S., Hassan, N., Coello, M., & Momartin, S. (2017). Relationship building, collaboration and flexible service delivery: The path to engagement of refugee families and communities in early childhood trauma recovery services. *Children Australia, 42*(3), 142–158.

Snyder, S. M., Hartinger-Saunders, R., Brezina, T., Beck, E., Wright, E. R., Forge, N., & Bride, B. E. (2016). Homeless youth, strain, and justice system involvement: An application of general strain theory. *Children and Youth Services Review, 62*, 90–96.

Stamm, B. H. (2005). *The ProQOL manual*. Pocatello: Idaho State University.

Stamm, B. H. (2009). *The concise ProQOL manual*. Pocatello: ProQOL.org.

Sundin, E. C., & Baguley, T. (2015). Prevalence of childhood abuse among people who are homeless in Western countries: A systematic review and meta-analysis. *Social Psychiatry and Psychiatric Epidemiology, 50*(2), 183–194.

Terr, L. C. (1991). Childhood traumas: An outline and overview. *American Journal of Psychiatry, 148*(1), 10–20.

Tsai, J., Rosenheck, R., Decker, S., Desai, R., & Harpaz-Rotem, I. (2012). Trauma experience among homeless female veterans: correlates and impact on housing, clinical, and psychosocial outcomes. *Journal of Traumatic Stress, 25*(6), 624–632.

Tummala-Narra, P., Li, Z., Liu, T., & Wang, Y. (2014). Violence exposure and mental health among adolescents: The role of ethnic identity and help seeking. *Psychological Trauma: Theory, Research, Practice, and Policy, 6*(1), 8.

Turgoose, D., & Maddox, L. (2017). Predictors of compassion fatigue in mental health professionals: A narrative review. *Traumatology, 23*(2), 172–185.

van der Kolk, B. A. (1994). The body keeps the score: Memory and the evolving psychobiology of posttraumatic stress. *Harvard Review of Psychiatry, 1*(5), 253–265.

van der Kolk, B. A., McFarlane, A. C., & Weisaeth, L. (Eds.). (1996). *Traumatic stress: The effects of overwhelming stress on the mind, body, and society*. New York: Guilford Press.

van der Kolk, B. A., Roth, S., Pelcovitz, D., Sunday, S., & Spinazzola, J. (2005). Disorders of extreme stress: The empirical foundation of a complex adaptation to trauma. *Journal of Traumatic Stress, 18*(5), 389–399.

Walker, L. (1979). *The battered women*. New York: Harper & Row.

Webster, D. C., & Dunn, E. C. (2005). Feminist perspectives on trauma. *Women & Therapy, 28*(3–4), 111–142.

Wilson, C., Pence, D. M., & Conradi, L. (2013). Trauma-informed care. *Encyclopedia of Social Work*. http://socialwork.oxfordre.com/view/10.1093/acrefore/9780199975839.001.0001/acrefore-9780199975839-e-1063. Accessed 22 June 2018.

Wolf, M. R., Green, S. A., Nochajski, T. H., Mendel, W. E., & Kusmaul, N. S. (2014). 'We're civil servants': The status of trauma-informed care in the community. *Journal of Social Service Research, 40*(1), 111–120.

Woolrych, R., Gibson, N., Sixsmith, J., & Sixsmith, A. (2015). "No home, no place": Addressing the complexity of homelessness in old age through community dialogue. *Journal of Housing for the Elderly, 29*(3), 233–258.

Yu, H., Jiang, A., & Shen, J. (2016). Prevalence and predictors of compassion fatigue, burnout and compassion satisfaction among oncology nurses: A cross-sectional survey. *International Journal of Nursing Studies, 57*, 28–38.

Chapter 14
Homeless Street Outreach: Spark for the Journey to a Dignified Life

Linda Plitt Donaldson and Wonhyung Lee

Introduction

Street outreach is a critical component in the constellation of services provided to people who are homeless. Researchers have found street outreach to be an effective strategy for connecting people who are homeless to housing and health care (Lettner et al. 2016; O'Toole et al. 2015; Slesnick et al. 2016). Street outreach is an important component in the implementation of Housing First (Padgett et al. 2016), a best practice for ending chronic homelessness that is promoted by the US Department of Housing and Urban Development and one that is central to strategies to chronic homelessness. Sixty communities across the United States have ended veteran homelessness by applying the Housing First strategy (US Interagency Council on Homelessness 2017). In President Obama's 2016 budget, street outreach was specifically identified as a core service in programs to help people who are homeless access health care, secure stable living conditions, and identify and support youth who are living on the streets (US Interagency Council for the Homeless 2016). As Housing First and Rapid Rehousing models continue to proliferate in various communities across the nation, the importance of street outreach in linking people to housing and other supportive services will continue to grow.

Although outreach involves the use of skills and behaviors that have been core to human functioning since the dawn of time (e.g., interacting with people, talking

---

Electronic supplementary material: The online version of this chapter (https://doi.org/10.1007/978-3-030-03727-7_14) contains supplementary material, which is available to authorized users.

L. P. Donaldson (✉)
Catholic University of America, Washington, DC, USA
e-mail: donaldson@cua.edu

W. Lee
University at Albany, Albany, NY, USA
e-mail: whlee@albany.edu

H. Larkin et al. (eds.), *Homelessness Prevention and Intervention in Social Work*, https://doi.org/10.1007/978-3-030-03727-7_14

with them, supporting them), street outreach has evolved into a practice that also draws on core social work values, practice methods, and evidence-based approaches to support people in their journeys out of homelessness. To introduce prospective social workers to street outreach practice in the field of homeless services, this chapter begins by defining street outreach and outlining its component parts and underlying values. Next, it describes various skills, methods, and approaches used in street outreach. It also describes evidence-based practices used in homeless services, such as Critical Time Intervention and the SSI/SSDI Outreach, Access, and Recovery (SOAR) program, which could be incorporated with outreach practice to improve outcomes for people who are homeless. The chapter concludes with a discussion of the future of street outreach as we enter into the third decade of the twenty-first century.

Street Outreach

Street outreach is a relational process between a street outreach worker and a person who is experiencing homelessness. It includes three core elements: (1) meeting people where they are, (2) building a trusting relationship overtime, and (3) connecting people to services (Connolly and Joly 2012; Lee and Donaldson 2018; Olivet et al. 2010). *Meeting people where they are* has two connotations. First, it means physically going into the community to places where the outreach worker might find people who are homeless (e.g., under bridges, alleyways, abandoned buildings, encampments, public parks, transit stations). Going out to meet people who are homeless in the community is in direct contrast to traditional social services where people who are homeless might seek services, such as drop-in centers, health clinics, and soup kitchens. The purpose of street outreach is to connect with people who are homeless and who may not avail themselves of existing social services provided in the community.

Meeting people where they are also means accepting people, without judgment, where they are in their journey out of homeless, whether they are struggling with addiction, active in their mental illness, or resistant to moving into housing, receiving services, or engaging in a conversation. Street outreach involves going out into the community, finding people who are homeless, and letting them know that you see them and care about them. Street outreach involves making people who are homeless aware that services are available to make life a little better, or at least more secure than living on the streets, when they are ready for such services. Street outreach also involves exercising qualities of patience and persistence, which are important components of the second element of outreach.

Olivet et al. (2010) describe the second element of outreach, *building a caring and trusting relationship between the outreach worker and the person who is homeless*, as the "linchpin" (p. 67) in the process of helping people recognize their dignity, live in hope, and reconnect to housing, health care, and other types of services that could make a meaningful difference in their lives. Bassuk et al. (1994) describe street outreach as a process that "seeks to establish a personal connection that provides the spark for the journey back to a vital and dignified life" (p. 10). Rowe et al. (2016) note the wariness that many people who are homeless feel regarding professional providers due to "their past negative experiences, difficulty balancing the exigencies of homeless life with the requirements of public service bureaucracies, or other reasons" (p. 56). Consequently, outreach workers must have an approach to their practice that includes patience, compassion, flexibility, creativity, nonjudgment, truthfulness, persistence, and unconditional regard for the person who is experiencing homelessness. Street outreach workers who are able to cultivate and embody these characteristics may establish the trust necessary to help someone living on the streets envision living successfully in stable housing.

Linking people to services is the third element of street outreach. People who are homeless have varying degrees of connection to services in their community. However, most people with whom outreach workers engage are disconnected from traditional social services, either due to their mental illness, addiction, lack of awareness about the service context, or previous negative experiences with traditional systems (Olivet et al. 2010). Research looking at the effectiveness of outreach on service connection has found outreach to be successful in helping people access drop-in centers (Slesnick et al. 2016), primary health care (O'Toole et al. 2015), and housing (Lettner et al. 2016). In their study of street outreach workers, Lee and Donaldson (2018) found that outreach teams also helped people who were homeless meet basic needs (e.g., food, shelter), access vital records (e.g., birth certificates, photo ID), apply for benefits (e.g., SSI, SSDI, and SNAP), and seek employment.

It may seem obvious, but success in connecting people with services is entirely dependent on the availability of such services in local jurisdictions. Street outreach trainer Ken Kraybill (2002) notes, "One of the biggest obstacles to effective outreach work is the scarcity of resources to which people who are homeless can be referred once they are willing and ready to accept services" (p. 134). For example, the lack of affordable housing across the United States is a barrier to moving people off the streets. Even people with government-subsidized housing vouchers (i.e., Housing Choice Vouchers) often express difficulty in finding landlords willing to accept a housing voucher. In his review of studies examining the impact of housing vouchers on families and communities, Varaday (2010) found that, in tight housing markets, housing vouchers need to be coupled with the expansion of affordable rental housing, housing search assistance, and laws that prevent discrimination based on source of income. In addition, access to health care, addiction and mental health treatment, income supports, and other social services is largely defined by federal and state policy that establish eligibility criteria and funding levels for such programs; such policies vary and are subject to change based on the current political administration and its ideological views toward the role of government in providing social welfare.

The political context of 2017 provides a stark example of how changes in political administration can cause dramatic shifts in the breadth and depth of safety net programs available to vulnerable communities given a particular point in time. For example, the initial budget proposed by the Trump Administration reduced funding levels for Community Development Block Grants (CDBG), the HOME program, and the US Interagency Council on Homelessness (USICH) to zero (Ingold et al. 2017). The USICH coordinates the federal interagency response to addressing and ending homelessness, and CDBG and HOME are important funding vehicles for affordable housing for low-income people, a linchpin in the strategy to end homelessness. These are just three examples of long-standing programs facing elimination following the change in political administration. The elimination of these programs, particularly CDBG and HOME, could have devastating impacts on the supply of affordable housing and the prevalence of homelessness in the United States.

In summary, street outreach is a practice that includes three core elements: (1) meeting people where they are, (2) building a trusting relationship, and (3) connecting people to services. Embedded in each of these elements is a set of core values associated with this method of practice. For example, the second element of outreach, *building a trusting relationship,* is largely about practicing deeply held values of human dignity, nonjudgement, patience, and care. The box below presents a story that shows the elements of street outreach in practice. The next section makes explicit a discussion of values from which good street outreach practice emerges.

Breakfast in Bed: An Outreach Story

When I first met Shane, he had been experiencing homelessness for close to a decade. He slept outside in all kinds of weather, rarely washed, and often went days without eating. It had been years since he'd visited a doctor, and he was completely disinterested in social services. I began my work with Shane simply, by helping him get items he wanted, such as new socks and snack bars.

Soon after we met, Shane was matched with a permanent supportive housing voucher. In the weeks that followed, however, he missed multiple appointments and struggled to make progress. We talked at length about how I could best support him to participate in the housing process. I suggested that on the mornings of important appointments, I would meet him where he slept, so we could walk together. Shane is a very private person, and he didn't want people to know where he stayed, but eventually he agreed.

The first morning I went to his spot, I found him curled up in his blanket, sleeping peacefully. He slept under a bridge with traffic passing maybe 20 feet from where he lay. It was an unusual moment for me as I thought of the best way to wake him while respecting his privacy and dignity. I called his name a couple of times, and, when he didn't wake, I gently touched his shoulder. He slowly awoke and looked at me, bleary-eyed. At the time, I was struck by a sense of responsibility. This man had allowed me into his most private of moments. I was in his bedroom as he was at his most vulnerable, bare-chested and sleepy, lying on the ground. I tried to act as I would like someone waking me to act. I quietly reminded him why I'd come and said I would give him some privacy while he got himself together. I walked away toward the road, facing away from him, while he dressed and packed his things for the day.

(continued)

During those few minutes, I regretted not bringing Shane something to eat. The next time we had an appointment, I cooked bacon and eggs, poured hot coffee into a thermos, packed some serving utensils, and strapped the lot onto the back of my bike. When I arrived at Shane's spot, I woke him, as before, and, when he was ready, I put the plates down on the ground, served the food and coffee, and we sat together and had breakfast. I knew it had been years since he'd had breakfast-in-bed, and he seemed quite happy as we ate. We talked about his housing voucher and how nice it would be when he could cook for himself. After that morning, I always brought Shane breakfast on the morning of appointments, and it seemed to me that he began to look forward to the days when we had work to do together.

The process to obtain housing can be a long and bureaucratic one, and Shane's was no exception. It took several more months of having breakfast together on the ground before he finally had a place to call home. During that time, we were able to get his birth certificate, photo ID, and social security card and attend other appointments. At times, when there were setbacks, he would become quite despondent, believing that his getting an apartment might be "too good to be true" or that the world might somehow intervene and take it away from him at the last minute. On a couple of occasions, he wanted to quit and walk away. He needed a safe outlet for these feelings and reassurance that everything would work out. Throughout our time together, Shane and I developed a trusting relationship, and I believe that this bond provided Shane the support needed to overcome doubt and stick with the process until he was housed.

Shane now has an apartment, has obtained Supplemental Security Income through the SSI/SSDI Outreach, Access, and Recovery Program, and has begun the long journey toward recovery. He has started to take an interest in life again and seems more hopeful about the future.

Ger Skerrett
Outreach and Engagement Specialist
Miriam's Kitchen
Washington, D.C.

Values Underpinning Street Outreach

The NASW Code of Ethics (NASW 2017) identifies six core values that serve as an important starting point for a discussion of values in street outreach: (1) dignity and worth of the person, (2) importance of human relationships, (3) service, (4) social justice, (5) integrity, and (6) competence. Each of these values relates to the practice of street outreach.

Dignity and Worth of the Person

Social workers should strive to believe in the inherent dignity and worth of all people. For social workers of faith, this belief is often grounded in the sacredness of human life, seeing all people as children of God who are created in God's image. For secular and humanistic social workers, this belief comes from their own deeply held values of compassion, empathy, and care for others. It is important that this core value of recognizing the dignity and worth of the person be made visible in the affective, cognitive, and behavioral dimensions of street outreach practice.

In writing about the use of empathy in social work practice, King (2011) discusses the importance of the affective, cognitive, and behavioral dimensions of social work practice. The affective dimension refers to "an interactive process of emotional connection and concern for others" (p. 687) that relates to how one *feels* in the context of the helping relationship. He adds that empathy is supported by two constructs, caring and congruence, with congruence defined as "an ability to be open, nonjudgmental, and honest within helping relationships" (p. 688). Similarly, the literature on street outreach reflects the importance of the core elements of Rogers' (1965) person-centered therapy for street outreach practice, including empathy, congruence, trust, and being strengths-based. So, social workers doing street outreach must first make their belief in the dignity of each person concrete through an authentic feeling of care, concern, and empathy for the people they encounter on the streets.

The cognitive dimension refers to a "group of conceptual processing and thinking skills that emphasize a level of objectivity and distance from the emotional content evident in a client's presentation and a careful assessment of the contextual cues therein" (King 2011, p. 689). The cognitive dimension of street outreach requires that, in the midst of their feelings of empathy, care, and nonjudgement, the street outreach worker maintains an emotional distance, so they are able to listen, assess, and consider appropriate ways of responding that help build a bonding relationship. Through weekly or regular conversations, street outreach workers not only focus on the relational aspects of the exchange but also listen for cues or language that might suggest an approach that might create an opportunity to overcome or test a current source of resistance to a type of service. It is by listening with this cognitive dimension that the street outreach worker might detect that opportunity. The example presented in the text box above demonstrates the cognitive dimension of street outreach as the street outreach worker recognized Shane's long-term experience of homelessness as a barrier toward accepting social services and housing but sees opportunity in providing socks and snack bars and bringing him "breakfast in bed."

Finally, the affective and cognitive dimensions are ultimately expressed in the behavioral dimension of street outreach, which is the outwardly observable actions of the outreach worker, such as persistent engagement, the use of motivational interviewing techniques, going with the person to appointments, helping track down vital records, and introducing the individual to housing options. These behaviors could be summarized as companioning a person who is experiencing homelessness in their journey out of homeless. Nothing speaks to one's care and belief in their inherent dignity than sticking with the person to the end.

Importance of Human Relationships

Philosophical, theological, and scientific literature make clear that human beings are social beings. We are meant to be in relationships with each other; we thrive and flourish through relationships with others. As mentioned above, the caring relationship between a street outreach worker and a person who is homeless is the "linchpin" (Rowe et al. 2016, p. 67) of the street outreach process that bridges the steps between *meeting people where they are* and *connecting them to services.* In their literature review of street outreach with youth, Connolly and Joly (2012) found that "ten of the 26 articles emphasize that forming a bond with the youth is key to successful outreach" (p. 530), and "a long-term, caring relationship can help build hope and promote positive client outcomes" (p. 530). So, the core value, *importance of human relationships,* is made manifest in a profound way in street outreach practice.

Service

As important and central as the relationship is in street outreach, a hoped-for outcome in street outreach is to connect people to housing, health care, mental health and addiction treatment, or other social services that will help people with lived experience of homelessness use their capacities to the extent they desire. In their literature review of outreach and engagement in homeless services, Olivet et al. (2010) found that street outreach yielded positive outcomes in housing and health care. In qualitative interviews with outreach workers, Lee and Donaldson (2018) reported on other ways outreach workers provided service to their clients. One outreach worker described his outreach practice as breaking the ice by offering a meal, then helping with getting photo IDs and medical insurance, and eventually moving toward services and supports that are more sustaining. Another outreach worker told the story of building a relationship for 2 years with a person living on the street, trying to talk him into applying for social security and how, when it finally happened, it seemed like a real success. But street outreach workers caution that success should be measured in small increments. One outreach worker noted, "defining success is moving somebody in a positive direction, whatever that is" (Lee and Donaldson 2018). Although street outreach workers strive to connect people on the streets to services, they recognize that patiently building strong relationships over time is a way to live out the NASW core value of service and is an essential first step toward connecting people with concrete services that will improve the quality of life of someone experiencing homelessness.

Social Justice

The ethical principle undergirding social work's core value of social justice is "Social workers pursue social change, particularly with and on behalf of vulnerable and oppressed individuals and groups of people" (NASW 2017, para 14). People who are homeless are among the most vulnerable people in society. People who are chronically homeless experience mortality rates that are three to four times higher than the general population (Henwood et al. 2015) and chronic pain that is difficult to manage due to poor access to prescription medications, poor sleeping conditions, and the stress of living in shelters (Hwang et al. 2011). Homeless populations also experience high rates of personal crime and violence. Estimates of the prevalence of violence among people who are homeless range from 14% to 21% as compared to 2% of the general population who report experiencing a violent crime (Meinbresse et al. 2014). People who are homeless are also deeply stigmatized and often blamed for their homeless circumstance. Belcher and DeForge (2012) attribute much of this discrimination and stigma to a homeless system that is largely based on subsistence rather than justice, where people's basic needs are barely met, yet more robust investments in housing, treatment, and social supports are deeply lacking.

Social work was founded as a profession that engaged in micro and macro practice to alleviate human suffering (Rothman and Mizrahi 2014). Given their close proximity to people who are living on the streets, street outreach workers are in a unique position to understand and advocate against the environmental and structural circumstances that contribute to homelessness (e.g., lack of affordable housing; inaccessible physical health, mental health, and addiction treatment; the fragmented nature of social services; complicated application processes for SSI/SSDI and other benefits; lack of employment options for people with disabilities; and discriminatory practices that make it hard to access mainstream systems). Outreach workers can and should ally with their clients and other stakeholders to change these circumstances and break down systemic barriers to help people get off the street. Exercising the value of social justice through pursuing structural change is an essential component of street outreach work for social workers.

Integrity and Competence

These two final core values speak to the character of social workers—people who are honest and trustworthy and who strive to improve their knowledge and competence in practice. The literature on street outreach points to a general mistrust or wariness on the part of people who are homeless toward the services offered by street outreach workers (Kryda and Compton 2009; Lam and Rosenheck 1999; Rowe et al. 2016). These negative perceptions come from a variety of experiences, such as perceived inauthentic care or support provided by street outreach workers, empty promises being made, and a lack of follow-through.

People who are homeless have also shared the impression that street outreach workers generally only offer short-term solutions to their problems and seem to be in it for the paycheck (Kryda and Compton 2009). Therefore, to live up to the value of integrity and competence, social workers engaged in street outreach practice must be truthful with the people they serve about the current service context and what they can deliver within this context. Building knowledge about the service context is an ongoing process for street outreach workers. They must continue to deepen their knowledge about the various array of services and how to negotiate complex systems in their jurisdictions. Despite the reservations some studies shared about perceptions of street outreach workers, Rowe et al. (2016) found, through focus groups with people receiving outreach services, that clients marveled at the invaluable depth of knowledge about service systems held by outreach workers. Street outreach based on a solid foundation of values that are deeply felt, considered, and expressed in observable actions is an important form of practice for social workers. The next section describes specific techniques and practices to strengthen outreach practice.

Skills and Practice Models to Use with Street Outreach

Street outreach workers need to draw on a set of core skills and competencies to increase their effectiveness at helping people who are homeless overcome their ambivalence with accepting services or entering housing (e.g., engagement and motivational interviewing). In addition, several models complement street outreach practice and may enhance outreach practice (e.g., SSI/SSDI Outreach, Access, and Recovery (SOAR) and Critical Time Intervention (CTI)). This section describes several of the skills and practice models that can help facilitate and strengthen street outreach.

Engagement

Considering that the first dimension of street outreach is to meet people where they are, a core competency required for street outreach concerns the ability to engage people and build trust. Olivet et al. (2010) make distinctions between outreach and engagement. Outreach refers to the practice of going out, building relationships, and connecting people to services, whereas engagement refers to the overall process of meeting people and building relationship overtime through repeated interactions.

Engagement is a critical competency for all levels of intervention (i.e., micro, mezzo, macro) and is typically suggested as the first step in the generalist intervention model in social work (Corcoran 2011; Kirst-Ashman and Hull 2015). The core component of engagement is to begin communication and subsequently build a relationship with the client or collaborator. More specifically, Brill and Levine (2005) point out that during the engagement process, practitioners are expected to pursue four tasks: "(1) involve themselves in the situation, (2) establish communication with everyone concerned, (3) begin to define the parameters within which the worker and the client(s) will work, and (4) create an initial working structure" (Brill and Levine 2005, p. 132). The core content of engagement is generally applicable to the context of outreach to homeless populations. For example, communicating with empathy, respect, and authenticity is a common thread of engagement that is directly applicable to street outreach. Some specific engagement skills include listening (without thinking about what to say next), making eye contact, asking open-ended questions, allowing silence, talking about things people seem to care about, and paying attention to clients' reactions, responses, and actions.

The engagement process with homeless populations on the street, however, may differ from the engagement processes used with the general population in that street outreach requires a high degree of acceptance, patience, and flexibility in the helping relationship. Even if the clients do not greet or speak to the outreach worker, and even if they say something upsetting, outreach workers are expected to continuously look for them and engage with them with unconditional regard. In Lee and Donaldson's (2018) field research, many outreach workers shared similar stories of pursuing and serving the same person every day for more than several months, and often up to several years, regardless of the individual's mental health struggles, unwillingness to change, or hostile attitudes. In serving those clients, outreach workers need to demonstrate strong and consistent dedication to the engagement process by sending out messages including, "I will never give up on you," "I accept you as you are," "I do not expect you to change," and "I want you to tell me what you need or what you'd like to work on." In this regard, street outreach is a long-term engagement and relationship-building process.

Alongside the engagement process, outreach workers must be able to assess the needs of the client and the availability of long-term solutions. Identifying a manageable goal and prioritizing goals are critical for street outreach because street outreach typically consists of numerous brief encounters, instead of long therapy sessions. In this limited time, it is important for outreach workers to be prepared to make efficient assessments and connect clients to community resources when they show interest. Street outreach workers may use a vulnerability assessment, such as the Vulnerability Index – Service Prioritization Decision Assistance Tool (VI-SPDAT), to assess medical vulnerability and prioritize access among people living on the street for the most appropriate housing program (100,000 Homes n.d.). These determinations are typically fed into a coordinated assessment system used to ensure the most medically vulnerable are matched to the appropriate level of service as quickly as possible.

For communities to be successful in connecting homeless people with services and housing, Kraybill (2002) suggests focusing on specific tasks, such as developing housing options, streamlining the requirements for housing, and maintaining strong linkages with housing retention case management teams, potential landlords, and community supports. As these tasks often place outreach workers between their clients and service entities, skills related to negotiation, mediation, crisis intervention, and advocacy are crucial to developing long-term solutions for clients.

Motivational Interviewing

Motivational interviewing (MI) is a useful technique for engaging someone's ambivalence in an effort to open them to the possibility of doing something different. As previously mentioned, people who are homeless and living on the streets may have had negative experiences with professional service systems. They may also be in active struggles with mental illness, addiction, or both. People who are homeless have often established their own support systems, including a community of friends who are homeless with whom they have functional and emotional bonds. Any of these experiences could contribute to someone's ambivalence to, fear of, or resistance to seeking social services or moving into independent housing. MI is "a collaborative conversation style for strengthening a person's motivation and commitment to change" (Miller and Rollnick 2012, p. 12). It is grounded in a set of principles that align with the values of social work and street outreach practice, including acceptance, compassion, evocation, and collaboration. MI includes a set of four processes that comprise the interview experience: engaging, focusing, evoking, and planning.

In the past 10–15 years, MI has been used in a variety of settings to achieve behavioral change, such as compliance with HIV/AIDS and diabetes care, engaging in healthy nutrition and fitness behaviors, and improving study habits and other pro-learning school behaviors (Miller and Rollnick 2012). Although much of the research on MI in the homeless population examines its efficacy in curbing substance use, it is identified as an important technique and best practice to use in implementing the Housing First model (Tsemberis 2010). Furthermore, the National Alliance to End Homelessness and the Center for Social Innovation offer regular trainings on MI, at annual conferences and in stand-alone formats, as a best practice in working with people who are homeless.

Conversations About Change

In his Center for Social Innovation blog, Kraybill (2016) describes MI as "a conversational style that encourages people to take a closer look into the mirror of their lives and to consider what changes, if any, they might want to make" (para. 1). In short, MI is engaging in "conversations about change" (Miller and Rollnick 2012, p. 3). Miller and Rollick describe MI as taking the middle place between a directive style of conversation, where the helper is giving instructions or advice, and a following style, where the helper is mostly listening, reflecting back, and affirming. They refer to this middle place as a "guided style" (p. 5) where one listens to the person speaking and only offers expertise as needed. Key to good listening in MI is noting places of ambivalence in one's desire or motivation to change. The state of ambivalence is the place where MI can gently nudge one forward in the process of change, as ambivalence is often the place where one gets stuck in this process.

Transtheoretical Model of Change

Prochaska and DiClemente's (1984) transtheoretical model of change, illustrated in Fig. 14.1, is important to help explain MI and its place in addressing ambivalence. Prochaska and DiClemente (1984) identify five stages of the change process:

1. Precontemplation: The individual is not consciously aware that there is a problem or a need for change. At this stage, the street outreach worker's role is to build rapport, raise consciousness, and make the person aware of the good things that lie beyond life on the street.
2. Contemplation: The individual is beginning to think about the possibility of accepting services and beginning to imagine a life beyond the street, or maybe the hope offered by the outreach worker gives them hope that life beyond the street is even possible. There may certainly be resistance, mistrust, and an expectation for great disappointment that create barriers for contemplating life beyond the street. As outreach workers build trust, they must also use this time to explore and resolve ambivalence about moving into housing, accessing medical or behavioral health treatment, or accepting other types of social services. Miller and Rollnick (2012) offer many techniques and processes to use in MI to tilt the scale of ambivalence toward wanting change versus the status quo.
3. Preparation: After a person has moved beyond the contemplation stage, it's important to help them prepare for the next step in the change process. Therefore, the outreach worker's primary tasks include continuing to affirm and encourage the person in their decision and to help the person create a plan for change. For example, if the person expresses readiness for housing, the outreach worker's role might be to take the person to visit various housing units to identify preferences of location and to help solidify their vision of themselves as a housed person.

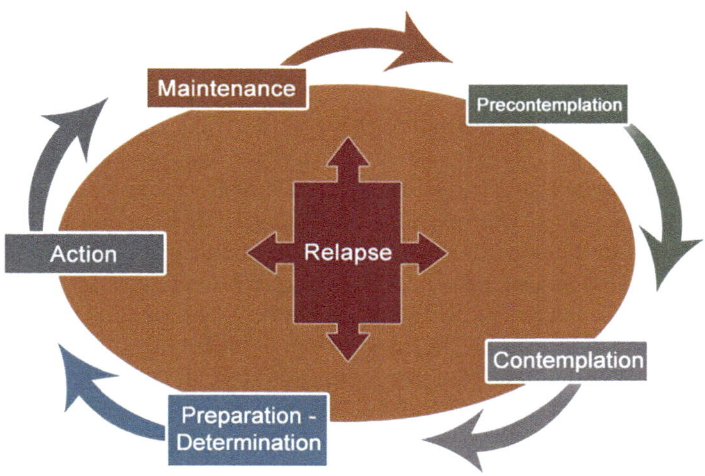

Fig. 14.1 Transtheoretical model of change. (Adapted Prochaska and DiClemente's 1984)

4. Action: In the action phase, the person is in the change process. The outreach worker's role at this stage is to offer support in the implementation of the plan that was developed in the preparation stage and to support the client in their transition to living in a new way. If the outreach worker is moving someone from the streets into housing, their role might be to take them shopping to select and buy needed supplies (e.g., bedding, cleaning supplies, furniture), to orient them to the neighborhood and transportation options, or to develop a plan to maintain medications and appointments or engage in treatment options. Outreach workers may also help individuals identify new sources of support (e.g., friends, churches, case managers) to whom the person can turn to maintain their new life situation.
5. Maintenance: At the maintenance stage, the individual is making efforts to sustain the change they have achieved. The role of outreach worker begins to diminish at this stage as the person gets more settled and is able to rely on other support networks.

At any point in the change process, an individual may relapse or return to previous behaviors. For example, those familiar with addiction know that relapse is part of the cycle of the disease. In the context of homelessness, sometimes people who have lived on the streets for many years may choose to sleep in a shelter or on the street, even after having moved into their own apartment, to spend time with friends or to be in a familiar, less isolating environment. Regardless of a return to old behaviors, street outreach workers never give up on the people with whom they have established a trusting relationship. They are patient with them as they transition from their old way of living to their new way of living. They never judge them or consider these moments of relapse a failure. It's all part of the journey, and MI is a useful tool in helping a person move forward on a path out of ambivalence (from contemplation, to preparation, to action). Social workers are encouraged to take a class or workshop on MI as it is an evidence-based practice that has applications far and wide, wherever one is seeking to foster a change in behavior.

Critical Time Intervention

This section provides a brief description of the Critical Time Intervention (CTI) model in relation to the goal of the outreach process and the skills that can be useful for outreach (for a fuller description of CTI, see Chap. 11). CTI is a homelessness prevention model that targets those going through critical periods of transition, such as going from a prison, shelter, or hospital back into society. The primary goal of the CTI is to use case management to connect people with community supports, so that those supports can remain in place after the transition. Although CTI has been implemented in multiple contexts, the origin of CTI began with the effort to help homeless individuals settle into housing after being discharged from shelters. The developers of CTI, in the mid-1980s, realized that clients often failed to navigate the system of care after having a place to live (Center for the Advancement of Critical Time Intervention n.d.). To prevent future homelessness, the CTI model offered systematic, client-focused support during the period of the transition. CTI aims to reduce the intensity of services over time while increasing the community supports for the client. Since its development, CTI has shown strong effectiveness for reducing recidivism to the shelter (Herman et al. 2011; Kasprow and Rosenheck 2007).

For people living on the street, street outreach could be considered an intervention that complements the implementation of CTI. First, CTI offers a concrete model for the next steps *after* street outreach for those exiting homelessness. Both CTI and street outreach share the overlapping goal of helping clients connect with permanent housing, establish needed service connections, and successfully transition out of homelessness.[1] To achieve this goal, outreach workers and CTI case managers work with clients through periodical engagements and encouragements – for example, developing a trusting relationship, engaging in collaborative assessments, connecting clients and caregivers, and monitoring client's progress during the transition. In terms of timeline, however, CTI has more concrete time limits and time-specific plans for the transition period that comes after the outreach. Specifically, CTI comprises three phases (i.e., transition, tryout, and transfer of care), each of which commonly takes 3 months. In this phased model, street outreach can be contextualized as "pre-CTI," the phase that occurs before the actual implementation of CTI but is critical for CTI workers (and outreach workers) to develop a trusting relationship with clients.

Both CTI and street outreach share a set of required skills. Broadly speaking, outreach is a core CTI skill that is critical for meeting people where they are (t3 2015). More specifically, active listening and motivational interviewing are two common engagement skills suggested for both CTI and street outreach (Kraybill 2002). These skills help CTI workers build a trusting relationship with clients and navigate unpredictable social interactions. In addition, it is noteworthy that both CTI and street outreach workers typically operate as a team. Therefore, understanding roles and responsibilities of each teammate and being able to work as a team are important skills for both practices. For example, a CTI team typically includes full-time CTI worker(s), a clinical supervisor, and a fieldwork coordinator. Depending on the role assigned to each member, the team's work will progress through case management and formal and informal services and supports in the community.

Technology for Street Outreach

Outreach workers commonly use basic technological tools, such as iPads or cell phones, to take notes, make referrals, text colleagues and clients, and look for information on the spot during the day-to-day work of outreach. Technological tools also

[1] Street outreach does not always seek connection to housing. Some street outreach is more focused on medical services, addiction services, or social services, in general.

help street outreach workers share data and coordinate services across agencies, which have been two important movements increasingly common in service delivery. A coordinated entry process is illustrative of such an attempt. Local homeless service systems are required to establish coordinated entry processes to help communities prioritize assistance and connect people with services in a timely manner (HUD 2015). In doing so, each local service system needs to establish as Homeless Management Information System (HMIS) that complies with HUD's data collection, management, and reporting standards (HUD 2017). This kind of information technology system requires homeless outreach workers to be familiar with the data entry and reporting systems they need to use at their own agencies. It is also helpful for them to have a general understanding of how the information they provide is used at the community level.

Attempts to connect resources among homeless service providers are also being tested at a municipality level. For example, New York City recently launched a new tool called *StreetSmart*, which provides city agencies and nonprofit groups with data on New York's homelessness on a daily basis (Lapowsky 2017). In addition, a recent phone app called *Street Reach* has been launched in Cincinnati, OH (Strategies to End Homelessness 2016). This app allows anyone who downloads the app to report the location and condition of a homeless person (either for one's self or for others) through submitting a brief report. This app also educates the public about basic information about homelessness and advice on how to approach homeless persons on the streets. Another app, *OurCalling*, based in Dallas, TX, helps people report homeless persons and find appropriate resources. To work with these systems, outreach workers need to be familiar with data entry and tool navigation processes on multiple platforms (e.g., computer, iPad, cellphone) as well as various ways of receiving and interpreting reports from the public.

SSI/SSDI Outreach, Access, and Recovery (SOAR)

The SSI/SSDI Outreach, Access, and Recovery (SOAR) program is a useful resource for street outreach workers for helping people living on the streets access cash income. SOAR is a federal initiative funded by the Substance Abuse and Mental Health Services Administration (SAMHSA), and its purpose is to increase access to two federal disability income benefit programs: Supplemental Security Income (SSI) and Social Security Disability Income (SSDI). SAMHSA initiated the SOAR program to address barriers to approval of disability benefits for eligible adults. To implement this program, they established a SOAR Technical Assistance (TA) Center to help local jurisdictions set up SOAR initiatives with three components (Dennis et al. 2011). The first component is to develop a SOAR community that includes service providers and staff from local Disability Determination and Social Security offices who receive and review applications. By establishing relationships and communication protocols, SOAR providers and federal staff can initiate phone calls and emails to streamline the application process. The second component is training. The SOAR TA Center offers a free, intensive online training program that requires 20–24 hours of time to complete. This training, along with the SOAR community, prepares case managers with the skills and techniques to develop more complete applications and therefore improve approval rates. The third component is ongoing technical assistance offered through the TA Center. This can take the form of helping jurisdictions address challenges in establishing or nurturing a SOAR community, expanding SOAR capacity through training and technical support and other ways unique to particular jurisdictions.

SOAR is specifically targeted to eligible adults who are homeless or at risk of homelessness and who also suffer from a medical or mental health disability. For people who are homeless and have disabilities, access to SSI and SSDI provides steady income and access to health insurance (i.e., Medicaid). In 2017, average benefit levels of SSI and SSDI were $735 and $1171 per month, respectively (Laurence 2017; SSA n.d.). Although these are very modest incomes that maintain an individual below the federal poverty level,[2] they can help people who are homeless secure housing, treatment, and other social supports (Rosenheck et al. 2000). In 2018, SOAR-assisted initial applications for SSI/SSDI received a 65% national approval rate as compared to the 29% application approval rate through the regular SSI/SSDI initial application process (SAMHSA 2018). SAMHSA estimates that SOAR brings in more than $406 million into the economy of participating states and communities.

Street outreach workers may want to go through the SOAR training or partner with a SOAR specialist to begin the SSI/SSDI application process for their clients. Since many people who live on the streets experience some level of disability, it is possible that SOAR could open doors to a whole new life that they never dreamed possible. The following story highlights how a street outreach worker partnered with a SOAR specialist to successfully help a client apply for Supplemental Security Benefits, which gave her some freedom to meet her modest needs.

Soaring with Tracy

When Tracy, a star student and basketball player, began experiencing the symptoms of schizophrenia, she felt her bright future slipping away. She began to hear voices that were not there and felt people were watching her through the television and radio. Tracy, previously a bubbly teenager, isolated herself and eventually stopped going to school. Her family, unable to cope with her auditory hallucinations, kicked her out. Tracy became homeless at age 15. She tried to work to support herself, but the voices always got in the way. She was unable to hold a job for more than a few months.

(continued)

[2] In 2017, the federal poverty level for a household of 1 was $12,060 per year (DHHS 2017).

Tracy experienced homelessness for almost 15 years. During her time on the streets, she spent many nights in the hospital. She checked herself into psychiatric wards when the voices became so unnerving that they pushed her to suicidal ideation, and sometimes she was involuntarily hospitalized when she was observed responding aggressively to her hallucinations. Once she left the hospital, Tracy always went back to the streets. Consequently, she received no consistent psychiatric treatment. When our outreach team met Tracy in the summer of 2016, she was downtrodden from years spent wandering the streets of Washington, D.C., without the care she needed.

As she started building trust with her outreach specialist, Tracy began to reclaim her future. Her outreach specialist made sure she always had clean clothes, a phone, and a safe place to go when she left the hospital (usually a crisis bed). Tracy applied for an apartment at a supportive housing facility for women and began to take medication that controlled her auditory hallucinations. Concurrently, she worked on an SSI application with a specialist who employed SOAR (SSI/SSDI Outreach, Access, and Recovery), a method of applying for income benefits that results in faster applications and higher success rates. The SOAR specialist worked with Tracy to collect medical records, communicate with the Social Security Administration, and compile a Medical Summary Report reflecting Tracy's medical, psychiatric, and personal history.

In November, all of Tracy's hard work came to fruition. The very day she met with her outreach specialist to pick up the keys to her new apartment, she got a call indicating that she was approved for SSI. Tears of relief streamed down her cheeks as she revealed a concern that had been eating at her: although she was ecstatic to be off the street, she worried that without any sort of income, she would go without food and home items. The Permanent Supportive Housing program helped Tracy get indoors, and the SOAR program secured a steady source of income for her. Just as winter's cold arrived, Tracy had the dignity of a home and the money she needed to build a life. Finally, she felt like she had a real chance to succeed.

Adriana Lopez-Piper
SOAR Specialist
Miriam's Kitchen
Washington, D.C.

Conclusion

Street outreach to people who are homeless is a complex and nuanced practice that social workers are uniquely prepared to undertake. Strategies to engage people in ways that communicate human dignity, care, empathy, and compassion are central to all forms of social work practice and are taught in all schools of social work. Social work programs can better prepare students for practice in the field of homeless services and for street outreach in particular, by incorporating the core skills, techniques, and intervention models described in this chapter. For example, schools could offer a 4-week, one-credit course on motivational interviewing. Schools could incorporate the SOAR online training as a component of a semester-long course on homelessness. In addition to MI and SOAR, faculty could get trained in and offer CTI as a component of homelessness curricula. The rapid pace of technology in social services requires faculty and social workers engaged in street outreach to remain current in new advancements in the field.

Street outreach workers must pay close attention to the policy decisions that impact the homeless service context. Declines in homelessness among singles and veteran populations give evidence that investments in housing, health care, and other social services make a difference in ending homelessness. However, shifts in political administrations often cause priorities, and therefore spending, to change. As mentioned above, President Trump's 2017 budget called for deep cuts in housing that would eliminate CDBGs and the HOME program and significantly reduce federal spending on Housing Choice Vouchers, public housing, and other housing subsidy programs (White House 2017). These programs are essential to the availability of affordable housing and strategies to end homelessness. Reducing these programs by billions of dollars would likely exacerbate homeless in communities across the country. Similarly, Congress continues to debate major changes in the US health-care system that could cut funding for Medicaid, add work requirements to Medicaid, and reduce access to health care for many vulnerable populations. Analyses from a range of groups, including the Congressional Budget Office, American Association of Retired Persons, Families USA, and other health advocacy organizations, have estimated that many low-income, disabled, and older adults would lose coverage as a result of proposed changes. One proposed change is to reduce the Affordable Care Act's essential benefits plan, which would likely make mental health, substance abuse, and other health-care services needed by people living on the streets more difficult to access.

Social workers must remain active in the fight against cuts to federal programs that could compromise the life, health, and safety of vulnerable populations. They must also work closely with state and local leaders to minimize the impact of these cuts on vulnerable populations at the local level. As these changes take place, street outreach processes will continue to function as a critical barometer to detect the hopes and despairs on the streets. Street outreach workers should monitor the impact of cuts and policy changes on people who are homeless and living on the streets and engage in social action against cuts and to promote investment in programs and services that support vulnerable populations. Social action strategies should include helping to organize people who are homeless to fight for their rights to housing, health care, and other supports.

References

1,000 Homes. (n.d.). Vulnerability index (VI) and service prioritization decision assistance tool (SPDAT): Prescreen assessment for single adults. http://dhhr.wv.gov/bhhf/Documents/2013%20IBHC%20Presentations/Day%203%20Workshops/VI-SPDAT%20Distribution%20Version%20August%202013.pdf. Accessed 30 June 2018.

100,000 Homes (n.d.). Vulnerability index (VI) & service prioritization decision assistance tool (SPDAT): Prescreen assessment for single adults. Retrieved from http://dhhr.wv.gov/bhhf/Documents/2013%20IBHC%20Presentations/Day%203%20Workshops/VISPDAT%20Distribution%20Version%20August%202013.pdf

Bassuk, E. L., Birk, A. W., & Liftik, J. (1994). *Community care for homeless clients with mental illness, substance abuse, or dual diagnosis*. Newton: The Better Homes Fund.

Belcher, J., & DeForge, B. (2012). Social stigma and homelessness: The limits of social change. *Journal of Human Behavior in the Social Environment, 22*(8), 929–946.

Brill, N. I., & Levine, J. (2005). *Working with people: The helping process* (8th ed.). Boston: Allyn and Bacon.

Center for the Advancement of Critical Time Intervention. (n.d.). Background of CTI model. https://www.criticaltime.org/cti-model/background/. Accessed 30 June 2018.

Connolly, J. A., & Joly, L. E. (2012). Outreach with street-involved youth: A quantitative and qualitative review of the literature. *Clinical Psychology Review, 32*, 524–534.

Corcoran, J. (2011). *Helping skills for social work direct practice*. New York: Oxford University Press.

Dennis, D., Lassiter, M., Connelly, W. H., & Lupfer, K. S. (2011). Helping adults who are homeless gain disability benefits: The SSI/SSDI Outreach, Access, and Recovery (SOAR) program. *Psychiatric Services, 62*, 1373–1376.

Henwood, B., Byrne, T., & Scriber, B. (2015). Examining mortality among formerly homeless adults enrolled in Housing First: An observational study. *BMC Public Health, 15*, 1209.

Herman, D. B., Conover, S., Gorroochurn, P., Hinterland, K., Hoepner, L., & Susser, E. S. (2001). A randomized trial of critical time intervention to prevent homelessness in persons with severe mental illness following institutional discharge. *Psychiatric Services, 62*(7), 713–719. https://doi.org/10.1176/appi.ps.62.7.713

Hwang, S. W., Wilkins, E., Chambers, C., Estrabillo, E., Berends, J., & MacDonald, A. (2011). Chronic pain among homeless persons: Characteristics, treatment, and barriers to management. *BMC Family Practice, 12*, 73.

Ingold, D., Whiteaker, C., Keller, M., & Recht, H. (2017). These 80 programs would lose federal funding under Trump's proposed budget. Bloomberg. https://www.bloomberg.com/graphics/2017-trump-budget/. Accessed 30 June 2018.

Kasprow, W. J., & Rosenheck, R. A. (2007). Outcomes of critical time intervention case management of homeless veterans after psychiatric hospitalization. *Psychiatric Services, 58*, 929–935.

King, S. H. (2011). The structure of empathy in social work practice. *Journal of Human Behavior in the Social Environment, 21*, 679–695.

Kirst-Ashman, K., & Hull, G. (2015). *Generalist practice with organizations and communities* (6th ed.). Stanford: Cengage Learning.

Kraybill, K. (2002). Outreach to people experiencing homelessness: A curriculum for training health care for the homeless outreach workers. National Health Care for the Homeless Council. https://www.nhchc.org/wp-content/uploads/2012/02/OutreachCurriculum2005.pdf. Accessed 30 June 2018.

Kraybill, K. (2016). Motivational interviewing: Salting the oats. Center for Social Innovation. http://us.thinkt3.com/blog/motivational-interviewing-salting-the-oats. Accessed 30 June 2018.

Kryda, A. D., & Compton, M. T. (2009). Mistrust of outreach workers and lack of confidence in available services among individuals who are chronically street homeless. *Community Mental Health Journal, 45*, 144–150.

Lam, J. A., & Rosenheck, R. (1999). Street outreach for homeless persons with serious mental illness: Is it effective? *Medical Care, 37*, 894–907.

Lapowsky, I. (2017, May 5). NYC's new tech to track every homeless person in the city. Wired. https://www.wired.com/2017/05/new-york-citys-businesslike-tech-fighting-homelessness/. Accessed 30 June 2018.

Laurence, B. (2017). Social security disability doesn't have a limit on unearned income, but there is a limit on how much you can make from working. Disability Secrets. http://www.disability-secrets.com/resources/social-security-disability/ssdi/income-limits-ssdi-benefits. Accessed 30 June 2018.

Lee, W., & Donaldson, L. P. (2018). Street outreach workers' understanding and experience of working with chronically homeless populations. *Journal of Poverty, 22*, 421. https://doi.org/10.1080/10875549.2018.1460737.

Lettner, B. H., Doan, R. J., & Miettinen, A. W. (2016). Housing outcomes and predictors of success: The role of hospitalization in street outreach. *Journal of Psychiatric and Mental Health Nursing, 23*, 98–107.

Meinbresse, M., Brinkley-Rubinstein, L., Grassette, A., Benson, J., Hall, C., Hamilton, R., Malott, M., & Jenkins, D. (2014). Exploring the experiences of violence among individuals who are homeless using a consumer-led approach. *Violence and Victimes, 29*(1), 122–136.

Miller, W. R., & Rollnick, S. (2012). *Motivational interviewing: Helping people change*. New York: Guilford Press.

National Association of Social Workers. (2017). *Code of ethics*. Washington, DC: Author.

O'Toole, T. P., Johnson, E. E., Borgia, M. L., & Rose, J. (2015). Tailoring outreach efforts to increase primary care use among homeless veterans: Results of a randomized controlled trial. *Journal of General Internal Medicine, 30*, 886–898.

Olivet, J., Bassuk, E., Elstad, E., Kenney, R., & Jassil, L. (2010). Outreach and engagement in homeless services: A review of the literature. *The Open Health Services and Policy Journal, 3*, 53–70.

Padgett, D. K., Hewood, B. F., & Tsemberis, S. J. (2016). *Housing first: Ending homelessness, transforming systems, and changing lives*. New York: Oxford University Press.

Prochaska, J. O., & DiClemente, C. C. (1984). *The transtheoretical approach: Crossing traditional boundaries of therapy*. Homewood: Dow Jones-Irwin.

Rogers, C. (1965). *Client-centered therapy: Its current practice, implications, and theory*. Boston: Haughton Mifflin Company.

Rosenheck, R. A., Dausey, D. J., Frisman, L., & Kasprow, W. (2000). Outcomes after initial receipt of social security benefits among homeless veterans with mental illness. *Psychiatric Services, 51*, 1549–1554.

Rothman, J., & Mizrahi, T. (2014). Balancing micro and macro practice: A challenge for social work. *Social Work, 59*, 91–93.

Rowe, M., Styron, T., & David, D. H. (2016). Mental health outreach to persons who are homeless: Implications for practice from a statewide study. *Community Mental Health Journal, 52*, 56–65.

Slesnick, N., Feng, X., Guo, X., Brakenhoff, B., Carmona, J., Murnan, A., et al. (2016). A test of outreach and drop-in linkage versus shelter linkage for connecting homeless youth to services. *Prevention Science, 17*, 450–460.

Social Security Administration. (n.d.). SSI federal payment amounts for 2017. https://www.ssa.gov/oact/cola/SSI.html. Accessed 30 June 2018.

Strategies to End Homelessness. (2016). One-of-a-kind outreach app developed locally. https://www.strategiestoendhomelessness.org/wp-content/uploads/2016-Spring-Summer-Newsletter-Web.pdf. Accessed 30 June 2018.

Substance Abuse Mental Health Services Administration (2018). SOAR Outcomes and impact. Retrieved from: https://soarworks.prainc.com/article/soar-outcomes-and-impact Accessed 30 June 2018.

t3. (2015). Understanding critical time intervention. Center for Social Innovation. http://us.thinkt3.com/courses-offerings/understanding-critical-time-intervention. Accessed 30 June 2018.

Tsemberis, S. (2010). *Housing first: The pathways model to end homelessness for people with mental health and substance use disorders*. Center City: Hazelden Publishing.

U.S. Department of Health and Human Services. (2017). U.S. federal poverty guidelines used to determine financial eligibility for certain federal programs. https://aspe.hhs.gov/poverty-guidelines. Accessed 30 June 2018.

U.S. Department of Housing and Urban Development. (2015). Coordinated entry policy brief. https://www.hudexchange.info/resources/documents/Coordinated-Entry-Policy-Brief.pdf. Accessed 30 June 2018.

U.S. Department of Housing and Urban Development. (2017). Homeless management information system. https://www.hudexchange.info/programs/hmis/. Accessed 30 June 2018.

U.S. Interagency Council on Homelessness. (2016). The president's 2016 budget: Fact sheet on homelessness assistance. https://www.usich.gov/resources/uploads/asset_library/2016_Budget_Fact_Sheet_on_Homelessness_Assistance.pdf. Accessed 30 June 2018.

U.S. Interagency Council on Homelessness. (2017). Mayor's challenge to end veteran homelessness. https://www.usich.gov/solutions/collaborative-leadership/mayors-challenge. Accessed 30 June 2018.

Varaday, D. (2010). What should housing vouchers do? A review of the recent literature. *Journal of Housing and the Built Environment, 25*, 391–407.

White House. (2017). FY 2018 budget. https://www.whitehouse.gov/omb/budget. Accessed 30 June 2018.

Chapter 15
Youth Homelessness: A Global and National Analysis of Emerging Interventions for a Population at Risk

Lauren Kominkiewicz and Frances Bernard Kominkiewicz

Youth Homelessness Stories

When Austin started his senior year of high school, his family was living out of their car. His mother and father had serious substance use issues, which made it difficult to pay rent for a house or an apartment. Austin was afraid to talk to anyone about being homeless because he did not want to be seen as different from his classmates. He would shower in the gym locker room before school every day and eat from friends' lunches during the week. However, Austin was often hungry and stole food from the cafeteria. Eventually, he was caught. Instead of punishment, Ms. Dunphy, the school social worker, intervened. After several one-on-one meetings, Ms. Dunphy built enough rapport with Austin to allow him to confide in her about his living situation. By this time, the family's car had been towed, and they were living in a tent. Over the course of a year, Ms. Dunphy helped the family relocate to a transitional housing program that provided supportive services for parents struggling with substance use issues, and she signed up Austin for the school's free lunch program. Although they still had not found permanent housing by the end of that year, Austin's parents were sober, and Austin was able to avoid stealing in order to eat.

Emma was 15 years old and living in a tent with her family when her city hosted the Olympic Games. She and her family had been living in the same area for over 2 years and had built significant relationships with individuals in their tent community. In an effort to improve the face of the city for an international audience,

Electronic supplementary material: The online version of this chapter (https://doi.org/10.1007/978-3-030-03727-7_15) contains supplementary material, which is available to authorized users.

L. Kominkiewicz (✉)
Children's Legal Services of San Diego, San Diego, CA, USA

F. B. Kominkiewicz
Saint Mary's College, Notre Dame, IN, USA
e-mail: kominkie@saintmarys.edu

H. Larkin et al. (eds.), *Homelessness Prevention and Intervention in Social Work*, https://doi.org/10.1007/978-3-030-03727-7_15

police in the host city conducted targeted cleanups to quickly remove large groups of homeless people. In the span of 3 days, Emma lost touch with the majority of her support network, causing her to turn to formalized social services. Emma and her family spoke to the emergency shelter social worker, Mr. Frank, about how they were asked to leave the area where most of Emma's peers were residing. Mr. Frank was sympathetic but was only able to provide referrals to programs in another community, far from everything Emma knew. Although her school provided bus services after her move to allow her to remain enrolled, the round-trip on the bus took several hours, and Emma began to fall significantly behind on her school work. Emma considered enrolling in a school closer to her, but after the trauma of her move and losing connections, she decided to drop out.

Chapter Outline and Goals

The two scenarios above reveal the vulnerability of homeless youth, a population often marginalized and facing daily obstacles that add complexity to their lives (Heerde et al. 2015). Where one youth attempted to keep his family together, the other was forced to separate from everyone she knows to obtain housing. Both leaned on their natural social supports before becoming involved with social workers. Austin benefited from Ms. Dunphy, realizing the significance and motivation of her support, whereas Mr. Frank simply moved Emma without regard for her concerns. Homeless youth can be the best teachers of what will help them succeed if practitioners take the time to listen.

How do social workers approach such diverse issues in a coherent way? This chapter outlines the causes and consequences of youth homelessness and reviews global and national policies, assessment approaches, and interventions. Through a thorough study of what causes homelessness, why definitions and policies can impact care, and how effective practice can change outcomes, you will become better equipped to manage cases involving youth homelessness.

Causes and Consequences of Youth Homelessness

The causes and consequences of youth homelessness are varied, and it can be difficult to differentiate between factors that preceded homelessness and factors precipitated by homelessness (Thompson et al. 2010). Overarching the causes and consequences of youth homelessness are the effects of poverty and racism. A lack of affordable housing intensified by the rising cost of rent, an increasing percentage of households who are renting, and dormant wage growth are contributing factors to homelessness (Damron 2015). Allocating a large percentage of income to housing leaves a household with limited resources for unexpected expenses, such as medical emergencies (Damron 2015).

Homelessness affects 2.5 million children in the United States annually (Sullivan-Walker et al. 2017). Moreover, youth between the ages of 12 and 17 are at a higher risk of becoming homeless than adults (National Conference of State Legislatures 2016). Sadly, that means 1 in every 30 children in the majority of public schools has experienced homelessness. We see the effects of this kind of stress when 75% of homeless youth drop out prior to graduation (Sullivan-Walker et al. 2017; National Conference of State Legislatures 2016).

Youth may develop problems with drug use or mental health, which contribute to leaving home or being forced out, and then further victimized while living on the street (Thompson et al. 2010). Additionally, youth experiencing homelessness frequently engage in substance use, but it is less clear regarding the direction of the relationship between youth homelessness and substance use (Thompson et al. 2010). It is difficult to delineate between pre-homelessness characteristics and those resulting from homelessness, such as substance use issues.

The federal strategic plan to end homelessness, *Opening Doors*, calls for an end to homelessness among unaccompanied youth by 2020 (US Interagency Council on Homelessness 2015). National estimates of homeless youth are ascertained through the US Department of Housing and Urban Development's (HUD) Point-in-Time (PIT) count conducted by communities across the country (HUD 2018). On a single night in January 2018, the PIT count located 36,361 unaccompanied homeless youth under the age of 25, which represents close to 7% of the total homeless population and 10% of people experiencing homelessness as individuals (HUD 2018). Homeless youth who are unaccompanied are more likely to be unsheltered (51%), living on the streets or in places not meant for habitation, as compared to all people who are experiencing homelessness (35%) (HUD 2018). Notably, almost a quarter (24.4%) of unaccompanied homeless youth are Hispanic or Latino (HUD 2018).

Poverty is a major factor in homelessness among youth. In 2012, the poverty rate among 18–64-year-olds was around 13.7% compared to 21.8% for youth younger than age 18 (DeNavas-Walt et al. 2013). Although children represent 23.7% of the total population, these statistics indicate that children comprise more than a third (34.6%) of individuals living in poverty (DeNavas-Walt et al. 2013). Moreover, the intersectionality of poverty and race continues to show a stark picture of youth homelessness. For example, the 2012 poverty rate for non-Hispanic Whites was 9.7%, lower than the poverty rates for other racial groups (DeNavas-Walt et al. 2013). Non-Hispanic Whites comprised 62.8% of the total population in 2012 and represented 40.7% of people in poverty (DeNavas-Walt et al. 2013). For reference, the poverty rate in 2012 for African-Americans was 27.2%, for Asians it was 11.7%, and for Hispanics it was 25.6% (DeNavas-Walt et al. 2013).

Lesbian, gay, bisexual, transgender, and queer (LGBTQ) youth are at a greater likelihood of experiencing homelessness than their heterosexual, cisgender peers (Gattis and Larson 2017). Youth who identified as transgender comprised approximately 1% of the unaccompanied youth population in 2018 (HUD 2018). People not identifying as male, female, or transgender accounted for a slightly larger percentage of the sheltered population than the unsheltered population (2% as compared to 1%) (HUD 2018). Women or girls comprised 38% of unaccompanied youth experiencing homelessness, which is a higher percentage than that of all individuals experiencing homelessness (28%) (HUD 2018). Compared to 27% of all unsheltered individuals, one-third of unaccompanied youth staying in unsheltered locations were female (HUD 2018).

Victimization during adolescence has been linked to homelessness (van den Bree et al. 2009). Many homeless youths are survivors of abuse during childhood and are likely to leave their home environments as a result of these adverse circumstances. Youth experiencing homelessness who have a history of physical abuse report more difficulty in finding basic necessities and feeling more anxious and depressed (Tyler and Schmitz 2018). Specifically, youth questioned while not living with a parent were more likely to have reported experiencing physical or sexual abuse while they were in the home (Substance Abuse and Mental Health Services Administration 2014). Threats and injuries were found to be most common, and one study found that 70% of youth living on the street reported that they were beaten, punched, hit, or burned (Kipke et al. 1997). The effects of victimization can remain for years and can increase the risk of substance use, psychiatric, or psychological issues, as well as further negative experiences while living on the streets (Whitbeck et al. 2004; D'Ercole and Struening 1990).

Homeless youth are also at higher risk for incarceration than their housed peers (Zhao et al. 2018). Youths who have a history of physical abuse and who are experiencing homelessness were almost twice as likely to be arrested and jailed in comparison to non-abused youth, controlling for the effects of drug use, interactions with deviant peer groups, and survival behaviors (Yoder et al. 2014).

Youth experiencing homelessness in late adolescence have demonstrated significant mental health challenges that could lead to major psychopathology if not treated (Parks et al. 2007). In order to determine the number of homeless youth with a DSM-IV-TR diagnosis, one study used the Mini International Neuropsychiatric Interview (MINI) with the population in San Francisco and Chicago; the study found that 87% and 81%, respectively, of the homeless youth participating in the study met the diagnostic criteria for a minimum of one MINI psychiatric diagnosis (Quimby et al. 2012). Homeless youth have also been found to have these psychiatric needs unmet within their communities (Saperstein et al. 2014).

Similar to the early onset of mental health impairments, homeless youth have been found to start using substances at a higher rate and at a much younger age than housed youth (Csiernik et al. 2017; Zhao et al. 2018). Across the nation, the percentage of substance use among homeless youth is estimated to be between 70% and 90% (Edidin et al. 2012). Moreover, research suggests that there is a special concern of hard drug use among these youth that resembles actions to self-medicate (Guo and Slesnick 2017).

A history of foster care also affects youth experiencing homelessness. Homeless youths who were formerly in foster care have demonstrated poor behavioral health outcomes and significant needs regarding mental health, substance use, education, and the ability to make an adequate income (Yoshioka-Maxwell and Rice 2019). Moreover, these youths have reported a higher rate of childhood maltreatment and experienced a longer period of homelessness (Bender et al. 2015) while also being linked to a greater search for mental health assistance (Crosby et al. 2018). Finally, youth leaving foster care may find that they are unable to achieve self-sufficiency and independence due to decreased educational achievement, vocational skills, and financial assistance provided to them (Curry and Abrams 2015).

Cognitively, the consequences of childhood socioeconomic adversity can negatively affect social, emotional, and educational development (Saperstein et al. 2014). The trauma of abuse suffered while in their home may compound the cognitive problems of adolescents who become homeless (Parks et al. 2007). Over 50% of homeless youths who had a mental health diagnosis were also found to have cognitive deficits placing them at risk of earning a wage that will not support them when they reach the age of independent living (Saperstein et al. 2014). Therefore, the cycle of poverty cannot be broken without particular attention to cognitive and emotional health in homeless youth (Saperstein et al. 2014).

Childhood sexual abuse experiences are associated with additional sexual victimization while living on the street (Tyler and Schmitz 2018). While homeless, youths enter into and become victimized by different forms of sexual behavior (Heerde and Hemphill 2016). For example, results of one study found that 41.2% of the homeless youth participants were victims of sex trafficking (Middleton et al. 2018). Further, youths who experience sexual victimization prior to becoming homeless are at an increased risk for engaging in behaviors associated with contracting HIV (Harris et al. 2017). The longer they lived on the streets, youth experiencing homelessness had a greater likelihood of dying due to increased risk in such areas as substance use, HIV transmission, and sexual or physical violence (Crawford 2018).

Youth who are homeless become pregnant at higher rates than housed youth (Begun 2015; Greene and Ringwalt 1998; Tucker et al. 2012). To illustrate the scope of the issue, among females ages 14–17 years old, 48% of those who were living on the street and 33% of those who were living in shelters had been pregnant at least once in comparison to 7% of those who were living in stable housing (Greene and Ringwalt 1998). Around 73% of pregnancies experienced by homeless youth are unintended (Gelberg et al. 2001) and possibly connected to intrafamilial incest found at a high rate within the population (Haley et al. 2004; Saewyc and Edinburgh 2010). Moreover, youth may experience homelessness as a result of becoming pregnant, with parents or guardians not allowing them to remain in the home after sharing the news (Meadows-Oliver 2006).

Finally, academic issues can precede and follow episodes of homelessness. Problems in school, including a lack of educational goals, poor academic achievement, and behavioral difficulties, are significant risk factors for homelessness (van den Bree et al. 2009). These difficulties can be indicative of decreased intellectual functioning (Parks et al. 2007) and social difficulties, including problems in conforming to a structured school environment (Whitbeck and Simons 1993; Kingree et al. 1999). For runaway youth, adjustment issues, failing grades, and suspensions can contribute to a decision to leave the home (Whitbeck and Simons 1993; Rosenthal et al. 2006). While homeless, youth reported stigma and bullying associated with receiving additional educational services (Saldanha 2017).

In 2014, 16% of youth experiencing homelessness received services under the Individuals with Disabilities Education Act (IDEA) (Sullivan-Walker et al. 2017).

However, the same homeless youths described special education as a brief stop, with designs and benefits that lacked foresight into later issues and the long-term goal of employment, which demonstrates the intersectionality of homelessness, disability, and age (Saldanha 2017).

Policy

This section reviews several aspects of policy that affect the daily functioning of homeless youth. It is necessary to understand the causes of youth homelessness and the dynamics of family relationships in order to effectively assess specific policies and to advocate for policy development for youth experiencing homelessness (Parker and Mayock 2019). When policy development and implementation do not account for the causes and consequences of youth homelessness, the goals of the policy may not be met. Popple and Leighninger (2019) argue that when knowledge is incomplete, social policy is an experiment because little is known about cause and effect relationships.

Effective policy in working with homeless youth or youth at risk of becoming homeless involves a collaborative, multidisciplinary approach that funds and supports evidence-based interventions for prevention as well as short- and long-term goals (Kidd et al. 2019). Therefore, working with homeless or housing-insecure youth includes providing supportive services and funding for immediate assistance along with long-term housing resources that assist youth in exiting homelessness (Kidd et al. 2019). Factors such as child abuse and neglect, human trafficking, mental health, physical health, family dysfunction, and other root causes of youth homelessness and housing instability must also be handled with care to make policy interventions effective (Parker and Mayock 2019).

Since there is little evidence regarding the types of services and collaborations between systems integral to helping youth transition out of homelessness, current policy can be viewed as falling short of being evidenced-informed (Kidd et al. 2019). Thus, it seems important to ensure that policy development is sensitive to inclusivity and addresses the causes of youth homelessness from micro, mezzo, and macro levels. Lyon-Callo (2000) cautions against focusing on the "disease" model of homelessness, as it distracts from progress toward dealing with homelessness in the face of race, gender, or class dynamics. Properly evaluating access to and distribution of resources is necessary in developing and assessing effective policy.

Lightfoot et al. (2011) discuss policy implications for working with youth experiencing homelessness. For example, assisting youth in strengthening their coping, decision-making, and goal-setting skills could lead to a decrease in problem behaviors that are often found in homeless youth (Lightfoot et al. 2011). Goal setting is a significant skill for youth experiencing homelessness to build and would help transition youth into self-sufficiency toward exiting the cycle of homelessness. Data-driven policy development would therefore provide opportunities for programs to receive resources to be able to teach these skills to homeless youth.

It is imperative that policy reflects the realities of homeless youth in order to be effective, and policymaking benefits from including the voice of youth who have experienced homelessness (Gomez and Ryan 2016). It is recommended that policies be assessed for their holistic approach in order to guarantee homeless youth have access to services, such as emergency shelter, housing, mental or physical health care, education, and independent living supports. Additionally, policies would benefit from incorporating treatment for substance use disorders due to the high number of youths who have been identified as having problems in this area. Moreover, policies that utilize harm reduction are sensitive to the consequences of substance use and can help to minimize the related stress and risk behaviors exhibited by homeless youth (Rhule-Louie et al. 2008).

Definitions

Definitions are important to policy for two primary reasons: measuring the problem and dictating which groups are eligible for what resources. For example, if a definition is too narrow, whole groups of people who may benefit can be excluded. On the other hand, a definition that is too broad can render the policy ineffective. Therefore, understanding how different policymaking bodies define homelessness informs the policy analysis process.

Homelessness is not unique to one country, and definitions or ideas about homelessness permeate borders. Beginning with an examination of the United States, the Department of Health and Human Services (HHS), the Department of Education (ED), and the Department of Housing and Urban Development (HUD) have their own definitions of youth homelessness (Morton et al. 2018). First, HHS is governed by the Runaway and Homeless Youth Act (RHYA), reauthorized by the Reconnecting Homeless Youth Act of 2008, which is the only federal policy specifically focused on unaccompanied homeless youth (42 U.S.C. § 5701 et seq.). RHYA defines a homeless youth as an "individual who cannot live safely with a parent, legal guardian, or relative, and who has no other safe alternative living arrangement" (42 U.S.C. § 5732a(3)). RHYA funds multiple services for homeless youth, which are discussed in later sections.

Second, ED employs the definition from the Homeless Education of Children and Youth (EHCY) program, under Title VII-B of the McKinney-Vento Act (McKinney-Vento), most recently reauthorized in 1995 by the Every Student Succeeds Act (ESSA) (42 U.S.C. § 11431 et seq.). EHCY defines homeless youth as those without a "fixed, regular, and adequate nighttime residence" or whose primary nighttime residence ranges from sharing housing due to economic hardships, to motels, and to emergency or transitional shelters (42 U.S.C. §11434(a)). The EHCY definition attempts to capture the variety of locations that youth utilize for shelter in order to remove barriers to enrollment and promote school stability.

Finally, HUD incorporates a general definition for homelessness from McKinney-Vento as amended and reauthorized by the Homeless Emergency Assistance and Rapid Transition to Housing (HEARTH) Act of 2009 (42 U.S.C. § 11302). The general definition tracks the language used in EHCY, linking homelessness to sleeping arrangements with specific parameters to qualify. This includes, for example, an individual or family who is losing their primary residence in 14 days and lacks resources to remain in housing (National Network for Youth 2019). Youth are covered under the label "unaccompanied youth" as long as they meet another federal definition, such as RHYA, and have been in unstable living situations or fleeing unsafe circumstances (Administration for Children and Families 2016).

There is also no fixed definition of homelessness that encompasses the experiences of children globally. The United Nations Children's Fund has attempted to categorize homeless youth as "[a]ny girl or boy who has not reached adulthood, for whom the street in the widest sense of the word, including unoccupied dwellings, wasteland, and so on, has become his or her habitual abode and/or source of livelihood, and who is inadequately protected, directed, and supervised by responsible adults" (United Nations Human Rights Office of the High Commissioner 2012). Moreover, the United Nations narrowed their definition by adopting three categories. The first, "children of the street," are adolescents with little or no contact with their families. The second, "children on the street," refers to children who spend a majority or significant portion of their time on the street but return home to their families or guardians at night. "Children from street families," the third category, are those who live together with their families on the street (United Nations Human Rights Office of the High Commissioner 2012).

A definition of homeless youth is necessary to accurately locate and account for this population because the varying definitions between programs and agencies complicate research and impact usefulness (Jocoy 2013). Moreover, without a standard, results in research can vary depending on which definition is used (Brakenhoff et al. 2015). For example, Morton et al. (2018) reviewed studies where HUD documented homeless youth as those up to 24 years old, and RHYA collected data on youth between the ages of 13 and 25, while other national estimates only focused on adolescents (Morton et al. 2018). Researchers call for a more inclusive definition of homeless youth (Glassman et al. 2010) that captures the realities of homelessness, such as residing for long periods of time on the streets or couch-surfing (Bender et al. 2010).

No global estimates of homelessness can be provided due to inconsistent definitions and a lack of reliable data (Busch-Geertsema et al. 2015). Therefore, global statistics of youth experiencing homelessness and housing insecurity cannot be reliably provided. Busch-Geertsema et al. (2015) suggest a global definition of homelessness that "denotes a standard of housing that falls significantly short of the relevant adequacy threshold in one or more domains," including security, physical, and social (pp. 6–10).

International Policies

Examining global social policies related to youth experiencing homelessness is expected to advance critical thinking about domestic policy, in support of a holistic approach. Global policies affecting youth experiencing homelessness tend to fall into three categories: criminalization, welfare, and rights-based (Thomas de Benitez and Jones n.d.). Thomas de Benitez and Jones (n.d.) explore these categories to effectuate interventions with homeless youth within their cultural context.

When a country applies the criminalization approach, homeless youth are viewed as responsible for their street-based conditions and can be detained for forbidden activities, including drug use or informal work. The criminalization approach, therefore, places an expensive responsibility on law enforcement and the criminal justice system. For example, during the Vancouver 2010 Olympic Games, the city implemented a series of street cleanup activities that moved out the homeless or marginally housed in an attempt to market its city for a global audience (Kennelly 2015). In the 2012 Olympic Games, London carried on this "unintended legacy" (Kennelly 2017). Although each city made efforts to connect homeless people with services, the planned positive outcomes rarely came to fruition for street-involved youth (Kennelly and Watt 2011). Moreover, self-regulation often bolstered a city's ability to carry out these practices without recourse from marginalized groups (Kennelly 2015).

Thus, the criminalization of individuals experiencing homelessness includes and affects homeless youth. The primary goal of policies that criminalize seemingly benign behaviors, such as panhandling and sharing food with the homeless in public spaces, is to enable communities to use law enforcement to "clean" the streets without providing more costly or less expedient social services to treat the underlying housing and biopsychosocial problems. Anti-homelessness policies provide a formal social control that equates the lack of homeless individuals with the successful management of homelessness (Aykanian and Lee 2016).

Criminalizing acts inherent to homelessness, however, has not been shown to produce the intended results for communities. One study found that police officers had feelings of frustration and of being burdened, while those experiencing homelessness had feelings of being targeted and harassed (McNamara et al. 2013). Where criminalization measures exist, judicial actions do not always respect the rights of homeless individuals (Sheffield 2015). In their advocacy role, social workers have an opportunity to prevent and scrutinize existing criminalization measures as part of a holistic framework to practicing with homeless youth.

The welfare approach focuses on giving homeless youth fundamental services, including shelter, health, education, and job training, with the goal that the youth will take advantage of conventional opportunities if they have these needs met. However, the welfare approach does not factor in the many existing mental health issues and deprivations. On the other side of the coin, the rights-based approach emphasizes youth participation when connecting with basic services to motivate youth through an understanding that they have the right to thrive in their home country (Thomas de Benitez and Jones n.d.).

Through a review of American and South Korean research on youth homelessness, Kim (2014) found that theoretical approaches and the effect of policies that prevent or improve youth homelessness over the past decade have received minimal research attention. In discussing the increase in youth experiencing homelessness and the lack of funding for affordable housing and employment programs for youth in Canada, Dolson (2015) attributes such changes to a shift in Canadian federal welfare policy in which "the federal government has been withdrawing increasingly from universal social assistance programmes" (p. 135).

Although not directly impacting youth, comparing policies affecting the general homeless population in Japan and the United Kingdom illustrates how culture impacts law. Homelessness policies in Japan primarily involve employment support for "rough sleepers"—individuals living in public areas, such as along roads and in parks—and welfare assistance to counteract homelessness due to a disability. However, when Japanese citizens cannot work due to socioeconomic reasons, there is little help. The socioeconomically impoverished population is dominated by individuals over the age of 50, who are less likely to find employment. In the United Kingdom, individuals experiencing homelessness are more often in their 40s or younger, and policies to assist them include social security when they are unemployed for any reason (Okamoto 2007). Moreover, accommodations and other support for those experiencing homelessness in the United Kingdom are required by law to be provided by local government (Okamoto 2007). According to a study conducted in the United Kingdom, "Most interventions currently available to young homeless people focus primarily on the immediate housing crisis by providing temporary accommodation" (Hodgson et al. 2015, p. 322).

US Federal Policies

While there are a number of organizations serving homeless youth in the United States, RHYA and McKinney-Vento provide the basis for most programs that provide direct services, housing, and supports. RHYA has served as the major homeless youth social policy since 1974 (Glassman et al. 2010). RHYA provides the authorization for grant programs that support local interventions with homeless or runaway youth. The grants fund the Basic Center, Transitional Living, and Street Outreach programs, which are administered by the Family and Youth Services Bureau, the Administration on Children, Youth and Families (ACYF), and the Administration for Children and Families (ACF) within the Department of Health and Human Services (HHS). "For purposes of Basic Center Program eligibility, a homeless youth must be less than 18 years of age…For purposes of Transitional Living Program eligibility, a homeless youth cannot be less than 16 years of age and must be less than 22 years of age" (45 C.F.R. § 1351). The "Assessment and Intervention" section below discusses more details related to each program.

In terms of education, McKinney-Vento attempts to remove hurdles for youth experiencing homelessness and housing instability to accessing academic resources. With the goal of stabilizing education, legislation aims to lower the stress of enrollment for a homeless student and improve attendance by mandating schools to become involved in the process (Stone and Uretsky 2016). In order to accomplish these goals, McKinney-Vento provides guidelines for educating homeless children and youth administered by the Department of Education's Office of Elementary and Secondary Education and created state educational agencies (SEAs) and local educational agencies (LEAs) that must ensure homeless students have equal access to the same free, appropriate public education as is provided to housed youth (42 U.S.C. §§11431–11435). SEAs and LEAs are required to review and undertake policies and practices to identify homeless youth; provide age-appropriate services; offer care coordination with public and private agencies; train professionals working with this population; remove application fees, fines, or deadlines for enrollment; and promote school stability by maintaining a child's school of origin despite housing status (42 U.S.C. §§11431–11435).

The Department of Housing and Urban Development (HUD) provides the Continuum of Care (CoC) grants, which are homeless assistance grants (National Center for Homeless Education 2013). These competitive grants are awarded annually to nonprofit organizations, states, and/or local governments through the CoC Program for supportive services, safe havens, transitional housing, specific types of permanent housing, and the operation of a Homeless Management Information System (HMIS), a community-wide data system (HUD 2012; National Center for Homeless Education 2013). The original recipients of the grants are allowed to contract with other organizations or government entities in order to implement the grant's programs. The CoC Program helps individuals, including unaccompanied youth, and families experiencing homelessness and provides the necessary services to move youth and families into transitional and permanent housing toward long-term stability (HUD 2012).

Additionally, the CoC Program encourages planning that includes the whole community, with a focus on using resources strategically, strengthening the coordination of those resources, improving data collection and assessment, and encouraging communities to design programs according to the communities' strengths and needs (HUD 2012). HUD provides project awards through this collaborative process with the local community CoC that includes local government agencies, direct and indirect service providers, and client community members, who together decide on the community's priorities and apply to HUD for funding (National Center for Homeless Education 2013). Although the majority of urban areas have their own CoCs, suburban counties often collaborate to form CoCs (National Center for Homeless Education 2013). Since many rural and some suburban areas are sparsely populated or too small to develop individual CoCs, they can consolidate into larger CoCs; a few states have formed one statewide CoC (National Center for Homeless Education 2013).

These larger policy and funding mechanisms provide the context for the discussion of assessment and intervention that follows. Recognizing that the diverse population of homeless youth cannot be fully captured through the lens of federal rules, specific subgroups are featured to highlight how the outlined policies impact the provision of care to individual homeless youth.

Assessment and Intervention

Unique interventions for homeless youth are recommended to facilitate appropriate services that counteract known risk behaviors and keep youth from further victimization and its consequences (Slesnick et al. 2016b). In order to increase effectiveness, social workers and other helping professionals can utilize knowledge of the effects of socioeconomic adversity to increase the educational, social, and developmental opportunities for youth experiencing homelessness. Using the example of Austin in the youth story at the start of this chapter, Ms. Dunphy, the school social worker, was aware that socioeconomic adversity can negatively affect student learning. She applied this knowledge in conducting her assessment and intervention with Austin and his parents. Preventing victimization and providing immediate support for youth who have experienced victimization may decrease the possibility of later adverse outcomes, such as homelessness (van den Bree et al. 2009). By providing a path for Austin and his family to secure transitional housing, for his parents to receive supportive services to address their substance use issues, and for Austin to access the free lunch program at school, Ms. Dunphy increased Austin's educational, social, and developmental opportunities.

In the United States, programs often attempt to address multiple needs within single interventions and are guided by national policies that fund programs to achieve certain goals. Looking first at the process of locating homeless youth, this section outlines theory and assessment tools used to support effective interventions. At the end of this section, you will be able to see how federal law and funding streams can guide local program goals and service delivery options.

Locating Homeless Youth

As discussed earlier, advocating for homeless youth begins with accurately accounting for individuals and areas they access. One common method communities use is the annual Point-in-Time (PIT) count, which strives to locate homeless adults and youth. In the United States, the PIT count is considered to be the primary source of data regarding individuals experiencing homelessness (Schneider et al. 2016) and is collected and used by communities receiving federal funding from the Department of Housing and Urban Development (Agans et al. 2014).

These counts rely on street- and shelter-based identification. Youth who are couch-surfing, sleeping in hidden locations, or avoiding services or being counted are underrepresented in sampling (Auerswald et al. 2013). In addition to the PIT counts, the Department of Education's count efforts entail assessing for homelessness using the Youth Risk Behavior Survey, a school-based data collection method. Thus, youth who are not attending school are inherently excluded (Cutuli et al. 2015; National Center for Homeless Education 2016).

Those attempting to count youth experiencing homelessness find it difficult for a number of reasons. Youth experiencing homelessness may be located at different locations and times as compared to older individuals or families experiencing homelessness, and many youths do not want to be located or do not view themselves as being homeless (Horwitz et al. 2018). Therefore, homeless youth are not always in the places one may expect them to be, such as among homeless adults or in organizations serving the general homeless population. Moreover, there are questions about what month to conduct the count for the most accurate results. The PIT counts required by HUD are conducted in January (Horwitz et al. 2018), which is a time of year when weather may result in individuals not being counted through street- and shelter-based counts. Therefore, the data related to the numbers of homeless youth may not be an accurate depiction of the problem. Further, homeless youth may be unwilling to share information about their housing status with individuals they do not know or trust. Difficulties can also result from computing errors, such as faulty reports, database failures, incomplete reporting, poor records, and the inability of some systems to provide a count (Burt 1992; Cloke et al. 2001; Kidd and Scrimenti 2004). PIT counts have also been criticized for being unreliable due to inconsistent results (Schneider et al. 2016).

The Voices of Youth Count project developed a toolkit for communities conducting PIT counts for homeless youth that addresses the challenges in counting youth experiencing homelessness and housing insecurity (Horwitz et al. 2018). Applying the same techniques in counting unaccompanied homeless youth that are used for counting homeless adults and families has been difficult, and many communities have striven toward improving their methods for conducting a youth count (Horwitz et al. 2018). The Voices of Youth Count toolkit integrates many of those methods into constructing a youth-centered count to improve the accuracy of practices used in the youth count and to collect data that would build knowledge about youth experiencing homelessness who are disproportionately represented (Horwitz et al. 2018).

Finally, homeless families are often difficult to locate (Wright and Devine 1995). However, through assessment, support systems can increase networking with youth experiencing homelessness as part of a family in order to gain the information needed to conduct an accurate count. Strong interviewing skills for those conducting the counts is important in order to gain relevant information from youth experiencing homelessness.

Homeless youth have been found to use social relationships and physical environments for social networking and navigating life on the streets. Geographic information systems can be used to conduct participatory mapping research, which can be used to illustrate youths' activities, use of space, and involvement with community services, such programs related to their psychological and physical well-being (Townley et al. 2016). In one study, homeless youths were found to participate most often in homeless service-related activities, such as shelters, mental health agencies, and day programs, and their level of activity was significantly associated with a perception of community and psychological well-being (Townley et al. 2016).

Assessing a homeless youth's ability to network and interact in a social environment includes interview questions designed to gain knowledge of his or her applicable space, previous living conditions, and present accommodations. For example, youths experiencing homelessness who were previously in foster care occupied a particular social space in the larger homeless youth network when interacting with their physical environment. Moreover, they were found to connect at a lower rate and remained more isolated than homeless youth without a history in foster care (Yoshioka-Maxwell and Rice 2017).

Using Assessment to Inform Interventions

Homeless youth have been a chronically underserved population, and effective, specialized interventions are required to maintain their participation in services (Rhule-Louie et al. 2008). Assessing the needs of youth experiencing homelessness includes challenges to conducting research, such as the inability to remain in contact with the homeless youth, obtaining either consent or assent prior to interviews, and maintaining ethically sound research procedures established by Institutional Review Boards (IRBs) throughout the entirety of the study. When entering into research projects involving runaway and homeless youth, the youth's autonomy is best protected through the use of informed consent (Meade and Slesnick 2002). Clear ethical conduct guidelines for researchers and clinicians are not provided by federal regulations and court decisions to work with runaway and homeless youth (Meade and Slesnick 2002). Researchers seek approval from an IRB, who reviews the research proposal and verifies that ethical research practices involving human beings are followed. Youth can participate in research in most situations only with approval from a parent or legal guardian, although exceptions are made if the youth is emancipated or a waiver of parental consent is granted (Koller et al. 2012).

In practice and research, social workers often use assessment surveys to gain knowledge about populations. One assessment tool is the Adverse Childhood Experiences (ACEs) Questionnaire, which elicits information about whether a person experienced the following in childhood: physical abuse, sexual abuse, emotional abuse, physical neglect, emotional neglect, witnessing intimate partner violence, witnessing violence toward their mother/stepmother, substance misuse within the household, household mental illness, parental separation or divorce, and incarceration of a household member (Felitti et al. 1998; SAMSHA 2018).

The Adverse Childhood Experiences Questionnaire, however, is typically used with adults, often long after the events have occurred (Felitti et al. 1998). Given the correlational relationship between ACEs and problems occurring in later life, assessing for ACEs in youth may inform intervention strategies that focus on the mitigation or prevention of the long-term impacts of ACEs and help promote stability. This speaks to the value of trauma-informed care for youth. One study conducted in Tanzania included eight questions adapted from the ACEs survey as they sought to determine the causes of youth homelessness (McAlpine et al. 2010). The authors stated that the ACEs questionnaire is a retrospective survey created for adults and was "not validated as a freestanding psychological instrument for assessing abuse and support in youth in another culture" (McAlpine et al. 2010, p. 31). However, meeting the needs of homeless youth requires an understanding of adverse childhood experiences. Social workers gather important information from comprehensive psychosocial assessments that include ACEs, which then offers the opportunity to plan treatment with youth to address ACEs, supported by guidance from the ecosystems perspective and program contexts applying knowledge of trauma-informed care.

Figure 15.1 illustrates the application of the ecosystems perspective to conduct assessment and intervention with youth experiencing homelessness and housing insecurity and the variables included in an assessment. It is not an exhaustive list, as

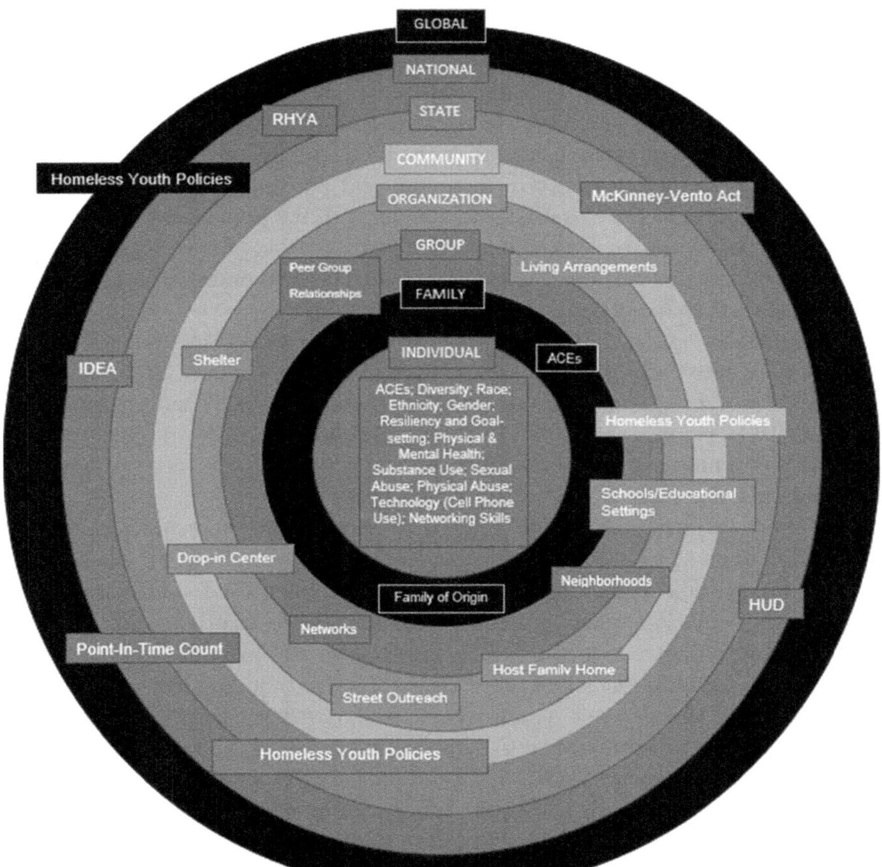

Fig. 15.1 Ecosystems perspective applied to assessment and intervention with youth experiencing homelessness and housing insecurity

application of the ecosystems perspective focuses on how each youth in their environment mutually reacts with the environment. Application of the ecosystems perspective assists the social worker in completing an assessment that results in effective and meaningful interventions with youth.

An ecosystems perspective focuses on the interaction between an individual and their environment. A focus on strengths and resiliency rather than a focus on a homeless youth's housing insecurity fits well with the application of the ecosystems perspective and utilizing biopsychosocial-cultural assessments in social work practice to assist the youth in locating strengths (Bender et al. 2007). Methods used by individuals, organizations, and societies to assess youth experiencing homelessness or housing insecurity are often guided by an ecosystems perspective. Using this approach as the theoretical basis for assessing, interviewing, and intervening with youth experiencing homelessness can strengthen practice and has been applied in studies of youth experiencing homelessness (Attar-Schwartz 2013; Crawford 2018; Slesnick and Prestopnik 2005; Thompson et al. 2008). Variables that may be assessed under an ecosystems approach include the following: housing status; demographics, such as race, ethnicity, socioeconomic status, and gender; presence of, consequences from, and responses to childhood physical or sexual abuse and violence in the family; relationships with family of origin; sexuality; physical and mental health, including access to treatment and prevention services; cognitive impairments; substance use issues; interactions with the juvenile justice or foster systems; sexual violence or trafficking issues; history of and present academic problems; support systems and identified strengths, such as networking skills, resiliency, and goal setting; and knowledge and use of technology.

The generalist approach in social work is based on systems theory and the ecosystems perspective (Suppes and Wells 2018). Applying the ecosystems perspective, social workers maintain a simultaneous focus on person and environments (Sommer 1995; Suppes and Wells 2018). In addition to assessment, social workers intervene on multiple levels: individual, family, group, organization, community, state, national, and global (Suppes and Wells 2018).

The levels of intervention impacting youth experiencing homelessness include an assessment and evaluation from the perspective of youth. These levels of intervention involve the individual, family, group, organization, and community (Kominkiewicz and Kominkiewicz 2008). Additionally, focus groups are a valuable tool for organizations conducting needs assessments and benefits the youths who participate by making them feel heard (Kominkiewicz and Kominkiewicz 2008). Empathy when working with youth who have experienced trauma increases the ability of the helping professional to gather all information needed for an accurate assessment (Kominkiewicz 2008).

Professionals gain clinical insight from examining aspects of daily life for youth experiencing homelessness and housing insecurity and benefit from incorporating their opinions (Robertson and Toro 1999). Assessing the variables above, practitioners can build a well-rounded action plan to best serve homeless youth in a timely and effective manner. This method can also be applied within organizations to fully encapsulate the biopsychosocial issues, as well as cultural and spiritual factors.

Knowledge of trauma-informed care, assessment, interviewing skills, and understanding how diagnoses impact care are vital to effectively working with youth experiencing homelessness. Social workers frequently assess individuals with a trauma history, including accumulated ACEs. Moreover, greater mental health symptoms were found in homeless youth with particular traumatic experiences that occurred before youth were homeless, such as sexual abuse, emotional abuse or neglect, and a toxic home environment (Wong et al. 2016). As noted earlier in the chapter, researchers have also found that exposure to physical abuse as a child accompanied higher arrest and incarceration rates even after correcting for any substance use, deviant peer group interactions, and survival behaviors while homeless (Yoder et al. 2014).

It is recommended that programs serving homeless youth address possible emotional, cognitive, or social issues related to trauma and offer programming focused on preventing delinquency (Yoder et al. 2014). Trauma-informed service delivery involves identifying early adversity in clients with an understanding of how trauma can affect a client's worldview and psychosocial functioning (Levenson 2017). The core principles of safety, trust, collaboration, choice, and empowerment are applied in trauma-informed social work while being sensitive to the type and level of trauma that has been experienced by the youth. This focus assists the social worker in addressing these issues through the interview process (Kominkiewicz 2008).

It is important that helping professionals working with homeless youth become knowledgeable about the extent of their clients' needs (Altena et al. 2010). Through building their base of understanding, helping professionals can work toward improving the quality of life of homeless youth and developing good working relationships that underlie successful interventions (Altena et al. 2010).

Understanding diversity within the homeless youth population improves assessment and overall services offered to assist them. For example, of the youth experiencing homelessness, 40% are estimated to identify as LGBTQ, which is significant when considering that only approximately 5–8% of the entire youth population in the United States identify as such (Durso and Gates 2012; Ray 2006). Agencies and organizations serving the LGBTQ community will often interact with LGBTQ youth experiencing homelessness, and policies affecting both populations may collide. For example, LGBTQ youths experience higher instances of HIV and suicidal behaviors in addition to being more likely to be victims of violence (Keuroghlian et al. 2014). Moreover, one study found that 39.3% of LGBTQ participants did not complete high school, and the majority did not request assistance from school staff or their local gay-straight alliance (Bidell 2014). The intersectionality of identities and experiences are often not accommodated by systems, and LGBTQ homeless youth of color can be negatively affected, particularly in achieving permanency in housing (Robinson 2018). Through provision of well-rounded care, homeless youth services have an opportunity to bridge the gap between meeting immediate housing needs and long-term mental health and stability.

Recognizing the capacity for children to problem-solve and plan can potentially help clinicians to build on protective factors that the child already possesses (Lightfoot et al. 2011). Vitopoulos et al. (2017) researched the importance of helping homeless youth develop strength-based coping skills and discuss their experiences. The researchers implemented interventions based on the rates of abuse and trauma in homeless youth and cited the need for a trauma-informed approach in working with this population, especially in a group setting (Vitopoulos et al. 2017). Effective assessment considers these multiple and varied experiences of homeless youth, including the ability of homeless youth to network with organizations and programs providing services, with the end goal of assisting helping professionals in building an effective intervention plan. Evidence clearly suggests that homeless youth require significant community-based resources that are responsive to the needs of the population.

A team approach to working with homeless youth with special education needs helps to achieve the most success by opening and maintaining clear lines of communication among youth as well as between youth and school officials, maximizing student supports, evaluating and monitoring student needs, and supporting students and their families (Sullivan-Walker et al. 2017). Moreover, since many youths may not return home, education and training are important for activating self-sufficiency after interventions have ended.

To an alarming degree, studies have found that children who have experienced homelessness demonstrate greater disruptions throughout their lives as compared to children who are low-income without housing instability (Buckner 2008). Although the immediate priorities for youth experiencing homelessness are shelter, food, mental health, and physical health, the long-term components of living stable lives must be addressed if these youths do not return home. Research has shown a higher severity of depressive symptoms in runaway and homeless youth was significantly related to family maltreatment (Lim et al. 2016) and running away from home more often (Tyler et al. 2018). As Anda et al. (2006) state, "extreme, traumatic, or repetitive childhood stressors such as abuse, witnessing or being the victim of domestic violence, and related types of ACEs are common, tend to be kept secret, and go unrecognized by the outside world" (p. 180). It is imperative to assess for adverse childhood experiences and articulate short- and long-term intervention goals.

Health issues, including physical and mental health issues, of youth experiencing homelessness and housing insecurity also call for multiple interventions by a social worker on various levels, including housing and medical resources. Homeless and housing-insecure youth are at greater risk to experience mental health issues, such as trauma, suicide attempts, and depression (Zerger et al. 2008). Furthermore, since a homeless youth's substance use is impacted by the larger social environment, treatment outcomes can be improved by supporting youth experiencing homelessness to gain employment, use educational opportunities, and become housed (Zhang and Slesnick 2018).

One study found that nearly half (49.8%) of the youth experiencing homelessness met the criteria for alcohol use disorder and 59.7% met the criteria of drug use disorder during the past year, with approximately 20% reporting that they used no substances (Thompson et al. 2015). Marijuana was the most commonly used drug, with 76% reporting that they used this drug, followed by 34.8% reporting use of prescription drugs, 25.8% reporting ecstasy use, 25.5% reporting cocaine use, 23.8% reporting use of hallucinogens, 19.3% reporting use of over-the-counter drugs, 17.1% reporting use of heroin or opiates, 16% reporting use of methamphetamines, and 16% reporting use of amphetamines (Thompson et al. 2015). Interventions differ according to the type of services sought by youth experiencing homelessness or housing insecurity and assessment findings. Ecologically based family therapy (EBFT) was found to be more successful in decreasing substance use with runaway youth than service as usual through a shelter (Slesnick and Prestopnik 2005).

Services for Youth Experiencing Homelessness

Theory guides practice and research with homeless youth, with practice wisdom and research findings in turn further informing how theory guides our work. Thus far, concepts and findings have been connected to assessment and direct practice implications. This section presents programs developed from US federal policies and funding streams. To gain additional benefits from this information, use the vignettes at the beginning of the chapter, and discuss how various interventions would best serve those clients.

Transitional Living and Basic Center Programs

The Transitional Living Program (TLP) provides significant support for youth who are in transition to self-sufficiency from the ages of 16 to 22 (FYSB 2018c). Through the Family and Youth Services Bureau (FYSB), services are provided for a period of time, generally up to 540 days, to remain in group homes, host family homes, supervised apartments, and maternity group homes (FYSB 2018c). These programs typically assist older youth experiencing homelessness (Giffords et al. 2007; Holtschneider 2016). TLPs offer housing and supportive services, such as mental and physical health care, training to achieve financial and interpersonal skills, and assistance to achieve educational and vocational goals, although the housing and supportive services are not guaranteed beyond 2 years (Curry and Petering 2017). A primary outcome of TLPs is to prepare youth for independence, although the structural causes of youth homelessness may still exist and impact long-term stability (Holtschneider 2016).

The Basic Center Program (BCP) is used by community-based and nonprofit agencies serving youth up to 18 years old to connect them with emergency shelter, food, clothing, counseling, and referrals to health care (FYSB 2018a). These programs can also provide up to 21 days of shelter for up to 20 youth and seek to reunite families or find alternative placements (FYSB 2018a). In terms of prevention, BCP grantees may offer in-home services to alleviate issues that may impact youth who are at risk of separating from their families (FYSB 2018a).

Street Outreach

The Street Outreach Program (SOP), operating in collaboration with provisions of the Violence Against Women Act (VAWA) (42 U.S.C. § 13701 et seq.), was developed to assist homeless youth between 14 and 21 who have become victims of sexual exploitation and abuse. The major objective of SOPs is to prevent the sexual abuse or exploitation of youth experiencing homelessness or housing insecurity (FYSB 2018b). To accomplish this goal, grantees offer supportive services, such as street-based education, access to emergency shelters, survival aid, and assessment and counseling. FYSB also requires the incorporation of the Positive Youth Development (PYD) approach that offers youth the opportunity to build leadership and other skills necessary to thrive in their community (FYSB 2018b). SOPs empower organizations to assist youth experiencing homelessness to leave the streets and give support services to youth for stable housing in order to achieve independence (FYSB 2018b).

Culturally, homeless youth adopt certain characteristics tailored to help them survive in their environment, such as moving locations frequently and sleeping during the day. As a result, using an outreach model can be most helpful for practitioners to reach youth within the context of their lives (Thompson et al. 2010). Studies define outreach as "contacting/engaging individuals within non-office settings, with successful outreach defined as service linkage" (Slesnick et al. 2016a, p. 451). Connecting with youth on the street, offering flexibility in hours of operation, and assessing the individual needs of youth experiencing homelessness or housing insecurity increase the success of street outreach programs (Baer et al. 2004). Limited research exists that documents services and programs focused on reintegrating youth who have a history of homelessness back into housing situations with stability and structure (Slesnick et al. 2016a).

Host Homes

A host family home entails a family or single adult home that provides shelter to a homeless youth (45 C.F.R. § 1351). Historically, in a host home arrangement, a youth experiencing homelessness moves into the home of a single adult, married couple, or couple with children (Kroner 1988). The youth can function independently and receives additional supervision to that of the host (Kroner 1988). Selection, training, and monitoring of host homes are vital to this process, with referring agencies involved in the home inspection as well as screening and supervision of the host home (Kroner 1988). One such referring agency was the Empire State Coalition of Youth and Family Services, which collaborated with the New York State Division for Youth to provide youth experiencing homelessness with emergency shelter through paid and volunteer "host" foster homes (Freudenberger and Torkelsen 1984, p. 135).

Host home programs provide support to hosts and case management to youth after matching youth with a host (Washington State Department of Commerce 2017). Families in host homes act as hosts for youth who require temporary emergency shelter (Naidich and Covenant House Nineline 1988). The need for a host home exists if a youth runs away from home due to such situations as the need for relief from family tension that might escalate into a physically or emotionally dangerous crisis or if a youth may not be wanted in the home (Naidich and Covenant House Nineline 1988). The host home gives youth and their families an opportunity to deescalate the situation and work with helping professionals in problem-solving and developing a plan that can be implemented after the host home placement (Naidich and Covenant House Nineline 1988). Youth are provided family-like environments by the hosts, which includes housing, food, transportation, mentoring and support, and coordination with the host home program to provide additional services needed by youth (Washington State Department of Commerce 2017).

Shelters and Drop-In Centers

Shelters and drop-in centers serve as entry to other support, such as medical, dental, and mental health services, and both provide specific services to youth experiencing homelessness (De Rosa et al. 1999; Mallett et al. 2004). Youth are connected to benefits, including Medicaid, cash assistance, food stamps, social security disability, and housing programs, and are provided with crisis intervention, educational support, employment resources, medical and mental health care, and HIV testing and counseling services (Guo and Slesnick 2017). To assist youth in exiting homelessness, both drop-in centers and shelters provide reintegration services, although youths are only allowed to stay overnight in shelters (Guo and Slesnick 2017).

Shelters have been promoted historically by the federal government as a means of assisting the homeless population. These shelters offer a variety of on-site programs, including tutoring and treatment (Pavlakis 2014). Shelters provide safety for youth experiencing homelessness by removing the dangers of living on the street and by assisting youth in locating stable housing that meets their needs (Dekel et al. 2003).

In one study, 78% of youth experiencing homelessness reported accessing drop-in programs, making them the service that homeless youth most often use (De Rosa et al. 1999). This may be due to the fact that drop-in centers have few restrictions in order to increase successful engagement with youth (Guo and Slesnick 2017). Drop-in centers usually provide specialized services, including substance use disorder counseling (Slesnick and Prestopnik 2005) and medical services to promote sexual health (Rew et al. 2002).

Drop-in centers are more often used by youth as compared to crisis shelters (Slesnick et al. 2015). Drop-in centers may have a greater ability to link homeless youth with community services through quick interventions with knowledgeable staff who can respond easily to obvious problems (Guo and Slesnick 2017).

Moreover, in a study of case management and individual therapy services offered through a drop-in center for homeless youth, it was found that substance use, mental health, and days housed were significantly improved for homeless youth up to 12 months following the baseline (Slesnick et al. 2008).

Housing Models and Programs

Housing First, a model of housing intervention, provides immediate access to housing without the requirements of psychiatric treatment or sobriety (Gulcur et al. 2003). The Housing First program has been found to increase housing stability and decrease hospitalizations for mental and physical health issues. It has also been shown to be effective in decreasing homelessness and can be utilized in suburban areas or in populations of the chronically homeless with multiple disorders (Gulcur et al. 2003; Stefancic and Tsemberis 2007).

The Continuum of Care of the Department of Housing and Urban Development (HUD), authorized by the McKinney-Vento Act, provides the funding for permanent supportive housing (PSH) and requires that the recipient of the service has a disability in order to be eligible (HUD 2012; HUD 2019). PSH programs were found to vary according to the type of housing configuration used, such as whether the placement was among nonprogram housing units or an all-in-one location, and by the type of service provision model that was applied, such as low-intensity case management, intensive case management, and behavioral health (Dickson-Gomez et al. 2017). In addition to case management, services provided by supportive housing programs varied, and the extent to which the supportive housing programs applied harm reduction versus abstinence policies also varied (Dickson-Gomez et al. 2017).

Youth who participated in PSH programs, however, were found to have increased costs for inpatient, crisis residential, and mental health outpatient services (Gilmer 2016). PSH programs may give more access to specialized inpatient services for youth, or the greater inpatient admissions may be indicative of a positive approach for youth (Gilmer 2016). It is important that PSH programs for youth are developed and implemented to increase their effectiveness on youth outcomes given the financial investment to this approach (Gilmer 2016).

Youth-oriented housing programs differ from adult programs in various areas, such as treatment, referral sources, and housing strategies. For example, youth more commonly make self-referrals as compared to adults. Additionally, housing resources for youth are more often initially considered transitional and provided more supervision and support and then moved toward a more permanent housing plan involving roommates and financial independence. Moreover, housing services greatly focused on maintaining educational opportunities for youth as a way to attain gainful employment (Gilmer et al. 2013).

Technology and Intervention

As with any youth, the Internet and social media play an important role in navigating everyday experiences while homeless. In the homeless population, the Internet can be a significant stabilizing force. For example, homeless youths who attribute their homelessness to mental illness are five times more likely to conduct an Internet search for health services as compared to other homeless youth (Curry et al. 2016). This lifeline allows an instant connection when physical proximity is an issue. Over the next few years, the research will likely be more pronounced in offering mental health or direct links online between service providers and homeless youth. However, ethical and legal questions are still being explored.

Because access to services is still limited, therapists who become involved with homeless youth are encouraged to examine how use of resources found via the Internet can help to manage mental health (Adkins et al. 2017). First, the youth population may be better able to manage appointments with reminders through their phone and achieve better outcomes through consistency. Second, youths could access apps that track their mood between sessions with a clinician and recall more behaviors that can be monitored. Third, communication over the phone could help youths feel less isolated by their label as "homeless" and help them establish normalcy through social interactions. Homeless youth have been found to use email in order to maintain contact with parents, caseworkers, and potential employers but use social networking sites most often to connect with nonparental family and peers (Rice and Barman 2014).

Moreover, research is improved through utilization of these tools. To increase our understanding of risk factors that affect psychiatric and substance use disorders in homeless youth, researchers have used social networking tools, such as email, cell phones, and Facebook, not only to give information to youth experiencing homelessness but also to increase the possibility that the youth will continue to participate in the study long-term (Quimby et al. 2012).

The benefits of Internet access need to be balanced with an awareness of the pitfalls. Cell phones may be available to homeless youth, but paying for coverage can become a family conflict, and financial limitations make access nearly impossible without Wi-Fi. However, youth can use conflict and financial limitations as motivators to mend relationships or engage with services that offer Internet access. Additionally, as practitioners, we need to understand our role in using cell phones for sharing information. Homeless youths are most interested in information related to their mental, sexual, and reproductive health if the source is confidential, truthful, and crosses over into other mediums, such as in-person interactions (Jennings et al. 2016).

Among self-reporting homeless youth, cell phones can assist with stability and support (Bender et al. 2014). However, practitioners and researchers are also tasked with being responsible for the youth's confidential information. Therefore, before using Internet resources for communication or clinical intervention, social workers are advised to speak with their supervisors and the youth to establish appropriate boundaries.

Youth Supporting Youth

Youth experiencing homelessness may often be hurt and angry at family or adults who have victimized them during their lives. Youths learn to avoid or show reluctance to engage with services meant to help them and will often rank self-sufficiency higher than the need for services to treat underlying issues. Homeless youths most often search for assistance from individuals they view as trustworthy, caring, and empathic (Collins and Barker 2009). However, when youth originate from families where neglect and abuse occurred regularly, they cannot be expected to easily develop a trusting relationship with another adult (Craig and Hodson 1998). Therefore, finding avenues to strengthen trust in a clinical relationship is important (Bruce et al. 2015).

Spending time on rapport building with clients has a significant impact on interventions with youth experiencing barriers to accessing mental health services (Adkins et al. 2017). However, rapport building can also mean utilizing resources around providers to build trust in the clinician as a teacher or service broker. Building rapport with youth experiencing homelessness and establishing trust prior to initiating the interview are vital to make certain that responses are truthful rather than given in response to what is socially acceptable (Pears and Noller 1995). Due to the complexity of issues presented to the social worker and other helping professionals by youth experiencing homelessness, the ability to provide highly specialized services and high-quality practice skills is necessary (van den Bree et al. 2009).

Incorporating peer relationships as part of clinical work can help deepen youths' relationships with services and will likely impact how youths perceive their involvement or possible outcomes of participation. Peer support has been found to be very promising, especially to confront social isolation and increased hopelessness among homeless youth (Kidd et al. 2016). By engaging individuals who have overcome homelessness in youth, currently homeless youths benefit through viewing the spectrum of outcomes their present situation can yield (Kidd et al. 2016). As an example of the effect of peer groups, youth experiencing homelessness in a social group of mainly unemployed, street-based peers may exhibit similar behaviors, such as failing to attend school regularly (de la Haye et al. 2012).

Peer support is an internationally utilized framework for interventions with homeless youth but must mirror the society in which it is meant to evoke change. For example, we can look to studies on peer relationships of homeless youth abroad. Thompson et al. (2007) found that even though some characteristics of street life transcended the culture of homeless youth, the home country's ideas on individualism or collectivism affected behaviors related to how the homeless youth viewed their experience. Moreover, the researchers found that service delivery systems for homeless youth could be strengthened by the development of culturally-specific interventions (Thompson et al. 2007). Therefore, building effective peer supports means understanding the cultural context of the social environment.

Finally, studies involving homeless youth can often be complicated by factors such as trust and rapport building. However, researchers have attempted to confront this issue by providing opportunities for youth to run and facilitate studies related to homeless youth in general. Gomez and Ryan (2016) found that youth-led research has resulted in richer interviews from the participants. Moreover, the youth researchers felt empowered and perceived their assistance as positive (Gomez and Ryan 2016). The symbiotic relationship in this system benefits the research on homeless youth and provides a venue for verbalizing personal information, validating and empathizing what is expressed by homeless youth, and focusing on the needs of homeless youth (Adkins et al. 2017).

Conclusions

Practitioners working with homeless youth have an opportunity to make a significant impact on the lives of their clients if they possess the appropriate skills. This chapter sought to demonstrate how assessment, intervention, and policy analysis are all important practice skills in order to comprehensively serve youth experiencing homelessness. The use of surrounding resources strengthens services and helps to build trust with the youth served. Applying knowledge in the context of a stable, consistent relationship can increase effectiveness and build on the strengths of youth experiencing homelessness.

References

Adkins, E. C., Zalta, A. K., Boley, R. A., Glover, A., Karnik, N. S., & Schueller, S. M. (2017). Exploring the potential of technology-based mental health services for homeless youth: A qualitative study. *Psychological Services, 14*(2), 238–245.

Administration for Children and Families. (2016). Definitions of homelessness for federal program serving children, youth, and families. https://www.acf.hhs.gov/sites/default/files/ecd/homelessness_definition.pdf. Accessed 1st Aug 2017.

Agans, R. P., Jefferson, M. T., Bowling, J. M., Zeng, D., Yang, J., & Silverbush, M. (2014). Enumerating the hidden homeless: Strategies to estimate the homeless gone missing from a point-in-time count. *Journal of Official Statistics (JOS), 30*(2), 215–229.

Altena, A. M., Brilleslijper-Kater, S. N., & Wolf, J. L. (2010). Effective interventions for homeless youth: A systematic review. *American Journal of Preventive Medicine, 38*(6), 637–645.

Anda, R. F., Felitti, V. J., Bremner, J. D., Walker, J. D., Whitfield, C., Perry, B. D., et al. (2006). The enduring effects of abuse and related adverse experiences in childhood. *European Archives of Psychiatry & Clinical Neuroscience, 256*(3), 174–186.

Attar-Schwartz, S. (2013). Runaway behavior among adolescents in residential care: The role of personal characteristics, victimization experiences while in care, social climate, and institutional factors. *Children and Youth Services Review, 35*(2), 258–267.

Auerswald, C., Lin, J., Petry, L., & Hyatt, S. (2013). *Hidden in plain sight: An assessment of youth inclusion in Point-in-Time counts of California's unsheltered homeless population.* Sacramento: California Homeless Youth Project. https://www.streetchildren.org/wp-content/uploads/2015/03/Hidden-in-Plain-Sight_FullReportFINAL.pdf.

Aykanian, A., & Lee, W. (2016). Social work's role in ending the criminalization of homelessness: Opportunities for action. *Social Work, 61*(2), 183–185.

Baer, J. S., Petersen, P. L., & Wells, E. A. (2004). Rationale and design of a brief substance use intervention for homeless adolescents. *Addiction Research and Theory, 12*(4), 317–334.

Begun, S. (2015). The paradox of homeless youth pregnancy: A review of challenges and opportunities. *Social Work in Health Care, 54*(5), 444–460.

Bender, K., Thompson, S., McManus, H., Lantry, J., & Flynn, P. (2007). Capacity for survival: Exploring strengths of homeless street youth. *Child & Youth Care Forum, 36*(1), 25–42.

Bender, K., Cook, M. S., Thompson, S., Williams, T., & Windsor, L. (2010). Homeless youth: Characteristics, contributing factors, and service options. *Journal of Human Behavior in the Social Environment, 20*(2), 193–217.

Bender, K., Begun, S., DePrince, A., Haffejee, B., & Kaufmann, S. (2014). Utilizing technology for longitudinal communication with homeless youth. *Social Work in Health Care, 53*(9), 865–882.

Bender, K., Yang, J., Ferguson, K., & Thompson, S. (2015). Experiences and needs of homeless youth with a history of foster care. *Children and Youth Services Review, 55*, 222–231.

Bidell, M. P. (2014). Is there an emotional cost of completing high school? Ecological factors and psychological distress among LGBT homeless youth. *Journal of Homosexuality, 61*(3), 366–381.

Brakenhoff, B., Jang, B., Slesnick, N., & Snyder, A. (2015). Longitudinal predictors of homelessness: Findings from the National Longitudinal Survey of Youth-97. *Journal of Youth Studies, 18*(8), 1015–1034.

Bruce, M., Chance, R., & Meulemans, L. (2015). Joining forces for families: An embedded response to neighborhood poverty. *International Journal of Qualitative Studies in Education (QSE), 28*(6), 750–756.

Buckner, J. C. (2008). Understanding the impact of homelessness on children: Challenges and future research directions. *American Behavioral Scientist, 51*, 721–736.

Burt, M. R. (1992). *Alternative methods to estimate the number of homeless children and youth*. Washington, DC: Urban Institute.

Busch-Geertsema, V., Culhane, D., & Fitzpatrick, S. (2015). A global framework for understanding and measuring homelessness. Institute of Global Homelessness. http://docs.wixstatic.com/ugd/d41ae6_97a693a1aba845058f91e9cf38f7c112.pdf. Accessed 2 July 2018.

Cloke, P., Milbourne, P., & Widdowfield, R. (2001). Making the homeless count? Enumerating rough sleepers and the distortion of homelessness. *Policy and Politics, 29*(3), 259–279.

Collins, P., & Barker, C. (2009). Psychological help-seeking in homeless adolescents. *International Journal of Social Psychiatry, 55*(4), 372–384.

Craig, T. K. J., & Hodson, S. (1998). Homeless youth in London: Childhood antecedents and psychiatric disorder. *Psychological Medicine, 28*, 1379–1388.

Crawford, M. (2018). Runaway sexual minority youth: Comparative analysis using Bronfenbrenner and Foucault. *Theory in Action, 11*(2), 51–71.

Crosby, S. D., Hsu, H.-T., Jones, K., & Rice, E. (2018). Factors that contribute to help-seeking among homeless, trauma-exposed youth: A social-ecological perspective. *Children & Youth Services Review, 93*, 126–134.

Csiernik, R., Forchuk, C., Buccieri, K., Richardson, J., Rudnick, A., Warner, L., & Wright, A. (2017). Substance use of homeless and precariously housed youth in a Canadian context. *International Journal of Mental Health and Addiction, 15*(1), 1–15.

Curry, S., & Abrams, L. (2015). Housing and social support for youth aging out of foster care: State of the research literature and directions for future inquiry. *Child & Adolescent Social Work Journal, 32*(2), 143–153.

Curry, S., & Petering, R. (2017). Resident perspectives on life in a transitional living program for homeless young adults. *Child & Adolescent Social Work Journal, 34*(6), 507–515.

Curry, S. R., Rhoades, H., & Rice, E. (2016). Correlates of homeless youths' stability-seeking behaviors online and in person. *Journal of the Society for Social Work & Research, 7*(1), 143–176.

Cutuli, J. J., Steinway, C., Perlman, S., Herbers, J. E., Eyrich-Garg, K. M., & Willard, J. (2015). Youth homelessness: Prevalence and associations with weight in three regions. *Health & Social Work, 40*(4), 316–324.

D'Ercole, A., & Struening, E. (1990). Victimization among homeless women: Implications for service delivery. *Journal of Community Psychology, 18*(2), 141–152.

Damron, N. (2015). *No place to call home: Child and youth homelessness in the United States [Poverty Fact Sheet]*. Madison: Institute for Research on Poverty, University of Wisconsin-Madison, Morgridge Center for Public Service.

De Rosa, C. J., Montgomery, S. B., Kipke, M. D., Iverson, E., Ma, J. L., & Unger, J. B. (1999). Service utilization among homeless and runaway youth in Los Angeles, California: Rates and reasons. *Journal of Adolescent Health, 24*(6), 449–458.

Dekel, R., Peled, E., & Spiro, S. E. (2003). Shelters for houseless youth: A follow-up evaluation. *Journal of Adolescence, 26*(2), 201–212.

de la Haye, K., Green, H. J., Kennedy, D. P., Zhou, A., Golinelli, D., Wenzel, S. L., & Tucker, J. S. (2012). Who is supporting homeless youth? Predictors of support in personal networks. *Journal of Research on Adolescence, 22*(4), 604–616.

DeNavas-Walt, C., Proctor, B. D., Smith, J. C., & Census Bureau, U. S. (2013). *Income, poverty, and health insurance coverage in the United States: 2012. Current population reports P60-245. U.S. Census Bureau*. U.S. Census Bureau.

Dickson-Gomez, J., Quinn, K., Johnson, A., Nowicki, K., Galletly, C., Bendixen, A., & Ko Ko, T. (2017). Identifying variability in permanent supportive housing: A comparative effectiveness approach to measuring health outcomes. *American Journal of Orthopsychiatry, 87*(4), 414–424.

Dolson, M. S. (2015). Trauma, workfare and the social contingency of precarity and its sufferings: The story of Marius, a street-youth. *Culture, Medicine, and Psychiatry: An International Journal of Cross-Cultural Health Research, 39*(1), 134–161.

Durso, L. E., & Gates, G. J. (2012). *Serving our youth: Findings from a national survey of service providers working with lesbian, gay, bisexual and transgender youth who are homeless or at risk of becoming homeless*. Los Angeles: The Williams Institute.

Edidin, J., Ganim, Z., Hunter, S., & Karnik, N. (2012). The mental and physical health of homeless youth: A literature review. *Child Psychiatry & Human Development, 43*(3), 354–375.

Every Student Succeeds Act, 42 U.S.C. § 11431 et seq.

Family and Youth Services Bureau (FYSB). (2018a). Fact sheet: Runaway & homeless youth – basic center program. https://www.acf.hhs.gov/sites/default/files/fysb/basic_center_program_fact_sheet_jan_2018.pdf

Family and Youth Services Bureau (FYSB). (2018b). Fact sheet: Runaway & homeless youth – street outreach program. https://www.acf.hhs.gov/sites/default/files/fysb/street_outreach_program_fact_sheet_jan_2018.pdf

Family and Youth Services Bureau (FYSB). (2018c). Fact sheet: Runaway and homeless youth – transitional living program. https://www.acf.hhs.gov/sites/default/files/fysb/transitional_living_program_fact_sheet_jan_2018.pdf

Felitti, V. J., Anda, R. F., Nordenberg, D., Williamson, D. F., Spitz, A. M., Edwards, V., et al. (1998). Relationship of childhood abuse and household dysfunction to many of the leading causes of death in adults: The Adverse Childhood Experiences (ACE) Study. *American Journal of Preventive Medicine, 14*(4), 245–258.

Freudenberger, H. J., & Torkelsen, S. E. (1984). Beyond the interpersonal: A systems model of therapeutic care for homeless children and youth. *Psychotherapy: Theory, Research, Practice, Training, 21*(1), 132–140.

Gattis, M. N., & Larson, A. (2017). Perceived microaggressions and mental health in a sample of black youths experiencing homelessness. *Social Work Research, 41*(1), 7–17.

Gelberg, L., Leake, B. D., Lu, M. C., Andersen, R. M., Wenzel, S. L., Morgenstern, H., et al. (2001). Use of contraceptive methods among homeless women for protection against unwanted pregnancies and sexually transmitted diseases: Prior use and willingness to use in the future. *Contraception, 63*(5), 277–281.

Giffords, E., Alonso, C., & Bell, R. (2007). A transitional living program for homeless adolescents: A case study. *Child & Youth Care Forum, 36*(4), 141–151.

Gilmer, T. P. (2016). Permanent supportive housing for transition-age youths: Service costs and fidelity to the housing first model. *Psychiatric Services, 67*(6), 615–621.

Gilmer, T. P., Ojeda, V. D., Hiller, S., Stefancic, A., Tsemberis, S., & Palinkas, L. A. (2013). Variations in full service partnerships and fidelity to the Housing First model. *American Journal of Psychiatric Rehabilitation, 16*(4), 313–328.

Glassman, M., Karno, D., & Erdem, G. (2010). The problems and barriers of RHYA as social policy. *Children & Youth Services Review, 32*(6), 798–806.

Gomez, R., & Ryan, T. (2016). Speaking out: Youth led research as a methodology used with homeless youth. *Child & Adolescent Social Work Journal, 33*(2), 185–193.

Greene, J. M., & Ringwalt, C. L. (1998). Pregnancy among three national samples of runaway and homeless youth. *Journal of Adolescent Health, 23*(6), 370–377.

Gulcur, L., Stefancic, A., Shinn, M., Tsemberis, S., & Fischer, S. N. (2003). Housing, hospitalization, and cost outcomes for homeless individuals with psychiatric disabilities participating in Continuum of Care and Housing First programmes. *Journal of Community and Applied Social Psychology, 13*, 171–186.

Guo, X., & Slesnick, N. (2017). Reductions in hard drug use among homeless youth receiving a strength-based outreach intervention: Comparing the long-term effects of shelter linkage versus drop-in center linkage. *Substance Use & Misuse, 52*(7), 905–915.

Haley, N., Roy, E., Leclerc, P., Boudreau, J. F., & Boivin, J. F. (2004). HIV risk profile of male street youth involved in survival sex. *Sexually Transmitted Infections, 80*(6), 526–530.

Harris, T., Rice, E., Rhoades, H., Winetrobe, H., & Wenzel, S. (2017). Gender differences in the path from sexual victimization to HIV risk behavior among homeless youth. *Journal of Child Sexual Abuse, 26*(3), 334–351.

Heerde, J. A., & Hemphill, S. A. (2016). Sexual risk behaviors, sexual offenses, and sexual victimization among homeless youth. *Trauma, Violence and Abuse, 17*(5), 468–489.

Heerde, J. A., Scholes-Balog, K. E., & Hemphill, S. A. (2015). Associations between youth homelessness, sexual offenses, sexual victimization, and sexual risk behaviors: A systematic literature review. *Archives of Sexual Behavior, 44*(1), 181–212.

Hodgson, K. J., Shelton, K. H., & van den Bree, M. B. M. (2015). Psychopathology among young homeless people: Longitudinal mental health outcomes for different subgroups. *British Journal of Clinical Psychology, 54*(3), 307–325.

Holtschneider, C. (2016). From independence to interdependence: Redefining outcomes for transitional living programs for youth experiencing homelessness. *Families in Society: The Journal of Contemporary Social Services, 97*(3), 160–170.

Homeless Emergency Assistance and Rapid Transition to Housing (HEARTH) Act, enacted as part of the Helping Families Save Their Homes Act (42 U.S.C. § 11302).

Horwitz, B., Hinsz, J., Karczmar, A., Matjasko, J. L., Patel, S., & Vidis, J. (2018). *Conducting a youth count: A toolkit* (2nd ed.). Chicago: Chapin Hall at the University of Chicago. http://voicesofyouthcount.org/wp-content/uploads/2018/07/Voices-of-Youth-Count-Toolkit-2018-FINAL.pdf. Accessed 30 Mar 2019.

Jennings, L., Lee, N., Shore, D., Strohminger, N., Allison, B., Conserve, D. F., & Cheskin, L. J. (2016). U.S. minority homeless youth's access to and use of mobile phones: Implications for mHealth intervention design. *Journal of Health Communication, 21*(7), 725–733.

Jocoy, C. L. (2013). Counting the homeless: The culture of quantification in American social policy. *Cultural Geographies, 20*(3), 397–403.

Kennelly, J. (2015). 'You're making our city look bad': Olympic security, neoliberal urbanization, and homeless youth. *Ethnography, 16*(1), 3–24.

Kennelly, J. (2017). Symbolic violence and the Olympic Games: Low-income youth, social legacy commitments, and urban exclusion in Olympic host cities. *Journal of Youth Studies, 20*(2), 145–161.

Kennelly, J., & Watt, P. (2011). Sanitizing public space in Olympic host cities: The spatial experiences of marginalized youth in 2010 Vancouver and 2012 London. *Sociology, 45*(5), 765–781.

Keuroghlian, A. S., Shtasel, D., & Bassuk, E. L. (2014). Out on the street: A public health and policy agenda for lesbian, gay, bisexual, and transgender youth who are homeless. *American Journal of Orthopsychiatry, 84*(1), 66–72.

Kidd, S. A., & Scrimenti, K. (2004). Evaluating children and youth homelessness. *Evaluation Review, 28*(4), 325–341.

Kidd, S., Frederick, T., Karabanow, J., Hughes, J., Naylor, T., & Barbic, S. (2016). A mixed methods study of recently homeless youth efforts to sustain housing and stability. *Child and Adolescent Social Work Journal, 33*(3), 207–218.

Kidd, S. A., Vitopoulos, N., Frederick, T., Leon, S., Karabanow, J., & McKenzie, K. (2019). More than four walls and a roof needed: A complex tertiary prevention approach for recently homeless youth. *American Journal of Orthopsychiatry., 89*(2), 248–257.

Kim, S. (2014). A review of research on runaway and homeless youth: A comparison of trends between American and South Korean journals from 2001 to 2010. *Child & Adolescent Social Work Journal, 31*(2), 107–118.

Kingree, J. B., Stephens, T., Braithwaite, R., & Griffin, J. (1999). Predictors of homelessness among participants in a substance abuse treatment program. *American Journal of Orthopsychiatry, 69*(2), 261–266.

Kipke, M. D., Simon, T. R., Montgomery, S. B., Unger, J. B., & Iversen, E. F. (1997). Homeless youth and their exposure to and involvement in violence while living on the streets. *Journal of Adolescent Health, 20*(5), 360–367.

Koller, S. H., Raffaelli, M., & Carlo, G. (2012). Conducting research about sensitive subjects: The case of homeless youth. *Universitas Psychologica, 11*(1), 55–65.

Kominkiewicz, F. B. (2008). Freeing children to tell their stories: The utilization of person-centered and experiential psychotherapy in child welfare investigations. In M. Behr & J. Cornelius-White (Eds.), *Person-centered work with children, adolescents, parents and families*. Herefordshire: PCCS Books Ltd..

Kominkiewicz, F. B., & Kominkiewicz, L. K. (2008). The dynamics and ethics of community focus groups: Exploring the social justice issues of homeless youth/Die Dynamik und Ethik von Fokusgruppen in der Gemeinwesenarbeit, die sich mit dem Thema sozialer Gerechtigkeit für obdachlose Jugendliche auseinandersetzen. In *30th international symposium of the association of social work with groups conference paper publication (CD)*. Cologne.

Kroner, M. J. (1988). Living arrangement options for young people preparing for independent living. *Child Welfare: Journal of Policy, Practice, and Program, 67*(6), 547–561.

Levenson, J. (2017). Trauma-informed social work practice. *Social Work, 62*(2), 105–113.

Lightfoot, M., Stein, J. A., Tevendale, H., & Preston, K. (2011). Protective factors associated with fewer multiple problem behaviors among homeless/runaway youth. *Journal of Clinical Child and Adolescent Psychology, 40*(6), 878–889.

Lim, C., Rice, E., & Rhoades, H. (2016). Depressive symptoms and their association with adverse environmental factors and substance use in runaway and homeless youths. *Journal of Research on Adolescence (Wiley-Blackwell), 26*(3), 403–417.

Lyon-Callo, V. (2000). Medicalizing homelessness: The production of self-blame and self-governing within homeless shelters. *Medical Anthropology Quarterly, 14*(3), 328–345.

Mallett, S., Rosenthal, D., Myers, P., Milburn, N., & Rotheram-Borus, M. J. (2004). Practicing homelessness: A typology approach to young people's daily routines. *Journal of Adolescence, 27*(3), 337–349.

McAlpine, K., Henley, R., Mueller, M., & Vetter, S. (2010). A survey of street children in Northern Tanzania: How abuse or support factors may influence migration to the street. *Community Mental Health Journal, 46*(1), 26–32.

McNamara, R. H., Crawford, C., & Burns, R. (2013). Policing the homeless: Policy, practice, and perceptions. *Policing: An International Journal, 36*(2), 357–374.

Meade, M. A., & Slesnick, N. (2002). Ethical considerations for research and treatment with runaway and homeless adolescents. *The Journal of Psychology, 136*(4), 449–463.

Meadows-Oliver, M. (2006). Homeless adolescent mothers: A metasynthesis of their life experiences. *Journal of Pediatric Nursing, 21*(5), 340–349.

Middleton, J. S., Gattis, M. N., Frey, L. M., & Roe-Sepowitz, D. (2018). Youth Experiences Survey (YES): Exploring the scope and complexity of sex trafficking in a sample of youth experiencing homelessness. *Journal of Social Service Research, 44*(2), 141–157.

Morton, M. H., Dworsky, A., Matjasko, J. L., Curry, S. R., Schlueter, D., Chávez, R., & Farrell, A. F. (2018). Prevalence and correlates of youth homelessness in the United States. *Journal of Adolescent Health, 62*(1), 14–21.

Naidich, W. B., & Covenant House Nineline. (1988). *The host homes model of temporary emergency shelter*. New York: Covenant House.

National Center for Homeless Education. (2013). Housing and education collaborations to serve homeless children, youth, and families. Best practices in interagency collaboration brief series. National center for homeless education at SERVE. National Center for Homeless Education at SERVE. https://nche.ed.gov/wp-content/uploads/2018/10/hud.pdf. Accessed 30 Mar 2019.

National Center for Homeless Education. (2016). *Federal data summary: School years 2012–13 to 2014–15: Education for homeless children and youth*. Washington, DC: U.S. Department of Education. Accessed 11 Mar 2019.

National Conference of State Legislatures. (2016). Homeless and runaway youth. http://www.ncsl.org/research/human-services/homeless-and-runaway-youth.aspx. Accessed 30 June 2018.

National Network for Youth (NN4Y). (2019). Public policy. https://www.nn4youth.org/policy-advocacy/public-policy/fed-definitions-homeless-youth/#_ftn1. Accessed 11 Mar 2019.

Okamoto, Y. (2007). A comparative study of homelessness in the United Kingdom and Japan. *Journal of Social Issues, 63*(3), 525–542.

Parker, S., & Mayock, P. (2019). "They're Always Complicated but That's the Meaning of Family in My Eyes": Homeless youth making sense of "family" and family relationships. *Journal of Family Issues, 40*(4), 540–570.

Parks, R. W., Stevens, R. J., & Spence, S. A. (2007). A systematic review of cognition in homeless children and adolescents. *Journal of the Royal Society of Medicine, 100*(1), 46–50.

Pavlakis, A. (2014). Living and learning at the intersection: Student homelessness and complex policy environments. *Urban Review, 46*(3), 445–475.

Pears, J., & Noller, P. (1995). Youth homelessness: Abuse, gender, and the process of adjustment to life on the streets. *Australian Journal of Social Issues (Australian Council of Social Service), 30*(4), 405–424.

Popple, P., & Leighninger, L. (2019). *The policy-based profession: An introduction to social welfare policy analysis for social workers* (7th ed.). Boston: Pearson.

Quimby, E. G., Edidin, J. P., Ganim, Z., Gustafson, E., Hunter, S. J., & Karnik, N. S. (2012). Psychiatric disorders and substance use in homeless youth: A preliminary comparison of San Francisco and Chicago. *Behavioral Sciences (2076-328X), 2*(3), 186–194.

Ray, N. (2006). *An epidemic of homelessness: Lesbian, gay, bisexual, and transgender youth*. Washington, DC: National Gay and Lesbian Task Force Policy Institute.

Rew, L., Chambers, K. B., & Kulkarni, S. (2002). Planning a sexual health promotion intervention with homeless adolescents. *Nursing Research, 51*(3), 168–174.

Rhule-Louie, D., Bowen, S., Baer, J., & Peterson, P. (2008). Substance use and health and safety among homeless youth. *Journal of Child and Family Studies, 17*(3), 306–319.

Rice, E., & Barman, A. A. (2014). Internet and social media use as a resource among homeless youth. *Journal of Computer-Mediated Communication, 19*(2), 232–247.

Robertson, M. J., & Toro, P. A. (1999). Homeless youth: Research, intervention, and policy. In L. B. Fosburg & D. L. Dennis (Eds.), *Practical lessons: The 1998 National Symposium on Homelessness Research* (pp. 3-1-3-32). Washington, DC: U.S. Department of Housing and Urban Development and U.S. Department of Health and Human Services.

Robinson, B. A. (2018). Child welfare systems and LGBTQ youth homelessness: Gender segregation, instability, and intersectionality. *Child Welfare, 96*(2), 29–45.

Rosenthal, D., Mallett, S., & Myers, P. (2006). Why do homeless young people leave home? *Australian & New Zealand Journal of Public Health, 30*(3), 281–285.

Runaway and Homeless Youth Act, as amended and reauthorized by Reconnecting Homeless Youth Act, 42 U.S.C. § 5701 et seq.

Saewyc, E. M., & Edinburgh, L. D. (2010). Restoring healthy developmental trajectories for sexually exploited young runaway girls: Fostering protective factors and reducing risk behaviors. *Journal of Adolescent Health, 46*, 180–188.

Saldanha, K. (2017). It should not be a pit stop: Voices and perspectives of homeless youth on labeling and placement in special education. *Journal of Mental Health Research in Intellectual Disabilities, 10*(2), 55–73.

Saperstein, A. M., Lee, S., Ronan, E. J., Seeman, R. S., & Medalia, A. (2014). Cognitive deficit and mental health in homeless transition-age youth. *Pediatrics, 134*(1), e138–e145.

Schneider, M., Brisson, D., & Burnes, D. (2016). Do we really know how many are homeless?: An analysis of the point-in-time homelessness count. *Families in Society, 97*(4), 321–329.

Sheffield, J. J. (2015). Homeless Bills of Rights: Moving United States policy toward a human right to housing. *Georgetown Journal on Poverty Law and Policy, 22*(2), 321–353.

Slesnick, N., & Prestopnik, J. L. (2005). Ecologically based family therapy outcome with substance abusing runaway adolescents. *Journal of Adolescence, 28*(2), 277–298.

Slesnick, N., Kang, M. J., Bonomi, A. E., & Prestopnik, J. L. (2008). Six- and twelve-month outcomes among homeless youth accessing therapy and case management services through an urban drop-in center. *Health Services Research, 43*(1), 211–229.

Slesnick, N., Guo, X., Brakenhoff, B., & Bantchevska, D. (2015). A comparison of three interventions for homeless youth evidencing substance use disorders: Results of a randomized clinical trial. *Journal of Substance Abuse Treatment, 54*, 1–13.

Slesnick, N., Feng, X., Guo, X., Brakenhoff, B., Carmona, J., Murnan, A., et al. (2016a). A test of outreach and drop-in linkage versus shelter linkage for connecting homeless youth to services. *Prevention Science, 17*(4), 450–460.

Slesnick, N., Zhang, J., & Brakenhoff, B. (2016b). Homeless youths' caretakers: The mediating role of childhood abuse on street victimization and housing instability. *Social Work, 61*(2), 147–154.

Sommer, V.L. (1995). The ecological perspective. In M.J. Macy, N. Flax, V.L. Sommer, & R. Stoessen (2004, July). Collaborating with faith-based services. NASW News, p. 4.

Stefancic, A., & Tsemberis, S. (2007). Housing First for long-term shelter dwellers with psychiatric disabilities in a suburban county: A four-year study of housing access and retention. *The Journal of Primary Prevention, 28*(3–4), 265–279.

Stone, S., & Uretsky, M. (2016). School correlates of academic behaviors and performance among McKinney–Vento identified youth. *Urban Education, 51*(6), 600–628.

Substance Abuse and Mental Health Services Administration. (2014). *Trauma-informed care in behavioral health services: Treatment improvement protocol (TIP) series 57* [HHS Publication No. (SMA) 13-4801]. Rockville, MD.

Substance Abuse and Mental Health Services Administration. (2018). Adverse childhood experiences. https://www.samhsa.gov/capt/practicing-effective-prevention/prevention-behavioral-health/adverse-childhood-experiences. Last updated July 9, 2018.

Sullivan-Walker, M. E., Rock, M. L., & Popp, P. A. (2017). Meeting the needs of students with disabilities experiencing homelessness: Federal, community, and educator roles. *Preventing School Failure, 61*(2), 155–162.

Suppes, M. A., & Wells, C. C. (2018). *The social work experience: A case-based introduction to social work and social welfare*. New York: Pearson.

Thomas de Benitez, S., & Jones, G. A. (n.d.). Youth and the United Nations: Briefing note on youth on the streets. United Nations. http://www.un.org/esa/socdev/unyin/documents/briefingnotestreetyouth.pdf. Accessed 30 June 2018.

Thompson, S., Kim, J., McManus, H., Flynn, P., & Kim, H. (2007). Peer relationships: A comparison of homeless youth in the USA and South Korea. *International Social Work, 50*(6), 783–795.

Thompson, S. J., Bender, K. A., Lewis, C. M., & Watkins, R. (2008). Runaway and pregnant: Risk factors associated with pregnancy in a national sample of runaway/homeless female adolescents. *Journal of Adolescent Health, 43*(2), 125–132.

Thompson, S. J., Bender, K., Windsor, L., Cook, M. S., & Williams, T. (2010). Homeless youth: Characteristics, contributing factors, and service options. *Journal of Human Behavior in the Social Environment, 20*(2), 193–217.

Thompson, S. J., Bender, K., Ferguson, K. M., & Kim, Y. (2015). Factors associated with substance use disorders among traumatized homeless youth. *Journal of Social Work Practice in the Addictions, 15*(1), 66–89.

Townley, G., Pearson, L., Lehrwyn, J. M., Prophet, N. T., & Trauernicht, M. (2016). Utilizing participatory mapping and GIS to examine the activity spaces of homeless youth. *American Journal of Community Psychology, 57*(3/4), 404–414.

Tucker, J. S., Sussell, J., Golinelli, D., Zhou, A., Kennedy, D. P., & Wenzel, S. L. (2012). Understanding pregnancy-related attitudes and behaviors: A mixed-methods study of homeless youth. *Perspectives on Sexual and Reproductive Health, 44*(4), 252–261.

Tyler, K. A., & Schmitz, R. M. (2018). Child abuse, mental health and sleeping arrangements among homeless youth: Links to physical and sexual street victimization. *Children and Youth Services Review, 95*, 327–333.

Tyler, K. A., Schmitz, R. M., & Ray, C. M. (2018). Role of social environmental protective factors on anxiety and depressive symptoms among midwestern homeless youth. *Journal of Research on Adolescence (Wiley-Blackwell), 28*(1), 199–210.

U.S. Department of Housing and Urban Development (HUD). (2012). HUD exchange. Introductory Guide to the Continuum of Care (CoC) Program: 2012 Understanding the CoC Program and the requirements of the CoC Program Interim Rule https://www.hudexchange.info/resources/documents/CoCProgramIntroductoryGuide.pdf. Accessed 30 Mar 2019.

U.S. Department of Housing and Urban Development (HUD). (2018). *The 2018 Annual Homeless Assessment Report (AHAR) to Congress. Part 1: Point-in-time estimates of homelessness.* Washington, D.C.: Office of Community Planning and Development.

U.S. Department of Housing and Urban Development (HUD). (2019). HUD Exchange. Continuum of Care (CoC) Program Eligibility Requirements. https://www.hudexchange.info/programs/coc/coc-program-eligibility-requirements

U.S. Interagency Council on Homelessness. (2015). Opening doors: Federal strategic plan to end homelessness. https://www.usich.gov/resources/uploads/asset_library/USICH_OpeningDoors_Amendment2015_FINAL.pdf. Accessed 30 Mar 2019.

United Nations Human Rights Office of the High Commissioner. (2012). Protection and promotion of the rights of children working and/or living on the street . http://www.streetchildrenresources.org/wp-content/uploads/2013/07/OHCHR-protection-promotion.pdf. Accessed 30 June 2018.

van den Bree, M. B. M., Shelton, K., Bonner, A., Moss, S., Thomas, H., & Taylor, P. J. (2009). A longitudinal population-based study of factors in adolescence predicting homelessness in young adulthood. *Journal of Adolescent Health, 45*(6), 571–578.

Violence Against Women Act, 42 U.S.C. § 13701 et seq.

Vitopoulos, N., Cerswell Kielburger, L., Frederick, T. J., McKenzie, K., & Kidd, S. (2017). Developing a trauma-informed mental health group intervention for youth transitioning from homelessness. *Professional Psychology: Research and Practice, 48*(6), 499–509.

Washington State Department of Commerce. (2017). Research and recommendations on host home programs report on host home licensing exemption per RCW 74.15.020 and RCW 24.03.550. http://www.commerce.wa.gov/wp-content/uploads/2015/11/Commerce-Host-Homes-Report-2017.pdf. Accessed 29 Mar 2019.

Whitbeck, L. B., & Simons, R. L. (1993). A comparison of adaptive strategies and patterns of victimization among homeless adolescents and adults. *Violence and Victims, 8*(2), 135–152.

Whitbeck, L. B., Johnson, K. D., Hoyt, D. R., & Cauce, A. M. (2004). Mental disorder and comorbidity among runaway and homeless adolescents. *Journal of Adolescent Health, 35*(2), 132–140.

Wong, C. F., Clark, L. F., & Marlotte, L. (2016). The impact of specific and complex trauma on the mental health of homeless youth. *Journal of Interpersonal Violence, 31*(5), 831–854.

Wright, J. D., & Devine, J. A. (1995). Housing dynamics of the homeless: Implications for a count. *American Journal of Orthopsychiatry, 65*(3), 320–329.

Yoder, J. R., Bender, K., Thompson, S. J., Ferguson, K. M., & Haffejee, B. (2014). Explaining homeless youths' criminal justice interactions: Childhood trauma or surviving life on the streets? *Community Mental Health Journal, 50*(2), 135–144.

Yoshioka-Maxwell, A., & Rice, E. (2017). Exploring the impact of network characteristics on substance use outcomes among homeless former foster youth. *International Journal of Public Health, 62*(3), 371–378.

Yoshioka-Maxwell, A., & Rice, E. (2019). Exploring the relationship between foster care experiences and HIV risk behaviors among a sample of homeless former foster youth. *AIDS & Behavior, 23*(3), 792–801.

Zerger, S., Strehlow, A. J., & Gundlapalli, A. V. (2008). Homeless young adults and behavioral health: An overview. *American Behavioral Scientist, 51*(6), 824–841.

Zhang, J., & Slesnick, N. (2018). Substance use and social stability of homeless youth: A comparison of three interventions. *Psychology of Addictive Behaviors, 32*(8), 873–884.

Zhao, Q., Kim, B. K. E., Li, W., Hsiao, H.-Y., & Rice, E. (2018). Incarceration history, social network composition, and substance use among homeless youth in Los Angeles. *Journal of Addictive Diseases*, 1–13. https://doi.org/10.1080/10550887.2018.1545555

Chapter 16
Incorporating Youth Voice into Services for Young People Experiencing Homelessness

Jonah DeChants, Kimberly Bender, and Kelsey Stone

Introduction

Who Are Homeless Youth?

Homeless youth are young people who have no safe, permanent place to live. The McKinney-Vento Act (2002) has defined this term more technically as young people who lack a fixed, regular, adequate nighttime residence (42 USC § 11434a [2] [B]). Young people who are unable to live safely at home with their families leave home to find alternative living arrangements. Some will find shelter in formal services, such as emergency youth shelters or in transitional housing; some will sleep on a friend's or acquaintance's couch; and some will live on the streets, sleeping in abandoned buildings, cars, or parks. The age range varies slightly across definitions, but homeless youth are typically defined as adolescents or young adults up to age 25 who are homeless and living without their families (76 Fed. Reg. 233). Although capturing the exact number of homeless young people is difficult, estimates suggest there are approximately 1.6 million homeless young people under the age of 21 in the USA (Hammer et al. 2002; Ringwalt et al. 1998). This means that nearly one-quarter of individuals who are homeless are adolescents or emerging adults (Cauce et al. 2000), a substantial group to be certain.

There are many reasons young people become homeless. Despite common depictions of the adventuresome or rebellious traveler, only a small proportion of young people choose to leave home for aspirational reasons, seeking adventure, and novel social situations (Lindsey et al. 2000). For most, the process of leaving home

---

Electronic supplementary material: The online version of this chapter (https://doi.org/10.1007/978-3-030-03727-7_16) contains supplementary material, which is available to authorized users.

J. DeChants (✉) · K. Bender · K. Stone
University of Denver, Denver, CO, USA
e-mail: jonah.dechants@du.edu; kimberly.bender@du.edu

H. Larkin et al. (eds.), *Homelessness Prevention and Intervention in Social Work*, https://doi.org/10.1007/978-3-030-03727-7_16

is often contentious and difficult. The majority of young people leave home as a last resort, due to family conflict, abuse, and neglect (Lindsey et al. 2000; Rosenthal et al. 2006). For others, leaving home is not a choice. Their families force them to leave or abandon them (Dadds et al. 1993), or they are placed in out-of-home care by child welfare authorities and then run away from their placements (MacLean et al. 1999). Clearly, youth are not typically leaving in stable or safe living environments; rather, they are seeking refuge with few resources.

Challenges and Adversities

After becoming homeless, young people face many challenges and adversities. Attending traditional schools becomes difficult while homeless; many young people do not graduate from high school and are unable to seek higher education degrees (Thompson et al. 2001). Lacking not only education but also basic job-hire requirements, like identification cards, a mailing address, and clean clothes, makes seeking and acquiring formal employment challenging. With few opportunities for formal employment, many young people turn to informal means of making money (Ferguson et al. 2012). They may panhandle on the corner, sell stolen goods or drugs, or engage in sex in exchange for food or money (Halcón and Lifson 2004; Watson 2011). These alternative ways of generating income are termed survival behaviors, because young people engage in them in order to gain resources to survive on the streets; yet, such behaviors often place young people in precarious and dangerous situations. Furthermore, youth often find themselves without safe places to stay. Relying on strangers for help or sleeping in public spaces is risky. Homeless young people often experience discrimination, stigmatization, and marginalization from broader society, including harsh treatment or invisibility in their communities (Kidd 2007). These factors often result in homeless young people experiencing high rates of physical and sexual victimization at the hands of strangers and acquaintances (Stewart et al. 2004; Tyler and Beal 2010).

Considering the great adversity faced by homeless young people, it is not surprising that this group often struggles with higher rates of substance use and mental health problems (Medlow et al. 2014). Between 48% and 98% of young people experiencing homelessness report symptoms of mental health problems (Hodgson et al. 2013), with rates varying by problem type, including depression (23%; Whitbeck et al. 2000), post-traumatic stress disorder (24%; Bender et al. 2010), anxiety (32%; Slesnick and Prestopnik 2005), and conduct disorder (76%; Whitbeck et al. 2004). Some homeless youth engage in substance use to cope with these mental health symptoms, as well as the experience of being homeless more generally, and traumas they have faced while homeless. Youth report that such substances numb their emotional pain, help them escape traumatic thoughts, and make life more bearable in the moment. However, young people acknowledge such coping is temporary and often leads to bigger problems in the long run, including crime and difficulty exiting the streets (Bender et al. 2014).

Unfortunately, many young people are not engaged in regular mental health or substance use treatment while homeless. Some report a distrust of formal social service systems that can be seen as inflexible (De Rosa et al. 1999). Others suggest that experiences of discrimination and stigma not only worsen mental health symptoms (Kidd 2007) but also serve as barriers to help seeking (Hudson et al. 2010). Many times, untreated mental health and substance use problems impede young people's exiting homelessness for more stable housing (Fowler et al. 2009). This relationship is often reciprocal, where symptoms prevent them from working through service steps to achieve housing while, at the same time, their inability to access a stable place to live may exacerbate symptoms (Hodgson et al. 2013).

Strengths and Resiliencies

Despite facing such adversity and challenges, homeless young people have many personal strengths and great resiliency, which help them navigate their homeless situations. Indeed, many of the survival behaviors described above may seem dangerous or illegal to the housed community, but in fact are resilient ways of getting needs met (Ungar 2004). Young people are quite resourceful; they are adept at finding services, such as free food or shelter, and are wise in pooling their resources (Roebuck and Roebuck 2016). Street smarts, developed through experiencing homelessness, involve skills and knowledge in navigating situations with scarce resources and little formal help. Young people rely on street smarts to efficiently find resources by determining who they can and cannot trust to help (Bender et al. 2007).

Young people experiencing homelessness often pride themselves on being self-reliant and taking care of themselves (Lindsey et al. 2000; Roebuck and Roebuck 2016). This often involves a great deal of self-confidence, or belief in themselves (Lindsey et al. 2000), as well as boosted self-esteem, or liking themselves (McCay et al. 2010). Indeed, young people are found to have advanced life skills, acting independently to locate resources, solve problems, and care for their own health and well-being (Roebuck and Roebuck 2016). Such independence requires balancing multiple services and unreliable transportation options (Bender et al. 2007). Furthermore, in the face of struggle, many young people strive for a better life, relying on a positive outlook to stay motivated and persevere (McCay et al. 2010). Many are also adept at using coping skills, like reading, writing, and creative work, when times are rough (Thompson et al. 2016). Such self-reliance is associated with social distancing (Kolar et al. 2012), or separating oneself from peer groups and formal sources of help due to distrust. Yet, some research suggests that loneliness is not, in and of itself, associated with reduced resilience and may be adaptive or protective for young people who lack safe people to rely upon (Perron et al. 2014).

In addition to self-reliance, many young people do rely on others as sources of support and resource. While service providers and housed friends and family sometimes serve as supports, other homeless peers often provide a supportive network, sharing resources (Rew et al. 2001) and providing protection from harm (Greenblatt and Robertson 1993). Young people will form street families, even labeling members as street moms, dads, brother, or sisters. In this way, more experienced peers offer younger or less experienced youth protection and connection (Roebuck and Roebuck 2016). When young people describe their street families, they discuss finding a group of peers that can understand and validate their struggles while also providing information, access to resources, and someone who has their back when in danger (Bender et al. 2007). In addition to peers, companion animals (most often dogs) are seen as a significant source of motivation and comfort (Rew and Horner 2003; Thompson et al. 2016). Young people describe their dogs as the closest thing they have to family and a source of stability in otherwise unpredictable lives (Bender et al. 2007).

It is clear that young people navigating homelessness bring (or develop) considerable strengths and resiliencies that enable them to navigate tenuous and dangerous situations without the traditional care of family and institutions. Recognizing some of these resiliencies is essential for developing programs and services that honor the whole youth and capitalize on their innate strengths.

Approaches to Working with Youth Experiencing Homelessness

Traditional Services for Homeless Youth

Traditional services for homeless youth reflect many of the challenges and adversities experienced by homeless youth. Most services aim to meet young peoples' basic needs, namely, providing housing and food. Housing is provided in the form of emergency shelters that offer temporary housing (often in the form of dormitories), regular meals, and case management to help identify other useful resources. Young people typically stay for a month or two in a shelter, with some youth stopping in only for a night or two and others staying until they can find longer-term housing. Transitional housing programs, often offered in apartment settings, are provided to a subgroup of youth, typically those who have been successful in shelter services and have moved up on established waitlists. Transitional housing offers longer-term housing, typically 1–2 years, with the expectation that young people will work toward transitioning to more independent (non-subsidized) living situations.

Aside from housing, basic needs are often met through drop-in centers or outreach programs. These are less structured programs that provide young people with things like food, socks, bus tokens, showers, laundry, and sometimes case management. Young people can drop in to a common space for a few hours and get these immediate needs met. Or, alternatively, outreach workers will visit common gathering places (e.g., parks or camps) and offer resources in the community, hoping to connect young people to services.

Beyond basic needs, some programs do offer treatment or training to young people. Treatment often takes place in the context of specialized housing programs that enroll young people with identified needs. Such programs target specific challenges, such as substance abuse, mental health, HIV prevention/treatment, and sexual health (Slesnick et al. 2009). In addition, training programs offer educational and employment programming, helping young people to study for equivalency exams (i.e., GED), enroll in formal or alternative education programs, search for jobs, develop resumes, and prepare for job interviews.

Traditional services are well-meaning and provide important resources, but they are limited in scope and approach. They tend to focus primarily on basic needs, offering housing, food, or clothing, rather than providing services more holistically by acknowledging other developmental needs, areas of personal growth, or the need for relationships and personal connection. In addition, traditional services tend to be provided from a deficit perspective, focusing on what youth lack or need help with rather than acknowledging and building upon their strengths, capabilities, or resiliencies. Such services also tend to be adult-led, with adults in charge of providing help or services to youth rather than young people sharing power and contributing to decision-making. These limitations are reflected in many service systems for marginalized or low-income youth. These systems tend to approach young people either as victims, who have faced adversity and need help, or as problems that require structure and consequences, rather than recognizing their strengths and resiliencies and promoting their holistic health and well-being (Cheon 2008).

Whether due to lack of funding to support alternative service approaches or difficulty breaking from the dominant service paradigm, limitations in traditional services can have significant consequences. It is often challenging to engage young people in these traditional services (Brooks et al. 2004; Feldmann and Middleman 2003), and such services are somewhat limited in their long-term effects (Pollio et al. 2006). This suggests room for improvement in the way most agencies approach youth homelessness. Young people are often hesitant to engage in traditional services (Hudson et al. 2010). After many negative or traumatic experiences with adults in their pasts, they may be distrustful of adults in authoritative positions (Collins and Barker 2009); such distrust leads to poor follow-through in attending services or completing tasks, power struggles, and frustration on the part of service providers (Auerswald and Eyre 2002). Furthermore, inexperience in the communication, organizational, or time management tasks required to engage in services effectively may lead to unsuccessful uptake of traditional case management approaches that can to be more task-oriented rather than relationship-based.

Limited research is available that examines the effectiveness of traditional programming. Some preliminary research suggests that drop-in centers may help to re-engage disconnected youth, but it is not clear whether such services truly reintegrate young people into mainstream society (Slesnick et al. 2009). Limited studies on traditional shelter services show that there are some immediate benefits on important outcomes, including education, employment, substance use, and emotional problems. However, these positive benefits may be short-lived, with some evidence that they fade over time (Pollio et al. 2006). These findings suggest that services that aim to meet the immediate needs (e.g., food, clothing, shelter) of young people are necessary and helpful, but other approaches may be important to truly engage young people in making real changes in their lives and their situations.

Such approaches, labeled as *youth voice* in this chapter, focus on developing young people holistically, recognizing their need for skill- and relationship-building, acknowledging the goals youth have beyond meeting their basic needs, and partnering with youth to accomplish those goals. Such approaches may prioritize building trust and rapport with young people by establishing them as partners in agency programming and processes. Three alternative approaches are particularly helpful in thinking about expanding youth voice in services for homeless young people: positive youth development, empowerment practice, and trauma-informed care.

Frameworks for Bringing Youth Voice into Services for Young People Experiencing Homelessness

Positive Youth Development

Positive youth development (PYD) is a framework that focuses on youth development through the promotion of positive experiences, assets, and opportunities. Typically, approaches to working with youth focus on deficits and risk factors rather than protective factors. Positive youth development aims to increase protective factors through a collaborative approach that involves a wide variety of relationships and support networks, including families, schools, and communities. The central theme of positive youth development is that "problem free isn't fully prepared" (Benson et al. 2006, p. 895). There are several features essential to carrying out services with a PYD approach, including physical and psychological safety, appropriate structure, supportive relationships, opportunities to belong, positive social norms, support for efficacy and mattering, and opportunities for skill building (Eccles and Gootman 2002).

Youth must feel *physically and psychologically safe* in a service setting for positive youth development to take place. PYD settings must be free of violence, unsafe behaviors, and health or environmental hazards and should provide structure and support to promote safe behaviors and positive peer interactions (Eccles and Gootman 2002). PYD programs must also provide appropriate structure, which consists of clear and consistent rules, predictability, and clear boundaries. Such structure helps to create a sense of safety for young people.

Supportive relationships, central to the PYD approach, consist of warmth, connectedness, good communication, responsiveness, and guidance. Research shows that supportive adult relationships can lead to an increase in motivation, self-esteem, and self-efficacy (Eccles and Gootman 2002). For young people experiencing homelessness, supportive, caring relationships with staff are key factors driving satisfaction with homeless services (Heinze and Hernandez Jozefowicz-Simbeni 2009). Young people search for meaningful connections with service providers, citing relationships with individual staff members as critical to their success (Gharabaghi and Stuart 2010).

It is also important for PYD programs to create *opportunities to belong* and *opportunities for skill building*. In order to create these opportunities, programs should strive to be inclusive spaces, regardless of youths' gender identification, sexual orientation, race, ethnicity, religious or spiritual affiliation, etc. Programs should also provide opportunities for youth to learn physical, social, and intellectual skills in order to adequately prepare them for adulthood. Opportunities to belong can also be promoted through positive social norms, another tenet of PYD programs. *Positive social norms* can be created through clear and consistent rules for behavior and through the creation of a clear group identity or culture. Finally, PYD programs should incorporate opportunities for self-efficacy and mattering (i.e., being taken seriously, having influence, feeling important). This can be achieved through allowing youth to have a voice in the structure of the program and encouraging youth to take an active role in making changes to their community. PYD programs can also provide youth with meaningful challenges and allow youth to take responsibility and be taken seriously by adults. These practices can empower youth and create an environment that encourages and supports youth voice (Eccles and Gootman 2002).

One key aspect of positive youth development is the focus on protective factors, rather than risk factors, and working to enhance those protective factors. This framework aligns well with the strengths-based perspective discussed above, as it asserts that all youth have the ability to achieve positive development. PYD also states that youth must have an active role in their development and, when given the opportunity, are often able to create the necessary environments for this positive development (Benson et al. 2006).

Positive youth development has been recognized as a key policy priority in recent years, although it has not been fully integrated into traditional services. The Administration for Children and Families, for example, has developed the National Clearinghouse on Families and Youth and resource guides (e.g., Putting Positive Youth Development into Practice) for implementing PYD in services to vulnerable youth and families, including runaway and homeless youth. Yet, more can be done. Homeless young people often score lower on domains of youth development compared to samples of youth who are housed (Heinze 2013). Whether due to the lack of training, resources, or priority, building youths' assets from a PYD perspective has not been fully embraced in services nationally.

Empowerment Practice

The core concepts of empowerment practice are equity, ownership, partnership, and accountability. When discussing empowerment practice, *equity* is achieved by establishing mutual respect for all individuals and valuing collective effort toward a shared goal; it can be achieved by providing youth with the opportunity to make an impact or contribution to their situation or environment (Larkin et al. 2008). The concept of *ownership* consists of the recognition that an individual or group of individuals is connected to their agency or environment and can make a lasting and impactful change to their environment. *Partnership* consists of mutual respect, communication, and collaboration. Finally, *accountability* is the willingness of an individual or group of individuals to take on responsibility for the collective functioning of their agency or environment (Larkin et al. 2008).

When working with youth, the goal of empowerment practice is to redistribute the power within the organization or agency, increase youth's belief in their ability to change their environment or situation, create shifts within the community, and allow youth to have a voice and an impact on their situation (Ferguson et al. 2011). Youth often feel that top administrative staff and key decision-makers do not truly understand them and their needs (Ferguson et al. 2011). Many youth report feeling frustrated that they have not met the top administrative staff at the agency (Ferguson et al. 2011). Unfortunately, ratings of empowerment are often significantly lower among youth experiencing homelessness compared to their housed counterparts in schools (Heinze 2013).

Strategies to increase partnership when working with youth could include establishing a youth mentorship program, having staff and youth work together on a council or advisory board, or allowing youth to participate in staff meetings at the agency. Such strategies allow youth to ask one another questions that they may not feel comfortable asking staff and allow youth to serve as resources for one another. Additionally, using these strategies could increase communication and collaboration between youth and program staff, as youth bring concerns to staff and administrators. This process may also increase a sense of community and collaboration between youth, as they are able to provide peer support to one another (Heinze et al. 2010).

Critical youth empowerment encourages young people to be involved in making changes in their environment, whether in organizations, neighborhoods, or the broader community, by challenging the power imbalances inherent in these systems. To engage young people in critical youth empowerment, adults must create a safe and welcoming environment that allows for meaningful participation by youth who partner with adults. As a team, they engage in critical reflection followed by participation in processes that effect change at the individual or community level (Jennings et al. 2006). Programs based on this model engage youth in social justice work, with young people thinking critically about the norms, values, structures, and root causes leading to inequalities. Critical empowerment practices move services from a focus solely on meeting basic needs to recognizing that homeless young people have many significant nonmaterial needs relating to facing exclusion from society and encountering regular experiences of stigma and blame (Watson and Cuervo 2017). Empowerment practice can help young people label these experiences and join others in acting against these injustices.

Trauma-Informed Care

The relatively recent movement toward trauma-informed care in services for homeless youth moves organizations beyond meeting crisis-oriented basic needs. Trauma-informed care involves recognizing the impact of trauma in young peoples' lives and structuring programming intentionally to address trauma symptoms through strengths-based, safe, empowering services (Hopper et al. 2010). One key principle of trauma-informed care is *trauma awareness*, which means that agency staff is aware of how young people's behaviors may represent symptoms in response to traumatic experiences. Agencies may screen for trauma experiences, may offer trauma-specific interventions, and may train all staff in the common symptoms of trauma and appropriate responses when faced with these symptoms. Another key principle, *safety,* emphasizes that organizations should strive to create physically and emotionally safe environments, including avoiding triggers and re-traumatization by having transparent boundaries and rules. Safety also involves developing mutually respectful, authentic, and nonjudgmental relationships, establishing privacy and confidentiality policies, and delivering culturally competent services (Hopper et al. 2010). Trauma-informed care also stresses the importance of *consumer control and empowerment*, creating predictable environments in which young people have a choice and efficacy to make decisions that they feel are best for them. To create this sense of control, trauma-informed care models encourage the sharing of power between staff and consumers in designing, running, and evaluating programming (Hopper et al. 2010). Finally, trauma-informed care models advocate for a *strengths-based approach* that, rather than focusing on deficits, helps youth identify and build upon their own strengths, building skills, and enhancing hope for the future (Hopper et al. 2010).

Overlap in Alternative Approaches

One may notice that there are commonalities across the three approaches described here. Indeed, these three approaches are not mutually exclusive; they overlap in several key ways (See Fig. 16.1). All three frameworks emphasize establishing a safe and welcoming environment as the foundation of all effective relationships and programming. Clients and staff cannot work together if youth do not feel safe in the program or physical space where services are offered. Safety includes psychological and emotional dimensions, with trauma-informed care placing special attention on minimizing reminders of past traumas. All three frameworks emphasize creating opportunities for authentic and nonjudgmental relationship building between youth, their peers, and adult staff. PYD and empowerment practice note that these relationships can be opportunities for adult staff to share power with youth clients, giving youth a stronger sense of belonging and investment in the program. These three models also all focus on individuals' skills and a sense of self-efficacy, while acknowledging the strengths and skills that youth already possess.

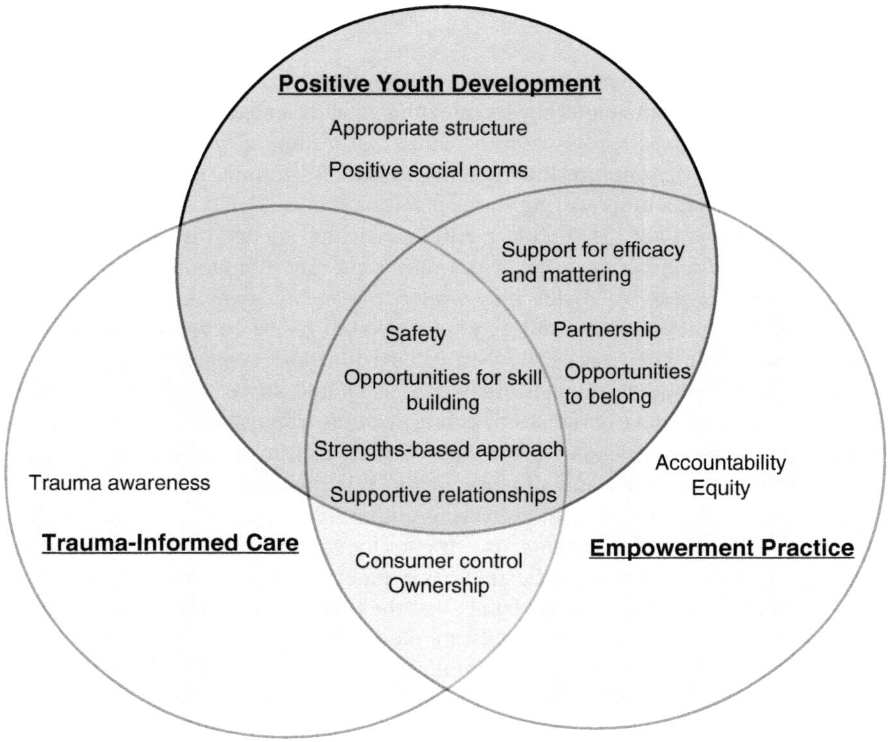

Fig. 16.1 Overlap of key constructs of positive youth development, trauma-informed, and empowerment frameworks

PYD and empowerment practice, however, extend trauma-informed care in several directions critical to serving young people experiencing homelessness. First, PYD emphasizes belonging and positive norms, stressing the importance of community to adolescents and emerging adults. Empowerment approaches broaden self-efficacy to include equitable power sharing and leadership on the part of young people. Both PYD and empowerment practice recognize the importance of giving youth opportunities for leadership and decision-making within any organization or program that serves them.

Thus, integration of these three frameworks may result in the most promising approach for working with homeless young people. Because these approaches are somewhat inconsistent with traditional methods of service-delivery, which have historically been deficit-based, individually-oriented, and adult-led, they may require adjustments to existing service models. Adults working with youth experiencing homelessness should make sure they are creating safe, welcoming environments. Adults should address youths' unique developmental needs to understand who they are in the context of others and to be nurtured through community building, skill development, and authentic relationship development. Programs for homeless youth should empower youth to build believe in themselves as individuals and to share power with adults, including the organization and broader society. With their own expert knowledge of life on the streets and their own needs, young people can inform programming and advocate for changes in policy and social climate.

Evidence Supporting Youth Voice Approaches

Existing research on youth voice approaches, including PYD and empowerment practice, have shown that these frameworks offer promise in promoting positive outcomes for youth in broad service settings (Jelicic et al. 2007). For young people who participate in PYD and empowerment programs, the psychological benefits include feelings of competence, autonomy, and the belief that one can have an impact (Larkin et al. 2008). Such benefits are associated with promotion of adolescent health and well-being (Gavin et al. 2010).

A relatively smaller, yet promising, body of literature examines youth voice practices in shelter and housing programs for youth. This research suggests that PYD programming with youth experiencing homelessness has been associated with higher levels of youth satisfaction with shelter services, greater self-esteem, and increased healthy behavior (Heinze et al. 2010). Specifically, Heinze and colleagues found that the PYD practices that provide appropriate structure (i.e., having clear rules and organized programs), a sense of belonging, and positive social norms (i.e., encouraging youth as they develop new skills or positive habits) were associated with higher reported client satisfaction with services (Heinze et al. 2010). These findings are similar to the work by Leonard et al. (2017), which found that service approaches that prioritize opportunities for youth to participate in governance are associated with greater program engagement. Given that youth experiencing homelessness are generally considered to be a difficult to reach population, increased client satisfaction may lead to greater engagement and retention in agency services and increased likelihood of reaching goals (Ferguson et al. 2011). Furthermore, young people who, through engaging with PYD and empowerment approaches, develop greater self-esteem may be less likely to engage in maladaptive coping behaviors, such as substance use (Dumont and Provost 1999).

One form of research that embraces a critical empowerment perspective, and has shown positive outcomes, is youth participatory action research (YPAR). YPAR is a research methodology that involves partnering with youth as co-researchers who collect information, analyze that information, and make recommendations for change (Cammarota and Fine 2010). Youth come together to determine a question about a social problem, gather and analyze information about that problem, and then share their results or advocate for action about the problem (Ozer and Douglas 2015). Photovoice, one YPAR method that involves collecting and analyzing data by taking photos of the community or surrounding environment, has been found to be a particularly useful way of engaging youth in research and social advocacy (Wang and Burris 1997; Wang 2006). Photovoice research gathers together members of a community and asks them to take photos of an issue within that community. Participants then analyze the photos through group discussion and collaboratively develop strategies for addressing the issue. Participatory action research and photovoice activities can also create opportunities for youth to take on leadership and decision-making roles within a project, organization, or broader social action in the community. These methods of engagement are particularly relevant for unstably housed youth who face the social problem of homelessness every day and who encounter a great deal of societal stigma and structural barriers to success.

While some may feel that homeless youth are too busy trying to meet their basic needs to engage in research or social advocacy, research indicates that homeless youth are in fact interested in, and motivated to participate in, research and social action (Gomez and Ryan 2016; Bender, Begun et al. 2018). Similar to other youth populations, young people experiencing homelessness are interested in having greater voice in both the agencies that serve them and the broader community (Ferguson et al. 2011). While it is certainly difficult to engage youth living in unstable housing in long-term research projects, evidence suggests that such research projects are feasible with youth living in emergency shelter (Bender, Barman-Adhikari et al. 2017). In fact, youth report that their interest in working toward social change is a key motivating factor to participate in a long-term project (Bender, Begun et al. 2018). Youth who participate in action research report feeling grateful for the opportunity to work toward social change and use their voices (Gomez and Ryan 2016).

Participation in photovoice is associated with positive outcomes for youth. One 3-month photovoice project found youth who participated showed improvements on standardized ratings of social connectedness and resiliency and reported increased ability to work through problems with others (Bender, Barman-Adhikari et al. 2017). Youth photovoice participants also report feeling empowered and respected when they present their research projects with people outside of the project (e.g., the general public, decision-makers) (Bender, Barman-Adhikari et al. 2017; Gomez and Ryan 2016). Such benefits are consistent with participatory methodologies that prioritize offering youth experiencing homelessness the opportunity to work together and build relationships with peers and adult facilitators while working toward change. An example of how photovoice has been used to empower homeless youth to engage in research and social action can be found in the text box below. While youth experiencing homelessness do face a variety of challenges in participating in research, participatory action research methodologies such as photovoice, which engage youth as co-researchers and co-creators of knowledge, offer exciting opportunities for youth to work together with their peers and adult facilitators to investigate problems and develop solutions, while gaining important skills and contributing to social change.

***Asking for Change*: A Photovoice Case Example**

Asking for Change is a collaborative project between Urban Peak, an agency that serves homeless youth, and the University of Denver's Graduate School of Social Work (GSSW). Faculty and students from GSSW work with Urban Peak's emergency shelter staff to run several photovoice projects for youth residents of the shelter. For 2 months, youth and adult facilitators met and collaborated on a photovoice project. Adult facilitators intentionally encouraged youth to lead the group whenever possible and empowered youth to make relevant decisions about the group's procedures and goals. Participants first established themselves as a group, setting group norms and participating in ice breaker activities to get to know one another. They then took basic photography classes, learning how to operate digital tablets, how to compose photographs, and about photographic ethics. The group then collectively decided on the themes they wanted to explore with their photography: barriers to services, stereotypes about homeless youth, feeling bored, and a sense of belonging. Each week, youth took photos and discussed how their photos represented the themes. Participants analyzed the photos collectively, discussing the root causes of the problems in their community. Youth prepared a public gallery event to showcase their work. They gathered and edited their photos, wrote captions explaining their relation to the themes, and prepared a short presentation. The gallery event was held at a local cafe and attended by many members of the larger Denver community. At the event, youth presented their photographs and talked about how it felt to be a homeless young person. They expressed gratitude that so many people were willing to listen to their stories and explained that participating in the *Asking for Change* project had given them more confidence to speak up on social issues, particularly homelessness. Youth participants also reported a significant increase in personal connections with their peers in the group and the adult facilitators (Bender, Barman-Adhikari et al. 2017; Bender, Begun et al. 2018). Urban Peak and GSSW continue to run the *Asking for Change* program, with hopes of integrating its elements of power sharing, empowerment, and social action further into shelter programming.

Figure 16.2 is a photo taken by an Asking for Change participant. The caption read, "I'm the chair, and I'm in the room, and I feel alone. I'm by myself, and no one understands me. The chair is dilapidated, and it's been worn, and that's how I feel. But at the same time, I'm still the chair that's able to stand whenever the weight drags down on me."

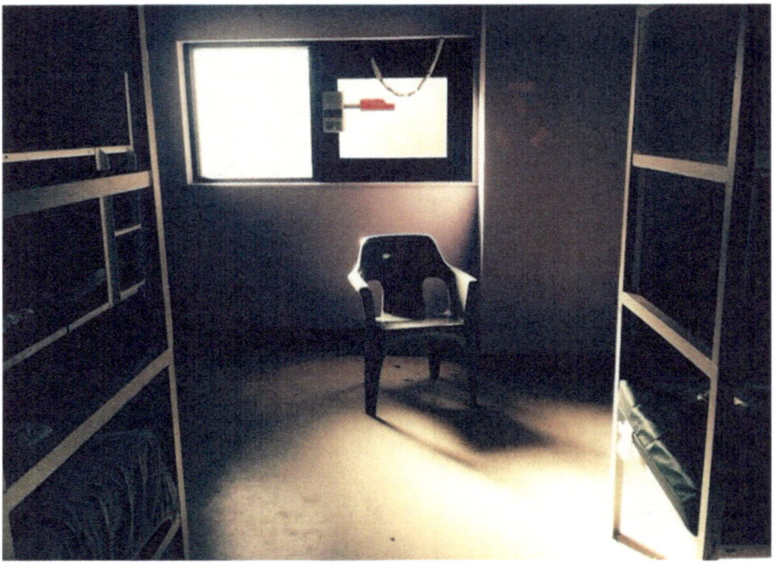

Fig. 16.2 Photo taken by *Asking for Change* participant

Practical Strategies for Empowering Homeless Youth

By now, one may be thinking that youth voice approaches, such as PYD, empowerment practices, and trauma-informed care, seem useful in working with young people experiencing homelessness. But, how does one go about integrating such practices into their work? A recent study investigated how PYD can be successfully implemented in a youth shelter setting and found three necessary ingredients: (1) the establishment of nonjudgmental, supportive relationships; (2) youth-driven goals and expectations; and (3) institutional practices and policies that prioritize safety and youth involvement (Leonard et al. 2017). According to Leonard et al. (2017), PYD can be successfully integrated when agency staff carefully develop supportive relationships with youth by respecting youths' autonomy by inviting youth to engage but not forcing or cajoling them. Youth appreciate staff's lack of judgment (Leonard et al. 2017). Furthermore, PYD can be successfully implemented when youths' needs are considered at all levels of policy and procedure development. For example, the agency under study decided to decline funding from certain sources that required the agency to describe their youth clients as "delinquent" (Leonard et al. 2017). Such decisions and priorities, supported by both agency staff and administration, allow for the implementation of the PYD framework in a hectic shelter environment with homeless youth.

There are a number of specific strategies individual providers, organizations, and policymakers can use to embrace and integrate youth voice practices into youth homelessness services. Table 16.1 provides some suggested strategies organized by

Table 16.1 Strategies for incorporating youth voice in services for homeless youth

Strategy	Description	Relevant constructs of PYD, empowerment practice, and trauma-informed care (see Fig. 16.1)
	Macro practice	
Funders require grantees to demonstrate incorporation of empowerment/PYD elements in services	Funders of homeless youth programming should require their grantees to incorporate elements of PYD into their agency services. Funders should offer technical assistance to help grantees implement these changes well	All constructs
Conduct organizational self-assessments	It is sometimes difficult for organizations to reflect accurately on the degree to which they are or are not empowering young people. Using standardized self-assessments can make this reflection more objective and informative. For example, the Youth Program Quality Assessment, published by the Forum for Youth Investment (Weikart 2012), provides questions that, through observation, can determine whether an agency is establishing a safe environment; a supportive environment; positive interactions of belonging, collaboration, and leadership; and engagement of youth in planning, choice, and reflection. Such assessments can help an agency identify areas of strength and areas for growth and to monitor progress over time	All constructs
Allocate more funding for staff time	Practicing PYD and building supportive relationships with youth requires significant time. Many current housing service agencies force front-line staff to be crisis-oriented, focusing on meeting basic needs. Providing funding for more staff would allow staff to dedicate time to getting to know youth and building relationships	Supportive relationships Opportunities to belong Emphasis on safety Safe and welcoming environment
Create physical spaces that are conducive to community building and privacy	Shelters and drop-in centers can be stressful places, as staff and youth work to address urgent needs in often cramped and crowded facilities. Service providers can consider the needs of youth clients as they design the layout of their physical plans. Does the agency feel inviting for youth as they enter? Are there communal spaces where youth and staff can congregate and socialize? Are there spaces where youth can have privacy when needed? Are sleeping spaces and bathrooms designed to create safe spaces for youth with various gender identities?	Physical and psychological safety Supportive relationships Opportunities to belong

Table 16.1 (continued)

Strategy	Description	Relevant constructs of PYD, empowerment practice, and trauma-informed care (see Fig. 16.1)
Develop youth councils or include youth in agency governance	Youth should have a say in how the agencies that serve them are governed. Youth councils, or spaces for youth to gather and discuss issues that are important to them and changes they would like to make to agency policies or practices, are one way to give youth voice. Youth representatives can also be included in existing agency boards or committees. Youth councils and representatives should be given real reasonability and power; they shouldn't simply be tokens whose opinions are not considered and put into action	Opportunities for efficacy and mattering Opportunities for skill building Authentic youth leadership and partnership Emphasis on equity and ownership
Assure that youth are involved in hiring decisions	In addition to youth councils or representatives, youth can provide input in who the agency hires. Whether the position is for a case manager who will be working with youth every day or for a marketing director who will present the face of the agency to the larger community, youth deserve the opportunity to assess candidates. Doing so is likely to result in selection of adult staff members who embrace a positive perspective of young people and their abilities; it will also likely disrupt the "us vs. them" mentality between staff and youth	Opportunities for efficacy and mattering Opportunities for skill building Power sharing
	Mezzo practice	
Require PYD and trauma-informed training for all agency staff	All agency staff should be trained in PYD, or other methods of youth empowerment, and trauma-informed care. This training should be ongoing so that new staff will be informed and issues that arise in the agency can be addressed. PYD practices may also be included in staff assessment and evaluation	Trauma awareness Awareness of adultism
Supports for staff	Working with youth in crisis is not easy. Practicing PYD can be difficult and emotionally tiring. Agencies should set up supports for staff, such as groups where staff can discuss their stressors and seek advice and support	Supportive relationships Positive social norms

Schedule time for informal staff-youth bonding	It takes time to build authentic, supportive relationships between adult staff and youth clients. Agencies can schedule time for youth and staff to "hang out" informally to get to know each other and develop those relationships. Examples could include watching a movie together, going on an outing, or playing board or video games. Youth should be consulted about how they would like to spend this time	Supportive relationships Opportunities to belong Positive social norms Community building
Give choice in assigning case managers	When possible, youth should be given a choice about which staff they work with most closely. While it is not always possible to honor every request, asking for input and preferences will give youth a sense of agency and can facilitate a stronger relationship between youth clients and adult staff	Appropriate structure Supportive relationships Opportunities for efficacy and mattering
Maximize contributions of volunteers	Staff members are not the only adults with whom youth can form meaningful relationships. Agencies can organize volunteer or mentor programs where adults regularly spend time with youth, getting to know them and forming relationships. Agencies should be sure to train these adults in PYD principles, ask that volunteers commit to a significant period of time (e.g., 6 months), and ensure that they are interacting with youth in a respectful and empowering way. Having "hang out" volunteers will increase positive interactions with adults in the context of the agency	Supportive relationships Opportunities to belong Positive social norms Community building
Provide opportunities for peer mentoring	Youth can be powerful supports and mentors for one another. Agencies can create programs where youth who have been engaged with the agency for an extended period of time take on leadership roles with increased responsibility. For example, youth who have been at a shelter for several months can provide tours or orientation for youth who have just arrived. For the more experienced youth, this is an opportunity to learn skills and have a sense of ownership. For new youth, this is an opportunity to feel welcomed, connected, and to learn about the norms of the agency	Appropriate structure Opportunities for efficacy and mattering Opportunities for skill building Authentic youth leadership and partnership
Involve youth in policy implementation	Youth can and should have leadership opportunities in implementing or enforcing agency policies. For example, some youth may be responsible for supervising other youth as they complete chores or other responsibilities. Agencies may create a restorative justice or peer mediation program where youth consider how to enforce consequences for violations of the rules. Again, this is an opportunity for youth who are peer leaders to gain important skills like communication and facilitation. For non-leader youth it is an opportunity to feel like they are being held accountable by their peers rather than by arbitrary rules or adults	Appropriate structure Opportunities for skill building Emphasis on equity and ownership

(continued)

Table 16.1 (continued)

Strategy	Description	Relevant constructs of PYD, empowerment practice, and trauma-informed care (see Fig. 16.1)
	Micro practice	
Create feedback check-ins during case management sessions	In addition to setting goals and making referrals, case managers should make a habit of starting sessions by checking in with the youth and asking for feedback. Asking how they feel their case management is going and if there is anything they would like to do differently signals to the youth that their opinions matter and that the case manager is there to listen to them and support them. It also serves to build relationship with young people	Opportunities for efficacy and mattering Supportive relationships Safe and welcoming environment
Share highs and lows	Agencies can incorporate the sharing of "highs and lows" (e.g., sharing one bad thing that happened that day and one good thing) into meal times or other regular gatherings. Giving youth a space to talk about their lives outside of their case plan or their housing needs helps everyone at the agency get to know one another and support each other. Agency staff should also, with intention, share *their* highs and lows so that youth can learn more about their lives outside of work	Appropriate structure Positive social norms Community building Opportunity to belong
Provide groups or social activities	Homeless youth are still youth. Like their housed peers, they should have opportunities to socialize or connect with one another. Housing agencies can organize groups (e.g., art workshops) or social activities (e.g., bowling, movies), which are opportunities to build skills, socialize, and connect. These groups or events give youth something to do, they allow youth and staff to get to know one another and build relationships, they help youth develop skills, and they allow youth to have some of the typical social experiences of other young people their age	Appropriate structure Opportunities to belong Positive social norms Opportunity for skill building Opportunity to belong
Use youth participatory action research projects to understand youths' needs and perspectives	Research projects co-led by youth and staff can help young people develop interpersonal and leadership skills while also providing valuable information to the agency. These projects offer a critical lens, helping youth analyze issues within their communities, or the organizations serving them, and develop recommendations for change. Such recommendations should be carefully considered by the agency and used to guide improvements in policy and programming	Critical analysis of sociopolitical and interpersonal process Opportunity for skill building

Recognize when youth are succeeding	Agencies should recognize youth who are making effort toward their goals (e.g., applying for a job), those who are succeeding in reaching accomplishments (e.g., getting a job), and those who are contributing positively to the agency culture (e.g., supporting a peer in their job search). This recognition can be formal, such as awarding a youth with a certificate for their accomplishments, or informal, such as thanking a youth for helping a peer. This positive recognition is a key component of PYD practice but can be difficult to implement in the rush of crisis-oriented services. Staff may need support and prompting from the agency in order to make time for this recognition	Appropriate structure Positive social norms Supportive relationships Opportunity to belong
Use person-first language	Because young people are more than their homelessness status, it is important to use language that recognizes them first as a person and secondarily as a person in a homeless situation. When addressing youth directly, or when discussing youth with others, say "youth or young adults experiencing homelessness" rather than "homeless youth"	Safe and welcoming environment Opportunities for efficacy and mattering Positive social norms

macro, mezzo, and micro practice levels. For each suggested strategy, a brief description is provided and the theoretical tenets underpinning this practice are noted. This list is by no means comprehensive. Strategies suggested here should be viewed as starting points for dialogues with colleagues and administrators about how their work with young people experiencing homelessness can incorporate youth voice principles in specific service settings. Strategies may need to be adapted, refined, or added in order to effectively integrate youth voice practices that fit the resources, missions, and clientele served in different settings.

Conclusion

Young people experiencing homelessness overcome great adversity by relying on internal strengths and adept navigation of resources and informal networks. The traditional services are set up to offer immediate resources that meet basic needs – important services that help young people eat, stay warm, and sleep in safe environments. Yet, expanding these service approaches to serve young people more holistically, harnessing strengths and partnering with youth as experts in their own lives, may serve to more deeply engage them in making longer-term changes in their lives. Together, positive youth development, empowerment practice, and trauma-informed care point to key principles for helping young people, including the importance of creating safe and welcoming spaces, developing authentic relationships, building skills and self-efficacy, focusing on strengths, and sharing power with young people. These approaches offer practical solutions for integrating youths' voices and perspectives into shelter, housing, and support services.

Agencies and individual providers can use a number of strategies to enhance their empowerment work with young people. They can begin on a macro level to establish systems of assessment, staff hiring, and governance that promote youth voice and choice. At the mezzo level, they can develop programming and policies that increase opportunities for adults to develop authentic relationships with young people and for young people to influence the workings of the agency. Finally, micro strategies allow empowerment through every individual interaction with young people, from how they are greeted and how they have fun to how adults notice their experiences and successes.

Implementing such strategies will require a committed, intentional process of organizational change. The process may begin by gathering adults with power and seeking partners invested in empowering young people. With investment of key administrators and staff members, a next step could be to assess the current organizational culture and services. Using standardized measures of program quality (e.g., Youth Program Quality Assessment; Developmental Assets Profile; Supports and Opportunities Scale) will help to identify ways the agency can grow to provide positive programming for youth. The agency should set goals related to areas of improvement. Key areas of growth should be targeted through organization-wide trainings in positive youth development, empowerment practices, and trauma-informed care.

Together, administrators, staff, and youth should then select strategies to meet growth goals and monitor progress toward reaching those goals over time.

Integrating a youth voice approach to working with young people experiencing homelessness represents a paradigm shift that requires a great deal of time, effort, and investment. Many adults will struggle to shift their goals and missions from fixing vulnerable youth or holding delinquent youth accountable to instead recognizing the strengths of young people and helping them to develop into powerful members of the society. Yet, research tells us that helping young people develop into adults sets them on positive life trajectories. Many adults may doubt that young people are capable of sharing power with adults and partnering with them on making key decisions in the agency. Yet, research suggests that young people do have incredible skills, are capable of gaining new skills, and are motivated to be seen and heard and to contribute. The potential benefits of making this shift to empowering young people (who are likely to feel respected, valued, connected, safe, and able to make change for themselves and others) and the potential benefits to agencies (who are likely see greater youth engagement, better long-term outcomes, and greater staff satisfaction) will likely far outweigh the costs.

References

76 Fed. Reg. 233 (2011). Rules and regulations. Federal Register: The Daily Journal of the United States. https://www.hudexchange.info/resources/documents/HEARTH_HomelessDefinition_FinalRule.pdf. Accessed 27 July 2018.

Auerswald, C. L., & Eyre, S. L. (2002). Youth homelessness in San Francisco: A life cycle approach. *Social Science and Medicine, 54*(10), 1497–1512.

Bender, K., Thompson, S. J., McManus, H., Lantry, J., & Flynn, P. M. (2007). Capacity for survival: Exploring strengths of homeless street youth. *Child and Youth Care Forum, 36*(1), 25–42.

Bender, K., Ferguson, K., Thompson, S., Komlo, C., & Pollio, D. (2010). Factors associated with trauma and posttraumatic stress disorder among homeless youth in three U.S. cities: The importance of transience. *Journal of Traumatic Stress, 23*(1), 161–168.

Bender, K., Thompson, S. J., Ferguson, K. M., Yoder, J., & Kern, L. (2014). Trauma among street-involved young adults. *Journal of Emotional and Behavioral Disorders, 22*, 53–64.

Bender, K., Barman-Adhikari, A., DeChants, J., Haffejee, B., Anyon, Y., Begun, S., Portillo, A., & Dunn, K. (2017). Asking for change: Feasibility, acceptability, and preliminary outcomes of a manualized photovoice intervention with youth experiencing homelessness. *Children and Youth Services Review, 81*, 379–389.

Bender, K., Begun, S., Dunn, K., MacKay, E., & DeChants, J. (2018). Homeless youths' interests in social action via photovoice. *Journal of Community Practice, 26*(1), 107–120.

Benson, P. L., Scales, P. C., Hamilton, S. F., & Sesma, A. (2006). Positive youth development: Theory, research, and applications. In R. M. Lerner & W. Damon (Eds.), *Handbook of child psychology: Theoretical models of human development* (pp. 894–941). Hoboken: Wiley.

Brooks, R. A., Milburn, N. G., Rotheram-Borus, M. J., & Witkin, A. (2004). The system-of-care for homeless youth: Perceptions of service providers. *Evaluation and Program Planning, 27*, 443–451.

Cammarota, J., & Fine, M. (Eds.). (2010). *Revolutionizing education: Youth participatory action research in motion*. New York: Routledge.

Cauce, A. M., Paradise, M., Ginzler, J. A., Embry, L., Morgan, C. J., Lohr, Y., & Theofelis, J. (2000). The characteristics and mental health of homeless adolescents: Age and gender differences. *Journal of Emotional and Behavioral Disorders, 8*(4), 230–239.

Cheon, J. W. (2008). Convergence of a strengths perspective and youth development: Toward youth promotion practice. *Advances in Social Work, 9*(2), 176–190.

Collins, P., & Barker, C. (2009). Psychological help-seeking in homeless adolescents. *International Journal of Social Psychiatry, 55*(4), 372–384.

Dadds, M. R., Braddock, D., Cuers, S., Elliott, A., & Kelly, A. (1993). Personal and family distress in homeless adolescents. *Community Mental Health Journal, 29*(5), 413–422.

De Rosa, C. J., Montgomery, S. B., Kipke, M. D., Iverson, E., Ma, J. L., & Unger, J. B. (1999). Service utilization among homeless and runaway youth in Los Angeles, California: Rates and reasons. *Journal of Adolescent Health, 24*(3), 190–200.

Dumont, M., & Provost, M. A. (1999). Resilience in adolescents: Protective role of social support, coping strategies, self-esteem, and social activities on experience of stress and depression. *Journal of Youth and Adolescence, 28*(3), 343–363.

Eccles, J., & Gootman, J. A. (Eds.). (2002). *Community programs to promote youth development*. Washington, DC: National Academy Press.

Feldmann, J., & Middleman, A. B. (2003). Homeless adolescents: Common clinical concerns. *Seminars in Pediatric Infectious Diseases, 14*(1), 6–11.

Ferguson, K. M., Kim, M. A., & McCoy, S. (2011). Enhancing empowerment and leadership among homeless youth in agency and community settings: A grounded theory approach. *Child and Adolescent Social Work Journal, 28*(1), 1–22.

Ferguson, K. M., Bender, K., Thompson, S. J., Maccio, E. M., & Pollio, D. (2012). Employment status and income generation among homeless young adults: Results from a five-city, mixed-methods study. *Youth and Society, 44*(3), 385–407.

Fowler, P. J., Toro, P. A., & Miles, B. W. (2009). Pathways to and from homelessness and associated psychosocial outcomes among adolescents leaving the foster care system. *American Journal of Public Health, 99*(8), 1453–1458.

Gavin, L. E., Catalano, R. F., David-Ferdon, C., Gloppen, K. M., & Markham, C. M. (2010). A review of positive youth development programs that promote adolescent sexual and reproductive health. *Journal of Adolescent Health, 46*(3), S75–S91.

Gharabaghi, K., & Stuart, C. (2010). Voices from the periphery: Prospects and challenges for the homeless youth service sector. *Children and Youth Services Review, 32*(12), 1683–1689.

Gomez, R. J., & Ryan, T. N. (2016). Speaking out: Youth led research as a methodology used with homeless youth. *Child and Adolescent Social Work Journal, 33*(2), 185–193.

Greenblatt, M., & Robertson, M. J. (1993). Life-styles, adaptive strategies, and sexual behaviors of homeless adolescents. *Hospital and Community Psychiatry, 44*(12), 1177–1180.

Halcón, L. L., & Lifson, A. R. (2004). Prevalence and predictors of sexual risks among homeless youth. *Journal of Youth and Adolescence, 33*(1), 71–80.

Hammer, H., Finkelhor, D., & Sedlak, A. J. (2002). *Runaway/thrownaway children: National estimates and characteristics (NCJ 196469)*. Washington, DC: U.S. Department of Justice, Office of Justice Programs, Office of Juvenile Justice and Delinquency Prevention.

Heinze, H. (2013). Beyond a bed: Support for positive development for youth residing in emergency shelters. *Children and Youth Services Review, 35*(2), 278–286.

Heinze, H. J., & Hernandez Jozefowicz-Simbeni, D. M. (2009). Intervention for homeless and at-risk youth: Assessing youth and staff perspectives on service provision, satisfaction and quality. *Vulnerable Children and Youth Studies, 4*(3), 210–225.

Heinze, H., Hernandez Jozefowicz, D. M., & Toro, P. A. (2010). Taking the youth perspective: Assessment of program characteristics that promote positive development in homeless and at-risk youth. *Children and Youth Services Review, 32*, 1365–1372.

Hodgson, K. J., Shelton, K. H., van den Bree, M. B., & Los, F. J. (2013). Psychopathology in young people experiencing homelessness: A systematic review. *American Journal of Public Health, 103*(6), 24–37.

Hopper, E. K., Bassuk, E. L., & Olivet, J. (2010). Shelter from the storm: Trauma-informed care in homelessness services settings. *The Open Health Services and Policy Journal, 3*(2), 80–100.

Hudson, A. L., Nyamathi, A., Greengold, B., Slagle, A., Koniak-Griffin, D., Khalilifard, F., & Getzoff, D. (2010). Health-seeking challenges among homeless youth. *Nursing Research, 59*(3), 212.

Jelicic, H., Bobek, D. L., Phelps, E., Lerner, R. M., & Lerner, J. V. (2007). Using positive youth development to predict contribution and risk behaviors in early adolescence: Findings from the first two waves of the 4-H Study of Positive Youth Development. *International Journal of Behavioral Development, 31*(3), 263–273.

Jennings, L. B., Parra-Medina, D. M., Hilfinger-Messias, D. K., & McLoughlin, K. (2006). Toward a critical social theory of youth empowerment. *Journal of Community Practice, 14*(1–2), 31–55.

Kidd, S. A. (2007). Youth homelessness and social stigma. *Journal of Youth and Adolescence, 36*(3), 291–299.

Kolar, K., Erickson, P. G., & Stewart, D. (2012). Coping strategies of street-involved youth: Exploring contexts of resilience. *Journal of Youth Studies, 15*(6), 744–760.

Larkin, M., Cierpial, C., Stack, J., Morrison, V., & Griffith, C. (2008). Empowerment theory in action: The wisdom of collaborative governance. *Online Journal of Issues in Nursing, 13*(2), 2–2.

Leonard, N. R., Freeman, R., Ritchie, A. S., Gwadz, M. V., Tabac, L., Dickson, V. V., Cleland, C. M., Bolas, J., & Hirsh, M. (2017). "Coming from the place of walking with the youth—That feeds everything": A mixed methods case study of a runaway and homeless youth organization. *Child and Adolescent Social Work Journal, 34*(5), 443–459.

Lindsey, E. W., Kurtz, D., Jarvis, S., Williams, B., & Nackerud, L. (2000). How runaway and homeless youth navigate troubled waters: Personal strengths and resources. *Child and Adolescent Social Work Journal, 17*(2), 115–140.

MacLean, M. G., Embry, L. E., & Cauce, A. M. (1999). Homeless adolescents' paths to separation from family: Comparison of family characteristics, psychological adjustment, and victimization. *Journal of Community Psychology, 27*(2), 179–187.

McCay, E., Langley, J., Beanlands, H., Cooper, L., Mudachi, N., Harris, A., Blidner, R., Bach, K., Dart, C., Howes, C., & Miner, S. (2010). Mental health challenges and strengths of street-involved youth: The need for a multi-determined approach. *Canadian Journal of Nursing Research, 42*(3), 30–49.

McKinney-Vento Homeless Assistance Act, Re-Authorized. (2002). 42 U.S.C. 11431 et seq 725.

Medlow, S., Klineberg, E., & Steinbeck, K. (2014). The health diagnoses of homeless adolescents: A systematic review of the literature. *Journal of Adolescence, 37*(5), 531–542.

Ozer, E. J., & Douglas, L. (2015). Assessing the key processes of youth-led participatory research: Psychometric analysis and application of an observational rating scale. *Youth and Society, 47*(1), 29–50.

Perron, J. L., Cleverley, K., & Kidd, S. A. (2014). Resilience, loneliness, and psychological distress among homeless youth. *Archives of Psychiatric Nursing, 28*(4), 226–229.

Pollio, D. E., Thompson, S. J., Tobias, L., Reid, D., & Spitznagel, E. (2006). Longitudinal outcomes for youth receiving runaway/homeless shelter services. *Journal of Youth and Adolescence, 35*, 859–866.

Rew, L., & Horner, S. D. (2003). Personal strengths of homeless adolescents living in a high-risk environment. *Advanced Nursing Science, 26*(2), 90–101.

Rew, L., Taylor-Seehafer, M., Thomas, N. Y., & Yockey, R. D. (2001). Correlates of resilience in homeless adolescents. *Journal of Nursing Scholarship, 33*(1), 33–40.

Ringwalt, C. L., Greene, J. M., Robertson, M., & McPheeters, M. (1998). The prevalence of homelessness among adolescents in the United States. *American Journal of Public Health, 88*(9), 1325–1329.

Roebuck, B. S., & Roebuck, M. M. (2016). The strengths of young people who are homeless. *Canadian Journal of Community Mental Health, 35*(2), 43–54.

Rosenthal, D., Mallett, S., & Myers, P. (2006). Why do homeless young people leave home? *Australian and New Zealand Journal of Public Health, 30*, 281–285.

Slesnick, N., & Prestopnik, J. (2005). Dual and multiple diagnosis among substance using runaway youth. *The American Journal of Drug and Alcohol Abuse, 31*(1), 179–201.

Slesnick, N., Dashora, P., Letcher, A., Erdem, G., & Serovich, J. (2009). A review of services and interventions for runaway and homeless youth: Moving forward. *Children and Youth Services Review, 31*(7), 732–742.

Stewart, A. J., Steiman, M., Cauce, A. M., Cochran, B. N., Whitbeck, L. B., & Hoyt, D. R. (2004). Victimization and posttraumatic stress disorder among homeless 364 adolescents. *Journal of the American Academy of Child and Adolescent Psychiatry, 43*, 325–331.

Thompson, S. J., Safyer, A. W., & Pollio, D. E. (2001). Differences and predictors of family reunification among subgroups of runaway youths using shelter services. *Social Work Research, 25*(3), 163–172.

Thompson, S. J., Ryan, T. N., Montgomery, K. L., Lippman, A. D. P., Bender, K., & Ferguson, K. (2016). Perceptions of resiliency and coping: Homeless young adults speak out. *Youth and Society, 48*(1), 58–76.

Tyler, K., & Beal, M. R. (2010). The high-risk environment of homeless young adults: Consequences for physical and sexual victimization. *Violence and Victims, 25*, 101–115.

Ungar, M. (2004). *Nurturing hidden resilience in troubled youth*. Toronto: University of Toronto Press.

Wang, C. C. (2006). Youth participation in photovoice as a strategy for community change. *Journal of Community Practice, 14*(1–2), 147–161.

Wang, C., & Burris, M. A. (1997). Photovoice: Concept, methodology, and use for participatory needs assessment. *Health Education and Behavior, 24*(3), 369–387.

Watson, J. (2011). Understanding survival sex: Young women, homelessness, and intimate relationships. *Journal of Youth Studies, 14*(6), 639–655.

Watson, J., & Cuervo, H. (2017). Youth homelessness: A social justice approach. *Journal of Sociology, 53*(2), 461–475.

Weikart, D. P. (2012) Youth program quality assessment. Center for Youth Program Quality. http://www.cypq.org/assessment. Accessed 27 July 2018.

Whitbeck, L. B., Hoyt, D. R., & Bao, W. N. (2000). Depressive symptoms and co-occurring depressive symptoms, substance abuse, and conduct problems among runaway and homeless adolescents. *Child Development, 71*(3), 721–732.

Whitbeck, L. B., Johnson, K. D., Hoyt, D. R., & Cauce, A. M. (2004). Mental disorder and comorbidity among runaway and homeless adolescents. *Journal of Adolescent Health, 35*(2), 132–140.

Chapter 17
"If I Don't Fight for It, I Have Nothing": Supporting Students Who Experience Homelessness While Enrolled in Higher Education

Rashida M. Crutchfield and Nancy Meyer-Adams

Introduction

> I think a lot of it too is that I don't want them to feel sorry for me…I guess now that I said it out loud, it is I don't want them to see me any different than the rest of the students. I am capable, just like everybody else. It is that my struggle is just a little bit bigger. (Yvette, age 24, four-year university undergraduate student)

Students who are homeless are part of a large, diverse student population served by colleges and universities in the USA. Although the benefits of earning a college degree are well known, research shows that children and youth experiencing housing instability have low college graduation rates (Dworsky and Perez 2009; Peters et al. 2009; Stagner and Lansing 2009). Students in higher education who experience homelessness know that earning a degree can expand their horizons, increase their likelihood of adult economic stability, and meet academic and social goals (Crutchfield 2016; Goldrick-Rab et al. 2017; Gupton 2017). Students have a wide range of strengths and aspirations to graduate from institutions of higher education, but they also navigate barriers inside and outside of the classroom that influence their participation in the college experience (Crutchfield and Maguire 2018; Goldrick-Rab et al. 2017; Gupton 2017; Tierney et al. 2008), and there is much to be learned about how to support them. College and university staff, faculty, and administrators across the country are gradually becoming more aware of homelessness within their student communities (Broton and Goldrick-Rab 2016; Crutchfield 2016). However, the narratives of students who are experiencing homelessness

Electronic supplementary material: The online version of this chapter (https://doi.org/10.1007/978-3-030-03727-7_17) contains supplementary material, which is available to authorized users.

R. M. Crutchfield (✉) · N. Meyer-Adams
California State University, Long Beach, Long Beach, CA, USA
e-mail: rashida.crutchfield@csulb.edu; nancy.meyer-adams@csulb.edu

H. Larkin et al. (eds.), *Homelessness Prevention and Intervention in Social Work*, https://doi.org/10.1007/978-3-030-03727-7_17

while seeking higher education have rarely been told, and there is minimal research on how to support them.

Research on homelessness for students in higher education is very limited (US Department of Housing and Urban Development [HUD] 2015b). There is some research that speaks to the pre-college experience of homeless youth (Buckner et al. 2001; Dworsky 2008; Hallett 2010; Hallett et al. 2015; Miller 2015; Murphy and Tobin 2011; Tierney et al. 2008). But, very little research addresses the experience of these students beyond admission into colleges and universities.

It is important to recognize that homelessness does not occur in a vacuum and must be embedded in a larger justice narrative that recognizes the economic and social marginalization that influences who, how, and how long people experience homelessness (Aviles de Bradley 2015). Further, the rising costs of tuition and housing, along with limited financial aid and public assistance programs, compound financial and emotional stress (Goldrick-Rab 2016). Recent and persistent state and federal government disinvestment in higher education has resulted in a higher burden on students and their families as state and federal financial aid programs have not increased to meet the rising costs (Goldrick-Rab 2016).

This chapter focuses on research, policy, and interventions to expand readers' knowledge of college students experiencing homelessness. It incorporates the voices of these students to enhance social workers' understanding of student experiences. Related policies and innovative practices are also discussed.

Overview of Homelessness in Higher Education

The McKinney-Vento Act, initially passed in 1987 and most recently reauthorized in 2015 by the Every Student Succeeds Act (ESSA), provides a definition for homelessness in education. The US Department of Education (DOE) uses the education subtitle of the McKinney-Vento Act's definitions of homelessness, which includes youth who lack a fixed, regular, and adequate nighttime residence and unaccompanied youth, which includes youth not in the physical custody of a parent or guardian. It also uses at risk of homelessness to refer to students whose housing may cease to be fixed, regular, and adequate (20 U.S.C. § 1001 et seq., 42 U.S.C. §11434a(2)(A); 42 U.S.C. §11434a(6). This definition, which is broader than what is used by the US Department of Housing and Urban Development (HUD), is the basis for homelessness determinations for K–12 students and in higher education, as it has been shown to be more commonly descriptive of young adult homelessness (Ausikaitis et al. 2015; Hallett and Skrla 2017; Mawhinney-Rhoads and Stahler 2006; Tierney et al. 2008).

Public school officials (K–12) identified 91,351 unaccompanied homeless children and youth for the 2013–2014 school year in the USA (US Department of Education [DOE] 2014). In higher education, according to the most recent data drawn in 2015–2016, 31,948 US college financial aid applicants were unaccompanied homeless youth, based on responses to questions required on federal financial aid forms or as determined by a college or university federal aid administrator (National Center for Homeless Education [NCHE] 2016). Both of these numbers are likely to be far smaller than the actual incidence of homelessness. Morton et al. (2017) report that a minimum of 700,000 adolescent minors (13–17 years) and 3.5 million young adults (18–25 years) experience homelessness in a 12-month period in the USA. Further, in terms of collegiate homelessness, many students are unaware of the status designation of homelessness or are sometimes unwilling to designate themselves as such (HUD 2015b). Beyond youth estimates, these numbers do not account for the number of college students who are above the age of 25, a number that continues to rise (National Center for Education Statistics 2016).

Growing evidence suggests that homelessness does exist on college campuses. Research at the University of Massachusetts Boston (Silva et al. 2015) found that 5.4% of their student population experienced homelessness. A study in the California State University (CSU) system found approximately 10.9% of CSU students experienced homelessness and housing insecurity (Crutchfield and Maguire 2018). A study at the City University of New York (CUNY) suggested that 40% of students experienced housing instability in the CUNY system (Tsui et al. 2011). Studies of community colleges suggest that the rate of student homelessness may be as high as 13–14% (Goldrick-Rab et al. 2015, 2017).

It is clear that homelessness in higher education is an issue across academic environments. Additionally, research suggests that students who experience homelessness struggle to meet a variety of competing needs, including management of many personal and financial responsibilities (including academic expenses) and accessing basic needs and medical care, all while navigating the college environment (Broton and Goldrick-Rab 2016; Crutchfield 2016; Goldrick-Rab et al. 2015, 2017; Gupton 2017). However, much work still needs to be done to develop a nuanced understanding of the complex experiences of students who experience homelessness.

Defining Homelessness in Higher Education

> But there's always like looming in the back of my head...Well, if I can ignore it, it's fine. But if I can't, then it's a really icy feeling in my heart and I just have to [say to myself], 'calm down, calm down, calm down.' (Monique, age 24, four-year university student)

HUD defines homelessness as sheltered (in an emergency shelter, transitional housing, or supportive housing) and unsheltered (on the streets, in abandoned buildings, or other places not meant for human habitation) (Homeless Emergency Assistance and Rapid Transition to Housing Act of 2009, P.L. 111-22, Section 1003). However, the US Department of Education (DOE) definition of homelessness includes youth, either unaccompanied or in the physical custody of a parent or guardian, who lack a fixed, regular, and adequate nighttime residence. The DOE also defines students as being at risk of homelessness when their housing may cease to be fixed, regular, and adequate (20 U.S.C. § 1001 et seq., 42 U.S.C. §11434a(2)(A); 42 U.S.C. §11434a(6)). This broader definition is used as the basis for homelessness determinations for K–12 students and has been shown to be more commonly descriptive of youth and young adult homelessness (Ausikaitis et al. 2015; Hallett and Skrla 2017; Mawhinney-Rhoads and Stahler 2006; Tierney et al. 2008). It is also used in higher education because it appears to mirror the housing instability and homeless experiences of college students (Crutchfield and Maguire 2017).

It is important to note that there is great diversity in the age and experience of college students. Not all college students are what most people think of as traditional-age students. In fact, the "traditional" college student, often thought of as coming directly from high school to college at 18 years old, continues to become a smaller proportion of the population of higher education (Broton and Goldrick-Rab 2013; Deil-Amen 2011; Goldrick-Rab 2016) as the number of undergraduate students over 24 continues to rise (National Center for Education Statistics 2016). This age trend warrants attention in relation to homelessness, since many of the policy protections for students experiencing homelessness end when they are in their early 20s. Older students may have compounding life circumstances, such as exiting foster care, having children or other dependents, working full-time, or other factors less common among "traditional" college-aged students that may influence their college experience.

A consistent and universally accepted definition of homelessness for higher education has not been developed since the awareness of homelessness in higher education is relatively new. However, researchers Ronald Hallett[1] and Rashida Crutchfield have developed a continuum of housing security to inform research, policy, and practice. The following describes in detail this model, which can be used to assist social workers and other student services personnel in understanding, utilizing, and further developing services to assist students experiencing housing insecurity.

Higher Education Housing Continuum

Often, homelessness on college campuses is identified by campus staff who may not have training in social work or experience working with people who experience homelessness (Broton et al. 2014; Broton and Goldrick-Rab 2016; Crutchfield 2016).

[1] Ronald E. Hallett is an associate professor of educational leadership in the Benerd School of Education at the University of the Pacific and research associate for the Pullias Center at the University of Southern California. For over 10 years, Hallett has been researching the intersections between homelessness and educational engagement. He has published a book that illustrates the social context of homeless teens – *Educational Experiences of Hidden Homeless Teenagers* (Routledge 2012). And, he coauthored a book that provides guidance for educators and educational leaders concerning how to address the issue of homelessness – *Serving Students Who Are Homeless: A Resource Guide for Schools, Districts, and Educational Leaders* (Teachers College Press 2017).

This identification is often reliant on what individuals may deem as homeless based on stereotypes one might develop about what someone who is homeless looks like or how they articulate their struggle. Hallett and Crutchfield (2018) constructed a theoretical continuum that can assist in identifying students in need of housing support. The continuum is inclusive, avoiding a binary approach of homeless or not, which oversimplifies the experiences of students living without housing security. Additionally, the continuum is constructed in a way that individuals can identify their housing arrangement without necessarily claiming the overarching identity of homeless, which carries social stigma (Barker 2015; Tierney et al. 2008).

The continuum presents categories within columns but also acknowledges the multidirectional movement within and between categories (see Fig. 17.1). This continuum acknowledges that students' experiences may overlap (e.g., they may sleep in a car when resident halls are closed during school breaks) and that gray areas exist (e.g., students may find what appears to be stable housing that then becomes precarious). Further, students may experience movement from left to right (toward housing security) and from right to left (away from housing security) as crises emerge or recede. For example, students who disclose their sexual orientation may move from housing secure to homeless as a result of being kicked out of their home by unsupportive family members, and students who are moving from friend's house to friend's house may find a living situation that becomes permanent. Table 17.1 provides details of categories; however, its authors strongly suggest that the continuum be used to acknowledge the gray areas that exist between each category and that each grouping is neither rigid nor hierarchical.

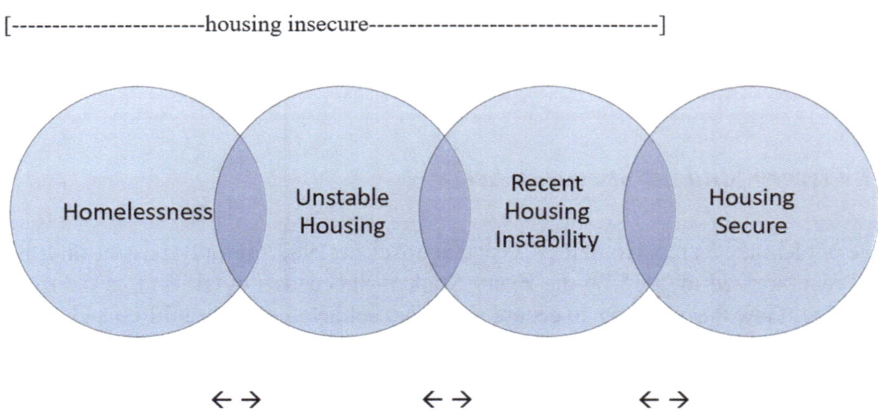

Fig. 17.1 Higher Education Housing Continuum (Hallett and Crutchfield 2018)

Table 17.1 Higher Education Housing Continuum (Hallett and Crutchfield 2018)

Housing insecure			
Homelessness	Unstable housing	Recent housing instability	Housing secure
Lacking housing that is fixed, regular, and adequate • Streets, parks, woods, and other public spaces • Vehicle or camper • Abandoned buildings, barns, or sheds • Garage or storage units • Homeless shelter • Religious institution • Domestic violence shelter • Hotel/motel • Couch surfing • Transitional housing program	Housing situations that may not remain fixed, regular, and adequate • Residence halls with no place to live during breaks • Over a month behind on rent (this could include the roommate not paying rent) • Nearing end of stable housing without viable options, including foreclosure • Doubled-up residences • Inability to pay utility bills and meet basic needs • Temporary substance abuse facility (if individual does not have stable residence to return to after treatment)	Stable housing but a recent history of housing insecurity within the past 3 years	Consistent, adequate, and safe housing with consistent funding to cover expenses Individuals have social connections and a safety net

Policy

Multiple federal laws impact the ability to apply for college and achieve a college degree. In this section, three laws are highlighted: the Every Student Succeeds Act of 2015, the Higher Education Opportunity Act of 2008, and the College Cost Reduction of 2007.

The Every Student Succeeds Act

The McKinney-Vento Homeless Assistance Act of 1987, initially passed in 1987 and reauthorized in 2015 by the Every Student Succeeds Act (ESSA), is the most prominent law that attempts to ensure academic achievement for children and youth who experience homelessness. ESSA provided guidance for the DOE's expansive definition of homelessness as someone who lacks *fixed*, *regular*, and *adequate* housing, allowing for the inclusion of those who may be temporarily housed in a home, motel, or any other location that is unstable. This acknowledges how housing instability impacts the educational experiences and overall well-being of a person.

ESSA revised McKinney-Vento to include college accessibility requirements, including the stipulation that McKinney-Vento district liaisons must notify unaccompanied youth, those not in the custody of their parents, of their rights as independent students for their financial aid applications. ESSA also specifically required that federal college access programs, like TRIO, give priority to students who are homeless. However, this legislation does not include any mandates or supportive services once students are enrolled in higher education.

Higher Education Opportunity Act

The Higher Education Opportunity Act (HEOA; Public Law 110-315) was enacted in 2008, amending and reauthorizing the Higher Education Act of 1965. Stipulations for students who are homeless under HEOA primarily address priority for federal college access programs. HEOA provides stipulations for federally funded programs to support college preparation and access for college to marginalized students. Under HEOA, these programs must prioritize students experiencing homelessness in high school. This includes programs such as TRIO, Upward Bound, Educational Opportunity Programs, and GEAR UP. The law also required the DOE to increase awareness of available financial aid for students and to develop grants for higher education institutions to provide temporary housing for students.

College Cost Reduction and Access Act

Historically, unaccompanied homeless youth have faced insurmountable barriers to attending college without some type of financial aid (HUD 2015b). However, in order to receive financial assistance, students must complete the Free Application for Federal Student Aid (FAFSA). In the past, this form required students to provide parental financial information to determine student eligibility for aid and mandated a parent or guardian signature. Although this requirement was appropriate for many college applicants, it created obstacles for unaccompanied homeless youth who were not supported by or in contact with parents or who did not have access to parental information (National Association for the Education of Homeless Children and Youth 2018).

Due to these concerns, Congress enacted the College Cost Reduction and Access Act (CCRAA 2012; P.L. 110-84) in 2007 to improve college access for unaccompanied homeless youth by defining the term "independent students" and encouraging federally funded college access programs to serve these students. Specifically, the law allows youth to be considered independent for the purpose of their FAFSA if they are verified as unaccompanied and homeless during the school year in which the application is submitted, or unaccompanied, at risk of homelessness, and self-supporting. This allows the student to complete the FAFSA without the use of parental information or signature. Verification of this status must be made by one of the following authorities: (a) a McKinney-Vento Act school district liaison; (b) a US Department of Housing and Urban Development homeless assistance program director or their designee; (c) a Runaway and Homeless Youth Act program director or their designee; or (d) a financial aid administrator at a college or university. In addition, this law requires youth who are homeless or at risk of homelessness to reapply each year. This means that the student must be interviewed, and provide the documentation that proves that the student is still considered homeless or at risk of homelessness (CCRAA 2012).

Research shows that there have been significant challenges to the implementation of CCRAA. Students are consistently required to prove they are homeless with additional documentation not required under the law (Cochrane and Szabo-Kubitz 2009; Cochrane et al. 2010; Crutchfield et al. 2016), which has led to long delays in obtaining financial aid and creates unnecessary barriers for students. Research also suggests that financial aid administrators responsible for FAFSA verifications are working to remove undue burdens for students, though there is room for continued development in collaborative work to ensure expediency in financial aid access (Crutchfield 2016).

State Policies

There are very few state-level policies that directly relate to homelessness in higher education. Colorado, Florida, Louisiana, Maryland, and Missouri have enacted some laws to support higher education for students; however, California has provided the most legislative direction.

Louisiana House Bill (HB) 906 requires public universities to house students experiencing homelessness over breaks and suggests institutions develop housing plans for unstably housed students. This law also encourages institutions to offer in-state residency status for students experiencing homelessness if they are under the age of 19. Colorado HB 16-1100 also allows for in-state residency for those under 22 years old. Florida Statute 1009.25 allows exemptions from tuition and fees for public institutions, and Maryland HB 482 makes students who are unaccompanied and homeless under the age of 25 exempt from tuition for 5 years of undergraduate study at public universities and community colleges.

California HB 801 provides priority registration and fee waivers for students experiencing homelessness and requires that the 23 public California State Universities and 114 community colleges designate a Homeless and Foster Youth Student Liaison to assist with access to financial aid and student support services. California Senate Bill 1068 requires homeless liaisons receive training and education, including training on educational rights, related state and federal law, and local resources. California Assembly Bill (AB) 1995 allows matriculated community college students experiencing homelessness access to shower facilities if they have paid school fees (or had them waived) and have a GPA of 2.0 or higher.

These federal and state laws directly affect whether or not students who are at risk for homelessness or are currently homeless can achieve a college degree. It is well documented that individuals with higher education are more likely to obtain higher paying jobs than people who have only a high school diploma (Pew Research 2014). Therefore, it is imperative that social workers in higher education are knowledgeable about these laws, can provide accurate information to students and administrators, and advocate for policy changes.

Experiences of Students Who Are Homeless

> So, I just started that, I guess, a little earlier than most young individuals. They have their parents as a crutch, and when something bad happens ... when something happens later on in their life, then they realize "oh my parents are not here anymore. Let me take care of myself". I just know that humans don't last forever, so let me just take care of myself now. That's really my motivation. (Charles, age 22, community college student)

Students who are homeless seek many of the same goals as their housed peers: to personally and socially grow and learn, to graduate from college, and to establish economic stability (Crutchfield 2012; Gupton 2017; Hallett 2012; Tierney et al. 2008). Students, passionate to participate in secondary education, straddle their place in temporary housing situations and in college settings, often feeling both disconnected from their homeless non-college-going peers and from college students they see on campus (Crutchfield 2012). Despite this, students' desire to earn a degree propels them to pursue higher education (Crutchfield 2012, 2016; Gupton 2017; Masten et al. 1993; Rafferty et al. 2004).

It is important to understand that students may not identify themselves as homeless, often avoiding the use of the word explicitly because of stigma or assumptions of what someone who is homeless might experience and how that might differ from their own experience (Farrugia 2011; Tierney and Hallett 2012; Toolis and Hammack 2015). Elias, who was living in a shelter for homeless youth and attending community college, suggested he had stereotypes about what homeless looks like and that he felt he did not fit that perception:

> I look at the next homeless man, and they're not like me. I see the next homeless man, he's walking, he's broke, he's on the streets, and I'm not like him. I'm a different type of homeless person. When I say different type, not just in where I'm living, but also in mindset. I haven't given up. I haven't decided that it's too late for me. I haven't gotten to that point where I've completely broken down and decided that there's nothing left for myself, for my future. I haven't gotten to that point. I refuse to get to that point.

Elias knew he was homeless. However, he also wanted to assert that he had his own path and had control over his destiny. Elias was acutely aware that he was homeless, but that was not his identity.

Researchers and practitioners may choose to ask explicit questions like, "Since starting college, have you ever been homeless?" However, other indicators may be used to assess housing security, such as where they live (e.g., in a car, shelter, place not intended for habitation), if their housing circumstance is reliable, the number of housing moves, the variety of places they have lived recently (e.g., with friends in dorms or from couch to couch). These indicators may be used to determine incidents of homelessness while avoiding stigmatizing students (Crutchfield and Maguire 2017). Thus, when working with students who are experiencing homelessness, practitioners and researchers must consider how, if, and when they choose to use the term homeless.

Aspirations and Ambitions

> And it's like, yeah all of this is happening, but I am one of those that's not going to let it get in the way of me getting somewhere, because you know all this will be temporary, you know. I'll be able to soon have like permanent housing, and I'll have transportation, and I'll have funding to be able to take care of myself. And, it'll all be because it worked out, and I kept pushing through it. (Ginny, age 21, community college student)

Much like other students, those who experience homelessness express a passion for learning and personal growth and also articulate the need for a college degree to gain economic stability (Crutchfield 2012; Gupton 2017; Hallett 2012; Tierney et al. 2008). Students experiencing homelessness express a great deal of motivation for going to college and staying in college, though it can be very difficult to do so. While in college, students describe facing unique obstacles as they attempted to manage academic demands while navigating housing insecurity. In many cases, students express fear and frustration that such barriers can result in failing to accomplish their educational goals and could result in long-term poverty.

Students may experience dual conditions of feeling different and alone in both shelter and college environments. Like Elias, students see themselves as unique among their shelter and transitional living peers in that they show determination, willingness, and ability and have opportunities to further their education. These students may perceive themselves as distinctively different from their housed peers in college environments (Crutchfield 2012). Students experiencing homelessness discuss being acutely aware that their experiences in community college are different than their housed college-going peers. As compared to those who have their needs met, students unable to access basic needs like food and housing are 80% less likely to participate in typical college social activities, 71% more likely to change or limit their food intake, 39% more likely to need to borrow money or use credit cards, 19% more likely to go without a computer, and 15% less likely to buy required textbooks (Broton and Goldrick-Rab 2016). Further, students experiencing homelessness are often working part- or full-time jobs alongside their many competing responsibilities (Broton and Goldrick-Rab 2016; Crutchfield 2012, 2016; Goldrick-Rab et al. 2017).

Moreover, students experiencing homelessness are likely to be under constant stress and to worry about their financial and housing stability (Broton and Goldrick-Rab 2016; Crutchfield 2012, 2016; Crutchfield and Maguire 2018; Gupton 2017).

Students experiencing homelessness speak about feeling alone, disconnected, and embarrassed in the college community because they are homeless. Vivian spoke about the differences between her and other students:

> [Other students] kind of idolize you with like being a transitional youth. But they're like, "Oh you work, and you're alone. You're doing this on your own. You're going to college. That's so cool." But like ... I don't know ... sometimes it's kind of like ... I kind of envy them, because they can focus on school, which I can't, because I have to think of other things, such as like maybe after I'm out of the program I'm going to be out on my own, so I have to pay bills ... knowing that we are all the same age, but I'm having a different experience.

Rachel built on this idea, speaking specifically about how her life is different:

> ... because I made a few acquaintances there [in college], and I would listen to them talk about them going home and getting in their bed in their room, where they're alone, you know, and watching TV, and it's like, I can't come back and do it, you know? It's no real relax time, you know, soon as I get out of school, I have to job search, and then from that I can't go upstairs until eight you know? So, if I'm tired, I just have to sit down here [in the shelter].

Students experiencing homelessness speak about feeling alone in college and often in the world as a whole. Many students who experience homelessness speak about a feeling of isolation in college. Teri spoke about being friendless at school:

> ... I'm 20, it's sad, and I don't have friends or anything. In school, I wasn't able to really be a social butterfly, because I was embarrassed of my situation. I mean, I can't really go out. Or, "Where do you live? Can we pick you up?" Like, I was really antisocial, and it really took a toll or whatever.

Students express never feeling completely "normal" as a homeless person or as a college student (Crutchfield 2012; Crutchfield and Maguire 2018). Despite these challenges, students express great motivation to graduate. Rachel realized that simply working without going to college would never pull her out of poverty:

> I was just like I can't just be here forever, and I know just getting a nine-to-five or an eight-hour job, minimum wage, wasn't what I wanted to do with myself. So...I have to go to school ... California is so high like to live here, I know a nine-to-five wasn't or just an eight-hour at $8.00 a job wasn't going to do it.

Similarly, Charles said he knows that college is a means to sustainable living. He pointed out that he had to grow up fast and become self-sufficient, and that if he does not achieve, there is no one to help him:

> So, I just started that, I guess, a little earlier than most young individuals. They have their parents as a crutch, and when something bad happens ... when something happens later on in their life, then they realize, "oh my parents are not here anymore. Let me take care of myself." I just know that humans don't last forever, so let me just take care of myself now. That's really my motivation.

Charles had to become an adult quickly, and with the maturity he had acquired at a very young age came the knowledge that he needed to strive to bring himself out of homelessness because no one else would. Others have support lines, or "a crutch," that he does not. Charles was motivated by the fact that there is no one else who will help him if he does not finish college. When asked who was the most important person that could help them stay in college, many of the students interviewed used the very same words, "it's me." Generally, they felt no one else could help them stay in college.

Homelessness in the Higher Education Environment

> …We understand that we can't solve everything for the students, but what we can do is provide a level of support that lets [students] know this university genuinely cares about their success and is willing to do something about it; build that trust. (a university Dean of Students)

In the last several years, there has been an emerging awareness among college and university staff, faculty, and administrators across the country that students in higher education experience homelessness (Broton and Goldrick-Rab 2016; Crutchfield 2016). However, these students remain largely hidden and underserved (Broton and Goldrick-Rab 2016; Crutchfield 2012, 2016; Gupton 2017). Broton and Goldrick-Rab (2016) explored staff, faculty, and administrator perspectives on students who were homeless and provided insight on the experiences of youth. Campus employees reported a growing change in practices to meet the needs of college students who are homeless, but this gradual process is impeded by college environments that have not been traditionally structured for students experiencing high levels of need for support of basic needs. These findings were consistent with those from other academic, agency, and government reports (Broton et al. 2014; Crutchfield 2016, Goldrick-Rab et al. 2015; HUD 2015b; National Association for the Education of Homeless Children and Youth 2014; Tsui et al. 2011).

Some staff, faculty, and administrators express hesitation to address these issues for fear of a mission drift, asserting that institutions of higher learning are not social service agencies. Others worry that, while this is an important issue, limited resources constrain the ability to address housing instability fully (Broton et al. 2014; Crutchfield 2016). Further, studies have found that some higher education employees aspired to serve students but were unclear on how to proceed (Broton et al. 2014; Crutchfield 2016). Although staff, faculty, and administrators may have a strong desire to support students experiencing housing insecurity, they often lacked the structural supports, funds, and information needed to best serve these students (Broton et al. 2014; Crutchfield 2016). As one university staff person said:

> A lot of these conversations take place inside our office with the door shut…I've seen over and over and over again the staff members take their own personal money and, many times hundreds of dollars, try to eliminate the food crisis or you know, whatever they can do. It's not really talked about… (a university support staff in a student equity program)

Some college and university staff, faculty, and administrators worry that responding to the needs of homeless students may be beyond their mission or capabilities. In a California State University system study (Crutchfield 2016), administrators at two campuses offered reports that contradicted statements from staff. While administrators reported a low incidence of housing insecurity, staff on those same campuses reported consistently providing case-by-case services to students. In some cases, there is a normalizing of the "starving student" as part of the college vernacular. This leads to a campus cultural belief that struggle in college is normal and that, outside of rare circumstances, students generally have the means to meet their needs but squander their resources with youthful behavior.

The California State University system has 23 campuses that serve over 470,000 students (California State University 2017). In 2015, five of 23 campuses in the CSU system had robust programs with a mission to serve students who were homeless or food and housing insecure (Crutchfield 2016). Campus leadership at those campuses chose to incorporate addressing students' basic needs as a part of the student success directives and the university mission.

Approaches to the development of programs and services at these campuses included establishing interdisciplinary advisory boards that included representatives from student affairs (student support programs), financial aid, housing, counseling, services for students with disabilities, food services, faculty, and others. Boards that reported greatest success recounted that they started campus initiatives with extensive research on the extent of the population on campus, exploration of current and needed resources and services, and emphasis on the development of relationships across the campus (Crutchfield 2016).

These advisory committees also sought to address the need to centralize services for students. This approach of a single point of contact (SPOC) has been a recommendation for students by several researchers and advocacy groups (Broton and Goldrick-Rab 2016; Crutchfield 2016; Goldrick-Rab et al. 2017; National Association for the Education of Homeless Children and Youth 2018; Tierney and Hallett 2012). This consolidation of services, often including linkage to financial aid administrators, support for emergency housing or food, referrals to on- and off-campus services, and other services, allows students to access services in one centralized location that is easy to find. At its best, a SPOC can also ensure that a student only has to tell their story to one person and is not required to disclose their circumstances repeatedly to access support from many different locations on campus. Similar to the McKinney-Vento liaison at the K-12 level, SPOCs implement a streamlined process to facilitate communication and quick referrals across the campus.

Financial Aid

One vital resource for student success is financial aid; however, students who are homeless often face obstacles to the financial aid they are eligible for (Crutchfield et al. 2016; Sackett et al. 2016). Studies indicate that students report burdensome verification procedures not required by law. Findings from Cochrane and Szabo-Kubitz (2009) also suggest that barriers to financial aid can delay or impede progress in college and that bureaucratic, cumbersome practices at all levels of college life can be an impediment to higher education for students experiencing homelessness.

Collaborative work with social workers, social service professionals, K–12 homeless liaisons, institutions of higher education, and college access program staff who wish to support college access for students who are homeless should receive training to facilitate the financial aid process. Homeless liaisons at the K–12 level and social workers should also build relationships with local higher education financial aid administrators to explore their respective roles and ways they might collaborate to improve access to financial aid. Many high schools have had success with an annual "McKinney-Vento FAFSA Week," a specifically designated week to ensure that schools identify and assist all youth experiencing homelessness to complete the FAFSA. Sample announcements, letters, presentations, and scripts are available as part of NAEHCY's Unaccompanied Youth Toolkits for Counselors and Liaisons.[2]

The Agency Experience for College Students Who Are Experiencing Homelessness

> Seriously, when I came to this program, I was telling [my case manager] like, I need a counselor now, 'cause I don't know why the fuck I have been crying so much. Like, I think this is the time where I am letting it out, like, all those years when I would suck it up … just like eat it and be stronger… But thank God I have the program… (Hailey, age 18, community college student)

Students experiencing homelessness often go unnoticed in college environments. If students find linkages with community-based agencies, they may receive support from these homeless service agencies rather than from on-campus college support services. These agencies can be a meaningful support for college students experiencing homelessness (Brooks et al. 2004; Slesnick et al. 2009). That said, the availability and capacity of housing agency support for young adults who are homeless vary greatly from region to region (Brooks et al. 2004; Esparza 2009). Many states have very few housing agencies, and those that do often have limited resources that only focused on basic needs, such as food, shelter, employment, and independent living skills, and often lack the capacity to address educational needs (Gharabaghi and Stuart 2010). A focus on immediate outcomes, such as low-wage employment, may be at odds with long-term goals for higher education.

If educational services are available at community-based agencies, students may find help that cannot be found on their campuses. Specifically, agency education specialists can provide advice, academic counseling, and access to financial aid and scholarships. Teri, a 20-year-old community college student, spoke about the

[2] For NAEHCY's Unaccompanied Youth Toolkits for Counselors and Liaisons, see http://naehcy.org/toolkit-high-school-counselors

importance of her education specialist. When asked to explain how her agency had helped facilitate her college process, she did not hesitate:

> A counselor that was assigned to me and could force them to really plan my schedule. That's what [my education specialist] did for me for 2012. She put all my prerequisites, and she's like, "You can take them this semester."... Why can't my counselor at school do that more professionally? (Teri, age 20, community college student)

At times, students seeking services from housing agencies may meet barriers to educational progress because of the seemingly incompatible demands of their housing agencies. To meet HUD-mandated indicators for success, some agencies require employment as a requirement for eligibility for continued services (HUD 2013, 2015a). This prioritization of employment can impede access to full participation in higher education. Teri was challenged by her agency case manager to focus on employment, but she chose to focus on college instead and lost her job. Her case manager informed her that she could not stay in the shelter if she did not maintain employment. She said, "I was going to take [a class] in winter, and I wasn't able to because they wouldn't let me go back to school... Oh yeah, I stopped going to school, because I didn't have a job, and they were like, 'your focus is too much on school'."

Nathaniel spoke about being discouraged from going to college by an agency representative whom he contacted to get public assistance. He said, "They recommended I didn't even go to school. Like, I just work [but]... if you just work, and you're living paycheck-to-paycheck... I'm never really going to make it to school if I don't start." Nathaniel, like many others, was advised by a service agency representative to focus on his immediate needs rather than attend college. While he understood the necessity of short-term income, Nathaniel chose to attend college to gain long-term economic well-being.

Temporary housing and services accessed by students are invaluable, in some cases allowing them to focus on their educational goals. Moreover, agencies provide support that students experiencing homelessness may not find on campus, including education specialists and case managers. Despite myriad barriers and financial shortfalls, young adults benefit from homeless agencies' programs and services (Esparza 2009).

Unfortunately, for students over the age of 24, no longer eligible for youth services, agency support sometimes stops prior to college completion. For instance, once a student enrolls in higher education, eligibility to programs like Supplemental Nutrition Assistance Program (SNAP), also known as food stamps, becomes more restrictive (Cady 2016; Goldrick-Rab et al. 2017). As Jasmine, a 32-year-old university student, said, "They don't expect us to get this far, and then when we get here it's like, what now? Like, you're going to cut off all my stuff, so now I have to fend for myself. So, when the subsidies got cut, rent stayed the same." Jasmine discussed how difficult it was for her once she "aged out" of much needed social services designed for young adults.

Conclusion

Housing, social service, and government agencies, in collaboration with colleges and universities, must collaborate to support students experiencing homelessness, developing policies and practices that support access to and progression through higher education. HUD (2015b) recommends that interagency working groups and higher education institutions explore effective strategies for this population. These recommendations are mirrored by the National Association for the Education of Homeless Children and Youth (2016), an agency that has been working at practice and policy levels to clear paths to higher education for homeless youth. However, long-term research on the outcomes of homeless youth who choose college over employment is necessary to ensure that resources for youth are directed at lasting self-sufficiency.

References

Ausikaitis, A. E., Wynne, M. E., Persaud, S., Pitt, R., Hosek, A., Reker, K., Turner, C., Flores, S., & Flores, S. (2015). Staying in school: The efficacy of the McKinney-Vento Act for homeless youth. *Youth and Society, 47*, 707–726.

Aviles de Bradley, A. M. (2015). *From charity to equity: Race, homelessness, and urban schools*. New York: Teachers College Press.

Barker, J. (2015). A habitus of instability: Youth homelessness and instability. *Journal of Youth Studies, 19*(5), 665–683.

Brooks, R. A., Milburn, N. G., Rotheram-Borus, M. J., & Witkin, A. (2004). The system-of-care for homeless youth: Perceptions of service providers. *Evaluation and Program Planning, 27*(3), 443–451.

Broton, K., & Goldrick-Rab, S. (2013). *Housing instability among college students*. Madison: Center for Financial Security.

Broton, K., Frank, V., & Goldrick-Rab, S. (2014). *Safety, security, and college attainment: An investigation of undergraduates' basic needs and institutional response*. http://www.wihopelab.com/publications/APPAM.Draft.10.28.2014.pdf

Broton, K., & Goldrick-Rab, S. (2016). The dark side of college (un)affordability: Food and housing insecurity in higher education. *Change: The Magazine of Higher Learning, 48*(1), 16–25.

Buckner, J. C., Bassuk, E. L., & Weinreb, L. F. (2001). Predictors of academic achievement among homeless and low-income housed children. *Journal of School Psychology, 39*(1), 45–69.

Cady, C. (2016). Starving for knowledge: Why campuses need to address student food insecurity. *About Campus, 21*(2), 27–31.

California State University (2017). *Facts about the CSU*. https://www2.calstate.edu/csu-system/about-the-csu/facts-about-the-csu

Cochrane, F. D., & Szabo-Kubitz, S. (2009). *Hopes and hurdles college foster youth and college financial aid*. http://ticas.org/blog/hopes-hurdles-california-foster-youth-and-college-financial-aid

Cochrane, F. D., LaManque, A., & Szabo-Kubitz, S. (2010). After the FAFSA: How red tape can prevent eligible students from receiving financial aid. The Institute for College Access and Success. http://ticas.org/sites/default/files/pub_files/AfterFAFSA.pdf. Accessed 8 July 2018.

College Cost Reduction and Access Act (CCRAA) of 2007, 20, §1001 et seq. (2012).

Crutchfield, R. M. (2012). "If I don't fight for it, I have nothing": Experiences of homeless youth scaling the collegiate mountain. PQDT Open. https://pqdtopen.proquest.com/doc/1112886563.html?FMT=ABS. Accessed 8 July 2018.

Crutchfield, R. (2016). *Serving displaced and food insecure students in the CSU*. California State University. http://www.calstate.edu/AcadAff/documents/ServingDisplacedandFoodInsecureStudetnsintheCSUJanuary20163.8.16.pdf. Accessed 8 July 2018.

Crutchfield, R. M., Chambers, R. M., & Duffield, B. (2016). Jumping through the hoops to get financial aid for college students who are homeless: Policy analysis of the College Cost Reduction and Access Act of 2007. *Families in Society: The Journal of Contemporary Social Services, 93*(3), 191–199.

Crutchfield, R. M., & Maguire, J. (2017). Researching basic needs in higher education: Qualitative and quantitative instruments to explore a holistic understanding of food and housing insecurity. California State University. https://www2.calstate.edu/impact-of-the-csu/student-success/basic-needs-initiative/Documents/researching-basic-needs.pdf. Accessed 8 July 2018.

Crutchfield, R. M., & Maguire, J. (2018). Report on CSU actions to support students facing food and housing insecurity. California State University. https://www2.calstate.edu/impact-of-the-csu/student-success/basic-needs-initiative/Documents/CSU-Basic-Needs-Action-Report.pdf. Accessed 8 July 2018.

Deil-Amen, R. (2011). *The 'traditional' college student: A smaller minority and its implications for diversity and access institutions*. Paper prepared for the Mapping Broad-Access Higher Education Conference, Palo Alto, CA: Stanford University.

Dworsky, A. (2008). *Educating homeless children in Chicago: A case study of children in the family regeneration program*. Chicago: Chapin Hall at the University of Chicago.

Dworsky, A., & Perez, A. (2009). *Helping former foster youth graduate from college: Campus support programs in California and Washington State*. Chicago: Chapin Hall Center for Children.

Esparza, N. (2009). Community factors influencing the prevalence of homeless youth services. *Children and Youth Services Review, 31*(12), 1321–1329.

Farrugia, D. (2011). Youth homelessness and individualised subjectivity. *Journal of Youth Studies, 14*, 761–775.

Gharabaghi, K., & Stuart, C. (2010). Voices from the periphery: Prospects and challenges for the homeless youth service sector. *Children and Youth Services Review, 32*(12), 1683–1689.

Goldrick-Rab, S. (2016). *Paying the price: College costs, financial aid, and the betrayal of the American dream*. Chicago: The University of Chicago Press.

Goldrick-Rab, S., Broton, K., & Eisenberg, D. (2015). Hungry to learn: Addressing food and housing insecurity among undergraduates. Wisconsin HOPE Lab. http://wihopelab.com/publications/Wisconsin_hope_lab_hungry_to_learn.pdf. Accessed 8 July 2018.

Goldrick-Rab, S., Richardson, J., & Hernandez, A. (2017). Hungry and homeless in college: Results from a national study of basic needs insecurity in higher education. Wisconsin HOPE Lab. http://wihopelab.com/publications/hungry-and-homeless-in-college-report.pdf. Accessed 8 July 2018.

Gupton, J. T. (2017). Campus of opportunity: A qualitative analysis of homeless students in community college. *Community College Review, 45*(3), 190–214.

Hallett, R. E. (2010). Homeless: How residential instability complicates students' lives. *About Campus, 15*(3), 11–16.

Hallett, R. E. (2012). *Educational experiences of hidden homeless teenagers: Living doubled-up*. New York: Routledge.

Hallett, R. E., & Crutchfield, R. (2018). *Homelessness and housing insecurity in higher education: A trauma-informed approach to research, policy, and practice [ASHE higher education report series]*. Boston: Jossey-Bass.

Hallett, R. E., & Skrla, L. (2017). *Serving students who are homeless: A resource guide for schools, districts, and educational leaders*. New York: Teachers College Press.

Hallett, R. E., Skrla, L., & Low, J. A. (2015). That is not what homeless is: A school district's journey toward serving homeless, doubled-up, and economically displaced children and youth. *International Journal of Qualitative Studies in Education, 28*(6), 671–692.

Masten, A. S., Miliotis, D., Graham-Berman, S. A., Ramirez, M., & Neemann, J. (1993). Children in homeless families: Risks to mental health and development. *Journal of Consulting and Clinical Psychology, 61*, 335–343.

Mawhinney-Rhoads, L., & Stahler, G. (2006). Educational policy and reform for homeless students: An overview. *Education and Urban Society, 38*(3), 288–306.

Miller, P. M. (2015). Families' experiences in different homeless and highly mobile settings: Implications for school and community practice. *Education and Urban Society, 47*(1), 3–32.

Morton, M. H., Dworsky, A., & Samuels, G. M. (2017). Missed opportunities: Youth homelessness in America. National estimates. Chapin Hall at the University of Chicago. http://voicesofyouthcount.org/wp-content/uploads/2017/11/ChapinHall_VoYC_NationalReport_Final.pdf. Accessed 8 July 2018.

Murphy, J., & Tobin, K. (2011). *Homelessness comes to school*. Thousand Oaks: Corwin.

National Association for the Education of Homeless Children and Youth. (2014). Financial aid for unaccompanied homeless youth: A survey report. Retrieved from http://www.naehcy.org/sites/default/files/dl/fafsasurvey-report.pdf

National Association for the Education of Homeless Children and Youth. (2016). Strategies for implementing HUD homeless assistance requirements to collaborate with schools and early learning programs. Retrieved from http://naehcy.org/educational-resources/housing

National Association for the Education of Homeless Children and Youth. (2018). Single Point-of-Contact Model. Retrieved from https://naehcy.org/wp-content/uploads/2018/08/SPOC-Model-Revamp-FINAL.pdf

National Center for Education Statistics (2016). Total fall enrollment in degree-granting postsecondary institutions, by attendance status, sex, and age: Selected years, 1970 through 2025. https://nces.ed.gov/programs/digest/d15/tables/dt15_303.40.asp?current=yes. Accessed 8 July 2018.

Pew Research Center (2014). The rising cost of not going to college. http://www.pewsocialtrends.org/2014/02/11/the-rising-cost-of-not-going-to-college/. Accessed 8 July 2018.

Peters, C. M., Dworsky, A., Courtney, M. E., & Pollack, H. (2009). *Extending foster care to age 21: Weighing the costs to government against the benefits to youth*. Chicago: Chapin Hall Center for Children.

Rafferty, Y., Shinn, M., & Weitzman, B. C. (2004). Academic achievement among formerly homeless adolescents and their continuously housed peers. *Journal of School Psychology, 42*(3), 179–199.

Sackett, C., Goldrick-Rab, S., & Broton, K. (2016). Addressing housing insecurity and living costs in higher education: A guidebook for colleges and universities. U.S. Department of Housing and Urban Development. https://www.huduser.gov/portal/sites/default/files/pdf/HousingInsecurityInHigherEd.pdf. Accessed 8 July 2018.

Silva, M. R., Kleinert, W. L., Sheppard, A. V., Cantrell, K. A., Freeman-Coppadge, D. J., Tsoy, E., & Pearrow, M. (2015). The relationship between food security, housing stability, and school performance among college students in an urban university. *Journal of College Student Retention: Research, Theory and Practice, 19*(3), 284–299.

Slesnick, N., Dashora, P., Letcher, A., Erdem, G., & Serovich, J. (2009). A review of services and interventions for runaway and homeless youth: Moving forward. *Children and Youth Services Review, 31*(7), 732–742.

Stagner, M., & Lansing, J. (2009). Progress toward a prevention perspective. *Future of Children, 19*, 19–38.

Tierney, W. G., Gupton, J. T., & Hallett, R. E. (2008). *Transitions to adulthood for homeless adolescents: Education and public policy*. Los Angeles: Center for Higher Education Policy Analysis.

Tierney, W. G., & Hallett, R. E. (2012). Social capital and homeless youth: Influence of residential instability on college access. *Metropolitan Universities Journal, 22*(3), 46–62.

Toolis, E. E., & Hammack, P. L. (2015). The lived experience of homeless youth: A narrative approach. *Qualitative Psychology, 2*, 50–68.

Tsui, E., Freudenberg, N., Manzo, L., Jones, H., Kwan, A., & Gagnon, M. (2011). *Housing instability at CUNY: Results from a survey of CUNY undergraduate students*. New York: City University of New York.

U.S. Department of Education (2014). Total number of homeless students enrolled in LEAs with or without McKinney-Vento Subgrants – Total: 2013–14. http://eddataexpress.ed.gov/data-element-explorer.cfm/tab/data/deid/5353/. Accessed 8 July 2018.

U.S. Department of Housing and Urban Development (2013). 2011 homelessness prevention and rabid re-housing program (HPRP): Year 2 summary. https://www.hudexchange.info/resources/documents/HPRP_Year2Summary.pdf. Accessed 8 July 2018.

U.S. Department of Housing and Urban Development (2015a). Rapid re-housing: Northwest youth services program profile. https://www.hud exchange.info/resource/4494/rrh-for-youth-northwest-youth-services-program-profile/. Accessed 8 July 2018.

U.S. Department of Housing and Urban Development (2015b). Barriers to success: Housing insecurity for U.S. college students: Insights into housing and community development policy. http://www.huduser.org/portal/periodicals/insight/insight_2.pdf. Accessed 8 July 2018.

Chapter 18
Practice Dilemmas, Successes, and Challenges in the Delivery of Homeless Services: Voices from the Frontline

Emmy Tiderington

Introduction

Frontline homeless service providers deliver services that address the needs of homeless individuals and families. They can be shelter staff, supportive housing case managers, or street outreach workers, among many other roles in a variety of settings. They come from different backgrounds and bring with them a range of experiences and competencies, from master's level clinical social workers to staff with no formal clinical training, but who have many years of experience in the field, to peers who provide support to those with mental illness, addiction, and a history of homelessness. These providers are often in jobs that pay little and work in settings that are less than glamorous. They have to negotiate their work roles in underfunded agencies and fight for resources in order to get the job done. They bear witness to the human condition and see resiliency and strength in action. Ultimately, they are frontline responders in the fight against one of the world's most wicked social problems.

Staff in homeless service settings are usually responsible for assisting individuals with basic needs (e.g., obtaining food, shelter, medical care) and are often directly or indirectly tasked with addressing clinical needs (e.g., intervening in mental health crises, providing medication monitoring, addressing substance abuse or other potentially harmful behaviors). These providers frequently need to work across systems. They may coordinate with child welfare agencies, the health-care system, entitlement programs, and other social services. Homeless service providers also need to

---

Electronic supplementary material: The online version of this chapter (https://doi.org/10.1007/978-3-030-03727-7_18) contains supplementary material, which is available to authorized users.

E. Tiderington (✉)
Rutgers, The State University of New Jersey, New Brunswick, NJ, USA
e-mail: emmy.tiderington@rutgers.edu

H. Larkin et al. (eds.), *Homelessness Prevention and Intervention in Social Work*, https://doi.org/10.1007/978-3-030-03727-7_18

work with a variety of other individuals and organizations within the service recipient's environment. You may find them working closely with a person's family, friends, and other natural supports, as well as interacting with the police, neighbors, religious leaders, and other community members in order to support an individual's tenure in the community. Through these many roles and responsibilities, homeless service providers can encounter challenges that originate at the individual, organizational, or system levels.

This chapter discusses the frontline work of homeless services. It draws on interviews and observations collected over a period of approximately 3 years from two homeless services agencies in a large urban area.[1] The intention of this chapter is to pull back the curtain on homeless service delivery and give the reader an in-depth and intimate portrait of this work. It is not a "how-to" guide to the provision of care in these service settings but a slice of life from the perspectives of those working in the field.

Homeless services are delivered in different ways in different settings. The providers whose words are included in this chapter come from two homeless service agencies. One is a permanent supportive housing program that utilized a Housing First approach. The other had both a transitional and permanent supportive housing program that operated from a more "treatment first" model, meaning that residents needed to demonstrate "housing readiness" through sobriety or treatment engagement in order to receive services. These candid accounts are the views of these providers only, and what they describe may not reflect practices found in other settings. However, many of the dilemmas described herein can be found in one form or another in other homeless service settings and may reflect larger issues at work within the homeless service system.

Like providers in other homeless services, the supportive housing providers heard from in this chapter are a diverse group – some had clinical degrees, and others had little to no clinical training or higher education. Some of them had their own experiences with homelessness, mental illness, and/or addiction and were self-identified "peers" working in a peer provider role. Others had the same type of lived experiences but chose not to disclose their background to employers. Some resided in or grew up in the neighborhood where they worked, while others were outsiders to the area. Some had been working in the field for a long time; others were fairly new. These are their descriptions of common practice dilemmas, successes, and challenges encountered on the frontlines *in their own words.*

A Day in the Life

A day in the life of a homeless services provider looks different depending on the setting. Shelter staff often work on-site at the shelter from day into night. Street outreach teams may walk the streets, subway tunnels, or tent cities to deliver services directly to individuals in the community. For providers of supportive housing,

[1] Frontline provider accounts in this chapter are derived from a National Institute of Mental Health-funded study of supportive housing for formerly homeless adults with co-occurring mental illness and substance abuse diagnoses (NIMH R01MH084903).

this work can involve being in the office, in service recipients' apartments, and other places in the community all in one day, as this permanent supportive housing provider explains:

> An ideal field day… I'll probably go to six apartments, see five or six people a day. I will go for a visit in their apartment. They need medication, I take their medication. Sometimes they need a check, I will take the check. I walk through the apartment and make sure everything's okay. Sometimes they have a lot of laundry, you know, you need to get it together so it can be washed. If they need to go outside…"Let's go to the store." … And then other days I might be sitting in a Social Security office, maybe for hours. I may be in court for maybe five hours or Public Assistance, Food Stamps office… It depends. I may take them shopping and buy stuff, if they need pots and pans. And I do a walk-through of the apartment. If I feel they need something like new curtains or maybe new furniture, I'll do a request and get them some new stuff. [2111]

Providing homeless services usually means being in people's homes and living spaces. Whether in a person's apartment, in the shelter or warming center where they lay their head at night, or being around the corner on the sidewalk or claimed space that they inhabit in the world, being in people's living spaces brings with it a degree of intimacy between service provider and recipient. If handled with care, this intimacy can lead to the possibility of a deeper working relationship or at least small steps toward closer engagement. And sometimes it is the little things that create intimacy and engagement between provider and service recipient:

> When I engage with consumers, I really just engage with them like I would an acquaintance or something at first. You know, just like "How is everything going? What's up? How are things in your life?" and whatever. And then sort of leave it casual, and so it's more comfortable. Especially since a lot of times I am in their house, so it's like, that's really a private space, and I'm intruding in that space, so…I always focus on what the consumer wants to talk about, and then I sort of guide it, you know? And with consumers that don't really want the service, but they are housed in our apartments, we keep continuing to go see them. That's a little more difficult. …I try various tactics. Like, in the past I have tried… like, if this guy was really interested in his health, I bought an orange for myself, and I bought him an orange, so he let me into his apartment. And sometimes that works. Sometimes it doesn't. Yesterday I tried to engage someone by bringing them a Thanksgiving meal that we had. And she was just like, "No, I don't want it." (laughs) She wouldn't let me come in. But I still talked to her about… I tried to get as much information about how she is doing without actually just forcefully putting myself in her space. Yeah, and it really just depends on…I think it's important in the engagement process to sort of like take it slow and focus not on like what we have to do – "Well we know she needs a medical appointment" or something like that...but more on just appreciating that having her engaged is part of the treatment and going and just not expecting a big success. You need smaller ones. "Oh, she let me put my foot in her doorway this time" (laughs), you know? [2103]

In homeless services, as in other direct service settings where service providers and consumers must work together, using humor and treating people with dignity and respect goes a long way, as this provider explains:

> …To have some banter, some regular real talk is always good. And it fosters a relationship. It fosters trust in both client to case manager and vice versa. So, I always try…and I have a really good sense of humor! …so, I always try to incorporate my sense of humor into all my visits with my clients. [2121]

The work of homeless services and being in people's homes and living spaces also means that providers encounter things they would not otherwise be privy to in an inpatient unit or outpatient clinic setting. Things like seeing photos on display of a person's family or friends whom they had not previously mentioned can provide openings for important discussions to take place. Clinical issues may be more apparent when visiting a person's home where a provider can see drug paraphernalia laying out, a service recipient sleeping for long stretches in the middle of the day, or the person living in unusually squalid conditions. Small clues like these can be used to piece together a larger picture of what is happening in a person's life:

> Like with the dishes, there is never no dishes in the sink. "Ok, so you know you have no dishes in the sink…is it put away? Let's see what's in the cabinets." You open the cabinets. There's no dishes in the cabinets. But there's no dishes in the sink. Where else could the dishes be? …So, you see, it's just like you have to kind of work your way in to it. I love Sundays the most because you get to spend more time with the clients because you have all day to be in the field. You get to see what's going on…. kind of get a feeling. You walk through the apartment, just kind of feeling… not go through their stuff, just kind of feel it. [2108]

Reading a person's surroundings is an important part of the job in homeless services, as this provider said, "Sometimes you can't even go by the services, sometimes you just have to go by what is in front of you when you get to the apartment. Like, you kind of just have to pick up on whatever energies, whatever's going on, you just pick up on that" [2112].

Overall, these intimate moments in someone's personal space – smelling their dinner cooking on the stove, meeting a loved one who has stopped by to visit, or finding a person in the middle of their favorite hobby – open a door to a private life that might not otherwise be on display in public settings. It is this privileged intimacy that can make the work in homeless services so rewarding, but bearing witness to these more mundane aspects of a person's life can also have some drawbacks.

> I have a shared apartment with three people and one of the girls accused the other one of eating some of her food. …The other roommate overheard. She got very upset, called the supervisor cursing and screaming about it and then her and the girl got into an argument. So, I came the next day, and everyone was in a bad mood, and she was screaming and cursing, and I was like, "What just happened here? I left on the weekend and everything was fine." So, it took a while to like calm them down, and they ended up making up the next day. And the girl, she admitted - she pretty much thought it was a mistake - she didn't think the other girl took her things. She just didn't realize it at the time, or she - I don't know. They're good now. But sometimes things happen that have like nothing to do with you and then you have to like do damage control. But it's like not part of your [client's service] goals, so it's just extra time taken out, because then it's like you do all that, then it's like, "Okay, now we have to talk about medication" after I spent 20 minutes trying to resolve this conflict and things like that. [2113]

Homeless service providers have to find ways to negotiate many different roles – conflict manager, confidant, recovery support, adviser, rule enforcer – and they have to find ways to negotiate the occasional conflicts that can arise between these roles. Sometimes supporting a person in maintaining their housing or shelter means enforcing rules with which the person may not agree, which can ultimately jeopardize engagement built from being their confidant and support. In cases where conflicts occur, it is important to draw on supervisors and other staff to help navigate these dilemmas.

Homeless service provision, by its very nature, involves being in individuals' personal living spaces, and this can create issues between service provider and recipient around privacy and ownership. In providing shelter or housing through a homeless assistance program, dilemmas often arise around who controls the living space and how it can be used, what the bounds of privacy are, and what rights the individual has as a tenant, resident, or overnight guest:

> I went into one of the clients' apartments. He didn't have a shirt on, and I told him that's inappropriate, and when counselors come to the apartment there, they have to be dressed properly. And he went on and on, he don't have to put a shirt on and this and that. And so, situations like that you're supposed to call your supervisor and let them know what's going on, and she advised me just to leave the apartment and not go back and forth with him about the situation. [2105]

The ways providers negotiate these dilemmas differ by setting and program rules. In shelters and transitional settings where the housing provided by the program is impermanent, and the person has no legal claim to the housing (e.g., through a lease), this can be particularly challenging. In fact, the place in which the service recipient resides and may call home is a temporary space offered and controlled by a service agency:

> So, like, when I go to see them, I try to be as like "this is your house" as much as possible. Like, I've seen some [case manager] people are a lot more, like they'll just use...like we have the keys, so they won't even ring. They just go in [the apartment]. And they have reasoning for that - they're like look, if people think that... It's almost like they just want them to just not get permanent, to know that this is transitional - do what you have to do and get out of here. But I want people to think that it's their house. [2107]

Thus, providers across homeless service settings face many challenges on the job day to day – from engaging with service recipients, to negotiating their many roles, to finding respectful ways to be present in someone's personal space and home.

Managing Risk

One of the more challenging aspects of the work in homeless services is managing risk and minimizing danger to self and others. Seeing vulnerable people with histories of substance abuse, mental illness, or criminal behavior in their homes and living spaces brings with it a degree of risk, and many times there is no security or police accompanying workers into these spaces. Working with this population can also mean that the service provider may be the first responder to crisis situations and one of the primary people making decisions around if and how to respond:

> I have called 911 twice. My most recent 911 [call] was because the person was living in the dark. The room was dark. He was never there. He had lost like 100lbs, you know, just really reclusive. Not meeting with me. He was using drugs heavily, but... because his psych

> history I had to call… First, we called a missing persons [report], because we hadn't seen him. Then we called the 911 again to get him to the psychiatric hospital. It was kind of scary, only because the person seemed scary when I went into the apartment. It was dark, and that stuff makes you more paranoid because you don't know whether… what they are capable of doing, because you are in their house. There is no security, you know? [2112]

Homelessness is often an extension of other social problems, like addiction, poverty, and mental health issues. Once housed or in shelter, these issues may improve, but for some individuals they may linger. Challenges associated with these problems can follow a person from the streets indoors. Bearing witness to all that comes along with the experience of homelessness then can also mean coming across a person using drugs, witnessing abuse and other illegal acts, and finding residents deceased, overdosed, or in medical distress. People experiencing homelessness have significantly higher rates of mortality than the general population (Barrow et al. 1999; Hwang 2001), and those who work with this population are frequently exposed to the deaths of service users (Lakeman 2011). All of this makes the work particularly challenging, and drawing on assistance from other supports is an essential part of the job.

However, bringing others in to help manage risk in these situations can also create additional problems. It is critically important to be thoughtful about when and if to intervene, and who to bring into a given situation, as these decisions can have enormous consequences:

> We caught him using in the apartment, and he gave us a hard time and the police a hard time. So that was something new that I've seen. They had to arrest him and put him in handcuffs. Before they went upstairs, we let them know what we found at his apartment, and how he was behaving with us, so they already knew what situation they was going into. [2105]

A person's tenure in the community rests not only on the person's own decisions but also on the decisions of others. This means that the job may involve dealing with guests, visitors, friends, and loved ones present in the person's space and knowing how and when to intervene in ways that are respectful of their decisions as well:

> Last week, when I went to go see my client in the Bronx, he wasn't there. There was some people in his house. When I was approaching the building, I saw his terrace door open, and there was a young man on the terrace, so I said, "Okay, I'm going up anyway." …And I knock, and I go, "[service recipient's name]?" No one says anything, but someone opened the peephole and blew marijuana smoke through the peephole. So, I go, "Is [service recipient's name] here?" No one said anything. Closed the peephole. It's those kind of encounters that's uncomfortable for me. It's not that it's a bad or good thing, but that's just really uncomfortable for me, you know? I asked him about it yesterday …He said, "Well, I wasn't home." I'm like, "Okay, when you're not home, to secure your housing, you need to clear your house. When you're not home, everyone should leave. Because I'm coming to your apartment thinking you're home. There could be danger just waiting for me. If you're not home, you got people and young kids in your house smoking marijuana. If they open the door and snatch me in, what's going to happen?" So, I just talk to him about, you know, safety and having people in your home when you're not there, putting your housing in jeopardy. Stuff like that. [2126]

Dealing with unfamiliar individuals can leave providers additionally vulnerable because, unlike a service recipient who the provider may know well, these individuals come without charts or detailed histories. Being in the person's space and surroundings while others are present can be even more risky:

> [This client]'s having company. I heard he's not having the right company in the apartment, which I agree. And ... I'm worried that it might escalate, because... for my safety, too. You don't know who these guys are dealing with and what they're doing, you know? And who may be living with their neighbor. And for me to come see them every day, it kind of puts me at risk. Because you have to come work with them every day to this apartment, and I don't know what they have going on. [2112]

Despite this additional risk, people have the right to a social life, and whether housed in a shelter, a supportive housing apartment, or other type of homeless assistance program, individuals may want others to visit or reside with them in their living space. Loneliness and isolation are well-documented issues for formerly homeless individuals in housing programs (Siegel et al. 2006; Stefancic 2014; Tsai et al. 2012), and having friends and family around can be a great benefit to recipients of homeless services. However, not all social relationships are healthy. Service recipients may find themselves vulnerable to exploitation in these settings, with providers in the awkward position of having to determine the fine line between healthy and unhealthy social relationships (Tiderington 2018):

> A lot of these clients, even the older ones that are estranged from their families, they get lonely, and they either want to suck you in – you know, meaning the worker – or they'll gravitate towards people who are just hanging out and about and seem to want to have some place to hang. "Well, come on, hang at my house." And it becomes a thing. I had a client where we actually—they, the drug dealers—and this was an older man with younger boys... These younger boys ran him out...he left the apartment and went to a shelter. But it started out with him not having anybody else and wanting to be around. And he smoked weed, and they had the weed, and one thing turned into another. I mean we literally had to turn the apartment over to the landlord because we couldn't get these guys out. They didn't care. We tried to change the lock, they broke back in. He went into a hospital. They still—they stayed in the apartment. They are living there, selling drugs, rent-free in our—you know? But that's basically the type of stuff that we deal with. [2118]

This type of risk extends beyond random people and drug dealers. Family and close friends can be equally as exploitative:

> He has family that visits his apartment. He has a group of friends that he keeps very distant from the team, which is fine. I think part of that though is when you come from more of a street homeless background, what tends to happen is you bring one friend, let's say, from a shelter, and they see how you're living, and then before you know it, everybody is like, "Oh, that's the new place to hang out"! So, like when they leave the shelter for the day, they have this great apartment they can come and hang out. So, there's always this concern that, you know, it only takes one person to sort of start to weasel their way sort of into the apartment and then not leave, and then it becomes really problematic. So, there's always concern around that. [2104]

The structure of services and program rules can also add challenges to the management of risk in these settings (Tiderington 2018). Guest and visitor policies, maximum occupancy standards, and service settings that allow only one gender or family type (e.g., men's shelters, family shelters, shelters that house only women and children) can put providers in the position to regulate the social lives of recipients in order to keep them in compliance with program rules and maintain them in housing. For example, a service recipient who wants their non-married partner to live with them in a single-room occupancy unit may find themselves in violation of the unit occupancy standard and/or the agency's guest policy. Ultimately, finding ways to minimize risk of eviction and keep service recipients, staff, and others safe from harm, while honoring service recipients' right to self-determination, can be a challenging task in homeless services.

Previous research has found that providers in homeless services employ certain tactics to manage this dilemma. In one study of frontline practice in supportive housing (Tiderington 2018), providers were found to surveil the unit, monitor for physical signs that a nonresident lived in the program apartment, and drop in on residents as a way to monitor potential risk via nonresident guests. They "turned a blind eye" to low-risk guests and encouraged service recipients to get married and formalize the tenancy of their nonresident guests as a work-around to the single-occupancy policies that hindered recipient's social, familial, and romantic lives. Homeless service provision then also means employing discretionary tactics like the ones above in order to juggle service recipient needs and agency expectations.

Reading a service recipient's surroundings and picking up on small clues in the person's living space, as previously discussed, can also be a useful tool for predicting and managing risk. However, not everything is as it appears, and understanding the limitations of this risk reduction strategy is important:

> He had drug dealers in the apartment, and I had no knowledge of that. I mean the last home visit I did, it looked so home-y. He was cooking a meal for his girlfriend and another guy who was there…it looked very domestic. But underneath it something else had been going on. Because that apartment was later raided by the SWAT team after he was incarcerated. They arrested two drug dealers in the apartment, armed! [2131]

Bringing in supervisors and other supports like the police, EMS, and crisis intervention teams can help frontline homeless service providers manage unsafe situations and determine when and if to intervene:

> I don't want to put myself in an unsafe situation. I also don't want to put the client in an unsafe situation. So, I would remove myself and I would go out and call the police. And go back in the apartment so this way I have the security that I need around me. And 911 would come in, they ask some questions, and they could see for themselves that the client is getting kind of violent. And if I explain what's going on with them, they'd ask me questions – "Have they been taking their medication? Have you seen the medications?" And sometimes [the service recipient] gets to the point, "I'm not showing you anything! I'm not going anywhere!" And [the police] said, "Well, we need to just go to a hospital, so you can be evaluated. And that's just…a couple times I had to do that situation. But I've never got physically harmed or anything like that. I just…because I know I remove myself before it gets to a point that I could be...there could be a chance that I'd be harmed, so I remove myself and just get the police involved. [2102]

Working with other staff or team members who are familiar with the service recipient can also be an effective tool for minimizing risk. Drawing on multiple perspectives in order to respond to crises and to develop and enact a plan for intervention can make a challenging situation a little easier and hopefully improve the final outcome.

In the end, crises can create opportunities for greater intimacy and depth in the working relationship between service provider and recipient, and even the most challenging situations can yield positive outcomes, as this provider describes:

> This guy who I was working really intensely with…he was convinced I was breaking into his apartment at night and raping him. He called me up and asked me to take money out of his account, and I asked him for what. And he said really nonchalantly, "Oh, I'm going to buy a gun and come down there and shoot you." And I was like, "Ok, well no. I'm not going to get you that money, and let's talk about this". And he was like, "No, I'll just come right now and kill you". And he was very…it was scary. It was a very sort of sociopathic-nonchalant "I'm about to kill you" thing. And that was the one time that I was really scared in like 12, 11 years. It's a pretty good record.
>
> So, the team…we had preemptively called the police, so they would be there outside when he showed up…to potentially hospitalize him because he was threatening. I was going to leave the office and go to a different place and then wait until the whole thing went down and then come back.…He usually came using this one train, so I went the other way and went towards the opposite train that he would never take. And as I'm walking by the train station, I see him coming up the stairs from that train that he never took. And he saw me, and he just started chasing me down the street. Thankfully I can run really fast, so I ran like nine blocks to the state building, because I knew there was security there.…So he got hospitalized. And weeks later I finally decided he was probably stable enough for me to go visit him in the hospital, because I stayed away. I didn't want to incite anything, and I wanted to see what was happening. And when I went he was blown away that I was even willing to talk to him ever again. It was like a switch went off in him, and like from that day on he was so engaged in treatment, so willing to do anything. Because he realized, "Oh my god, I really was going to hurt you", and yet you're here to say, "What do you need?" [2104]

These moments make clear the complications inherent in this work and demonstrate how the challenges and successes of practice in homeless services often overlap.

Letting Go of Control

Finding ways to let go of control in this work with high-risk homeless populations is another common practice dilemma in these settings. In delivering services, there is an expectation by programs and funders that frontline providers will do what they can to keep service recipients safe from harm and assist them in achieving positive outcomes. Frontline workers in these setting then find themselves with a sense of responsibility for recipients' safety, security, and well-being. But in programs serving homeless people, this expectation adds another challenging layer to the work:

> Working in social services, you just feel like you're there to fix a problem. Like you have this, "This should happen." You just look for the result. Especially when you've put time in it and all the work you've been putting in it. You can question yourself, like am I doing anything? I think I'm just accepting that you can't change people's lives; you're not here for that. You just have to accept them and respect their own decisions. [2112]

While putting a roof over someone's head may end their homelessness, other issues that can come along with homelessness, like mental illness, substance abuse, or chronic medical conditions, are not as easy to cure. Holding a sense of personal responsibility for fixing these complex problems can feel like a heavy burden:

> I get frustrated with them. Like you have all these doctors' appointments, I am busting my back to get you these appointments, you're not going to them, and it's like, you get frustrated! (laughs) Because they are not where you want them to be.... It's frustrating. Because you feel like, when you go to work you feel like your job is to problem solve, to solve people's problems. And that is not the reality of it. You can't. You can just put people in the right direction. And that is what I think. I get frustrated, because I think I kind of like to turn people around, make them do this, and make them do... But that's mostly where the frustration is, because you feel like you can't change people. (laughs) [2112]

Like providers in other high-risk fields (e.g., child welfare, substance abuse, domestic violence), frontline staff in homeless services are well aware of liability issues on the job:

> When I found a client dead, that was kind of "whoa." That was an eye opener at this job. This job, at any given time, anything could happen. So, you have to be on your Ps and Qs on how to do your job here....because a guy died. He was dead when I got there. He looked like he was sleeping. And I could have been another counselor, "Oh, he is sleeping, I'm not going to bother him", but then said that they saw him, and then this guy is dead on your time! And it's like, "Oh, where were you?" So that could have blown up, right? Because of you he died! You know what I am saying? So, it's a lot of unpredictability about this job. [2112]

And often, frontline staff work to ensure that they are protected when and if something happens to a service recipient on their watch: "We want to cover ourselves to make sure if anything happens. We are somewhat responsible for all the people on our caseload and stuff, so I guess it's like constant... It's like a lot of covering yourself" [2103].

While it is undoubtedly important that providers do their best to protect the individuals with whom they work and work with them to improve their lives, this sense of responsibility and liability can lead providers to "do for" the person, instead of with them, robbing the person of the opportunity for mastery and sense of accomplishment that comes with doing for oneself (Longhofer et al. 2010). It can result in providers overreacting to circumstances that could have benefitted from a more measured approach, and it can create a dynamic of imposed control that violates service recipients' right to self-determination and decision-making on their own behalf:

> It's overwhelming. I feel like sometimes to have all that responsibility over an adult's life, not only for me, it feels like maybe that shouldn't happen, but also for...I just always think about what it is like from the consumer's point of view to have so many people involved in their life and like controlling it basically and telling them what they can and can't do as an adult? And I feel like it should be a little more free. You know? ...You can help someone manage their symptoms and their mental illness without being controlling of their actions I guess. I think that happens sometimes, and I don't think we mean it. I just think that happens because we want to help and also, we are required to do so many things or we are afraid of something happening that um... you know, we don't want to be responsible for all that. [2103]

Consumer advocates have long argued for allowing service recipients' "dignity of risk and the right to fail" (Corrigan 2011). There is also increasing recognition of the need to integrate a client-centered, consumer-driven approach into homeless services (Gillis et al. 2010; Sheedy and Whitter 2009), and these principles are now considered important elements in regard to homeless policy, planning, research, and services (Barrow et al. 2007). But what does this mean for frontline providers? How do these workers navigate the expectation for consumer-driven care while also meeting funder and organizational expectations to keep people safe and on a positive trajectory? What if a person wants to use illegal drugs in their apartment or make other potentially harmful decisions? How can a worker relinquish control over individuals in these settings while also keeping people safe?

> I think staff can be a big barrier to engagement. If we jump in too soon, if we become too directive and not so consumer-driven, but more our own "You need to do this, this would help, you should be doing this" or any sort of judgmental talk about substance use especially, nobody wants to hear that. Everyone knows that crack is not good for you. Nobody thinks it's good for you. ... So, adults, who are... most of them are a lot older than the staff working for them...to be told by a youngster (laughs)...they shouldn't be smoking crack is kind of like..." Yeah, okay great. Thanks." And that can really... as simple as it may seem, can really shut people down. Because they have been told that their whole lives. Most of them, when we come into their life we are like the 10th or 20th social worker they have come across that they are now telling their whole life story again to. So, we have to be very vigilant about maintaining a supportive stance, even in the face of something so obviously not helpful.... because it's the long term, it's the bigger picture that matters. It's keeping that person engaged in treatment that's more important than making some point that is sort of meaningless. [2104]

Harm reduction, which is a nonjudgmental, pragmatic approach to working with individuals who engage in harmful behaviors (Marlatt 1996), is increasingly being employed in homeless services to limit or prevent negative consequences of harmful behaviors without exerting control over an individual's own decision-making (Pauly et al. 2013). It relies on the strength of the relationship between service recipient and provider and the service provider's ability to creatively engage with the person regarding their behavior (Tiderington et al. 2013):

> You have to be extremely empathic. You have to believe fully in harm reduction and understand what that means. That does not mean you are condoning drug use, doesn't mean you are telling somebody to go smoke crack. What it means is that you are able to sit with the uncomfortableness (sic) of other people's choices and understand that it is their choice and try to explore why they're doing the behavior that they're doing versus judging it or feeling hopeless about them because of their behavior. So, it really requires a lot of training and a certain ability I think that is just instinctual for some people. [2104]

This approach stands in contrast to the treatment requirements that some homelessness programs still have. Many programs require sobriety and/or psychiatric stability to receive services or at least mandate engagement in treatment programs; the rationale is the need for a safe environment and a greater likelihood of positive, long-term outcomes for individuals in care. Some homeless assistance programs also have requirements for participation in religious activities or work. In these programs, it usually falls on the frontline worker to enforce these requirements and report when the rules have been violated, which adds additional challenges to the work (Henwood et al. 2014):

> That's when we have the program director become involved, because we remind them that this is a drug-free program and that you can't be using drugs in the apartment or actively using because one, it's not safe for you, but also sending a message to the rest of the residents that it's okay to do it. It's against the program policy. And it depends how severe each case is. If they continue to use, we find places that are a more appropriate level of housing… maybe more supervised. No one is like, put out or anything like that, it's just that we'll find a placement… place them in maybe long-term care to address their sobriety issues. Place them in a more supervised setting where they can get extra support and um…you know, until they are strong enough to deal with their environmental issues, strong enough to deal with their relationships…you know, bring them back to an orientation to help them build back up to that level. [2102]

Whether employing a harm reduction approach or enforcing program requirements, workers in both types of programs can be challenged by the amount of control they are expected to have or to relinquish over another person's life. This can be a heavy burden, not easily navigated, but commonly faced in the delivery of homeless services.

Juggling Many Demands

Homeless service provision has been characterized as stressful and highly demanding work (Mullen and Leginski 2010; Olivet et al. 2010), as echoed by the providers in this chapter. Staff in the homeless service sector have many demands on their time and often meet these demands with very little support. Homeless assistance agencies, like other social services, often face staffing challenges and difficulties providing adequate supervision and support to frontline staff (Olivet et al. 2010):

> Interviewer: What's working here like for you? You have been here for 3½ years? 2113: Mm-hmm. God, it was unfortunate my first word that came is "stressful." It is stressful, because there is just not enough time to do what needs to be done, unfortunately. You know, one thing with this job that is maybe different from a lot of other positions like this is we do a lot of fieldwork and a lot of paperwork. And there is just never enough time for both. So, usually one gets sacrificed a little bit to finish the other, then you catch up on that one, and it goes back and forth. But it is frustrating because you sometimes kind of feel like you're always trying to catch up on one of those things. So that is part of it that kind of makes it stressful. [2113]

Homeless programs are funded through a variety of funding streams at the private, federal, state, and local level, with each funder usually requiring some type of documentation for quality assurance and/or billing purposes. The volume of this documentation can be onerous when agencies pull on multiple streams of funding. Documentation of the work also has its benefits. It helps the worker track progress with the service recipient and can be a tool for shared decision-making with the recipient around service provision goals. Thorough documentation can also help minimize liability and help a worker stay organized. However, juggling both the demands for keeping up with this paperwork and doing the "real work" with service recipients can become a major challenge in these settings (Tiderington et al. in press):

> It's also frustrating when I don't have the time to spend more time with the consumer because I gotta get my paperwork done. Yeah, it's a lot of paperwork. But being able to give the consumer the time to do the things that need to be done - like with benefits, sometime I could spend the whole day in the Social Security office. I go to housing court. I do a lot of things to keep them from being evicted ...yeah. We have some who have their own place, but they haven't paid their rent so, then I go become their payee. Go to court to stop eviction and run around to the Marshall and a lot of stuff just to keep them housed. Yeah, and then that's the only time I can do it is when I'm out doing the stuff [in the field]. But that's what I like to do. That's my specialty. But I need to balance it out. [2111]

Beyond juggling the work with service recipients and paperwork demands, providers in homeless services also need to find time to take care of themselves:

> ...The amount of work that is put into each individual, it's a lot of work. I feel like I have more to do with their lives than with my own. And that's what it is with this type of job. ... because you're accountable for everything that goes on with this person, you know their psychiatric needs, their medical needs, you're linked to everything that is going on with this person, and you have to try to get them in the right direction and the right services. And you... we're human too. We have our own needs, too. And it's like you don't even have time to gather what is going on with you, because you are so focused on meeting deadlines and fixing everyone else's problems. [2112]

Burnout, compassion fatigue, and secondary traumatic stress have been identified as particularly serious issues in the frontline work of homeless services (Baker et al. 2010; Bride 2007; Howell 2012; Mullen and Leginski 2010). Being exposed to traumatic events through work with high-risk groups, being around others experiencing trauma, or even just hearing others regularly describe traumatic events can result in secondary traumatic stress. Providers can also experience compassion fatigue and burnout, feeling hopeless and helpless regarding their ability to do good work. In one study of 245 homeless services staff, 25% of workers in these settings reported experiencing burnout and compassion fatigue to the point where job performance, as well as quality of life, decreased. In this same study, 36% of workers reported symptoms of post-traumatic stress disorder (PTSD), which the researchers indicate would very likely result in a diagnosis of PTSD (Waegemakers Schiff 2016).

Attending to self-care then becomes a critical strategy for doing effective work in homeless services. It is both the responsibility of the worker and the responsibility of the organization to infuse this into agency practices and the organizational culture:

> I feel like I'm (sighs) just all over the place sometimes. And when I get away from the office, and I get in their environment, I don't feel like that as much. But when I have to do—how many visits I have—70 visits? In 20 days? You don't feel so inspired, you know? And then often we don't have time for our own wellness, you know? One of my biggest problems is that we don't get to decompress. We're not invited to. And we have some days that are like, "Oh my god, like did I just go through this? (laughs) Did that just happen?"

> And it's just like, "Okay, just write a note. Alright, see you tomorrow." And then, you know, that takes the wind out of your sail. It really does. [2114]

Management needs to model self-care for staff (e.g., by taking lunch and mid-shift breaks and encouraging staff to do the same). They need to acknowledge and respond to traumatic events and monitor for signs of burnout, compassion fatigue, and secondary trauma (Newell and MacNeil 2010). For providers, use of direct supervisors can help minimize the risk of encountering these issues:

> I can meet with my supervisor once a month, sometimes twice a month. Whenever I feel like, you know, because I get stressed out sometimes. ... Or, you know, if things happen to [service recipients], I get emotional. So, we have supervision and I—we'll talk about it, you know, whatever I feel like I need to discuss with her. Anything I feel like I need to improve on or I feel like I'm not doing well, I'll talk to her about it. If I'm stressed out, if I need a mental health day, you know, I'll discuss all these things with her. [2111]

Keeping Hope Alive

Despite the many challenges described in this chapter, homeless service providers are often inspiring in their innovations and dedication. Despite the plethora of paperwork handed down by funders, the potentially spotty supervision and support, and the risky work environment, frontline providers of these services keep the home fires burning for hundreds of thousands of individuals and families every night. They keep hope alive when there may be little hope available to that person at that time:

> ...Empowering [service recipients'] that recovery is possible and that they can do things, valuable contributions to society. I think that that is the most...that is really effective. Because I've seen so many people just sort of... who had lost hope, gain it. ...So just giving people that hope that they can do something that they feel is valuable and they been told they couldn't do, is powerful. [2103]

Ultimately, these are the first responders to individuals in great need, often operating in high-risk, high-stress environments with few resources at their disposal. They provide an incredibly important service and, despite the challenges described above, find ways to offer hope to individuals and families in trying times – somehow hustling together what is needed to address one of today's most challenging social problems through innovative real-world solutions:

> I think everyone here does the best they can, and they do a lot. I think counselors wear a bunch of different hats. I think they're therapists, they're unlicensed therapists, they're counselors, they are emergency contacts, they're family, they do everything. And I think like, we're almost like hustlers, because we find a way to get things done within the red tape. So, it's definitely a lot of work, but somehow it gets done. I don't know how. Somehow it gets pieced together with tape and paperclips. [2117]

References

Baker, C. K., Billhardt, K. A., Warren, J., Rollins, C., & Glass, N. E. (2010). Domestic violence, housing instability, and homelessness: A review of housing policies and program practices for meeting the needs of survivors. *Aggression and Violent Behavior, 15*(6), 430–439.

Barrow, S. M., Herman, D. B., Cordova, P., & Struening, E. L. (1999). Mortality among homeless shelter residents in New York City. *American Journal of Public Health, 89*(4), 529–534.

Barrow, S., McMullin, L., Tripp, J., & Tsemberis, S. (2007). *Consumer integration and self-determination in homelessness research, policy, planning, and services*. Washington, D.C: Paper presented at the 2007 National Homelessness Conference.

Bride, B. E. (2007). Prevalence of secondary traumatic stress among social workers. *Social Work, 52*(1), 63–70.

Corrigan, P. W. (2011). The dignity to fail. *Psychiatric Services, 62*(3), 241–241.

Gillis, L., Dickerson, G., & Hanson, J. (2010). Recovery and homeless services: New directions for the field. *Open Health Services and Policy Journal, 3*, 71–79.

Henwood, B. F., Padgett, D. K., & Tiderington, E. (2014). Provider views of harm reduction versus abstinence policies within homeless services for dually diagnosed adults. *The Journal of Behavioral Health Services and Research, 41*(1), 80–89.

Howell, A. M. (2012). Working in the trenches: Compassion fatigue and job satisfaction among workers who serve homeless clients [Master of Social Work Clinical Research Paper 116]. St. Catherine's University. http://www.sophia.stkate.edu/msw_papers/116. Accessed 27 July 2018.

Hwang, S. W. (2001). Homelessness and health. *Canadian Medical Association Journal, 164*(2), 229–233.

Lakeman, R. (2011). How homeless sector workers deal with the death of service users: A grounded theory study. *Death Studies, 35*(10), 925–948.

Longhofer, J., Kubek, P. M., & Floersch, J. (2010). *On being and having a case manager: A relational approach to recovery in mental health*. New York: Columbia University Press.

Marlatt, G. A. (1996). Harm reduction: Come as you are. *Addictive Behaviors, 21*, 779–788.

Mullen, J., & Leginski, W. (2010). Building the capacity of the homeless service workforce. *Open Health Services and Policy Journal, 3*, 101–110.

Newell, J. M., & MacNeil, G. A. (2010). Professional burnout, vicarious trauma, secondary traumatic stress, and compassion fatigue. *Best Practices in Mental Health, 6*(2), 57–68.

Olivet, J., McGraw, S., Grandin, M., & Bassuk, E. (2010). Staffing challenges and strategies for organizations serving individuals who have experienced chronic homelessness. *The Journal of Behavioral Health Services and Research, 37*(2), 226–238.

Pauly, B. B., Reist, D., Belle-Isle, L., & Schactman, C. (2013). Housing and harm reduction: What is the role of harm reduction in addressing homelessness? *International Journal of Drug Policy, 24*(4), 284–290.

Sheedy, C. K., & Whitter M. (2009). *Guiding principles and elements of recovery-oriented systems of care: What do we know from the research?* [HHS Publication No. (SMA) 09–4439]. Rockville: Center for Substance Abuse Treatment, Substance Abuse and Mental Health Services Administration.

Siegel, C. E., Samuels, J., Tang, D., Berg, I., Jones, K., & Hopper, K. (2006). Tenant outcomes in supported housing and community residences in New York City. *Psychiatric Services, 57*, 982–991.

Stefancic, A. (2014). "If I stay by myself, I feel safer": Dilemmas of social connectedness among persons with psychiatric disabilities in Housing First. Columbia University Academic Commons. https://doi.org/10.7916/D83B5XSS. Accessed 27 July 2018.

Tiderington, E. (2018). The apartment is for you, it's not for anyone else: Managing social recovery and risk on the frontlines of single-adult supportive housing. *Administration and Policy in Mental Health and Mental Health Services Research, 45*(1), 152–162.

Tiderington, E., Stanhope, V., & Henwood, B. F. (2013). A qualitative analysis of case managers' use of harm reduction in practice. *Journal of Substance Abuse Treatment, 44*(1), 71–77.

Tiderington, E., Stanhope, V., & Padgett, D. K. (in press). "How do we force six visits on a consumer?": Frontline dilemmas and strategies for person-centered care under Medicaid fee-for-service. *American Journal of Psychiatric Rehabilitation.*

Tsai, J., Mares, A. S., & Rosenheck, R. A. (2012). Does housing chronically homeless adults lead to social integration? *Psychiatric Services, 63*(5), 427–434.

Waegemakers Schiff, J. (2016). Burnout and PTSD in workers in the homeless sector in Calgary. Calgary Homeless Foundation. calgaryhomeless.com/content/uploads/Calgary-Psychosocial-Stressors-Report.pdf. Accessed 27 July 2018.

Index

H. Larkin et al. (eds.), *Homelessness Prevention and Intervention in Social Work*, https://doi.org/10.1007/978-3-030-03727-7

Printed by Printforce, the Netherlands